Canine Parasites and Parasitic Diseases

Canine Parasites and Parasitic Diseases

Seppo Saari, DVM

Anu Näreaho, DVM, PhD

Sven Nikander, DVM, PhD

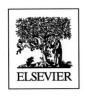 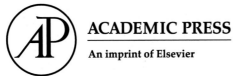 ACADEMIC PRESS

An imprint of Elsevier

Academic Press is an imprint of Elsevier
125 London Wall, London EC2Y 5AS, United Kingdom
525 B Street, Suite 1650, San Diego, CA 92101, United States
50 Hampshire Street, 5th Floor, Cambridge, MA 02139, United States
The Boulevard, Langford Lane, Kidlington, Oxford OX5 1GB, United Kingdom

Notices
Knowledge and best practice in this field are constantly changing. As new research and experience broaden our understanding, changes in research methods, professional practices, or medical treatment may become necessary.

Practitioners and researchers must always rely on their own experience and knowledge in evaluating and using any information, methods, compounds, or experiments described herein. In using such information or methods they should be mindful of their own safety and the safety of others, including parties for whom they have a professional responsibility.

To the fullest extent of the law, neither the Publisher nor the authors, contributors, or editors, assume any liability for any injury and/or damage to persons or property as a matter of products liability, negligence or otherwise, or from any use or operation of any methods, products, instructions, or ideas contained in the material herein.

Library of Congress Cataloging-in-Publication Data
A catalog record for this book is available from the Library of Congress

British Library Cataloguing-in-Publication Data
A catalogue record for this book is available from the British Library

ISBN 978-0-12-814112-0

For information on all Academic Press publications
visit our website at https://www.elsevier.com/books-and-journals

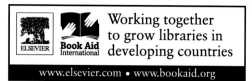

Working together
to grow libraries in
developing countries

www.elsevier.com • www.bookaid.org

Publisher: Andre Wolff
Acquisition Editor: Linda Versteeg-buschman
Editorial Project Manager: Carlos Rodriguez
Production Project Manager: Punithavathy Govindaradjane
Cover Designer: Victoria Pearson

Typeset by SPi Global, India

Contents

Preface

The dog is a habitat for some of the most amazing animals on the planet. If one has the opportunity to become more closely acquainted with parasites, natural disgust may slowly turn to admiration. The beauty of the refined structures in microscopy or the cleverness of the complicated life cycles astonishes the observer. We, the authors of this book, have been privileged to familiarize ourselves with parasites for decades in our daily work and have become big fans of them. We wanted to share our enthusiasm through this exceptionally visual book.

The book celebrates the wonder and complexity of nature, but also offers up-to-date information to veterinary professionals and dog owners regarding their parasitological questions. We hope that readers will push their prejudice away and enjoy the amazing world of canine parasites. The control of canine parasite infections through endoparasite and ectoparasite management has become a routine for veterinary professionals and dog owners. These treatments are often preventative measures and nowadays, the diagnosis of parasitic disease is based on detecting eggs, antigens from the parasite, seroconversion by the host, or finding molecular traces about the parasites. This means that the key player of the event, the parasite itself, is hardly ever seen. Thanks to effective control methods and narrow host range, many canine parasites are becoming rare or are even at risk of extinction. This gave us the motivation to portray such a wide spectrum of canine parasites, even the ones with lesser clinical importance.

Know Your Dog's Parasite Risks

Prevalence of parasites vary in different countries and areas; the risks are not the same everywhere. In addition, the availability of medications differ. Ask your own veterinarian about the canine parasites specific for your area, and the control practices that are at use. Check the legislation and the local recommendations in your country.

Acknowledgments

We thank all who in one way or another contributed in the completion of this project. Due to the beauty of parasites and their complicated life cycles, we wanted to invest in the visual content of this book. A major part of the figures originates from our own projects, including photographs and microscope and electron microscope figures, collected over decades. Many have been acquired through our international connections. We had the opportunity to portray some rare parasites thanks to helpful foreign colleagues, who sent them over to us. We thank all those people and institutions that helped us to gather the book's figures. It has been a joy to share our enthusiasm and interest in parasites with them. We would also like to show our gratitude to Pushpraj for sharing the pearls of his artistic talent by creating the illustrations for this book.

We are indebted to the Dean of the Faculty of Veterinary Medicine, University of Helsinki, Professor Antti Sukura, who has supported us from the very beginning of the project and enabled the writing and photographing of the material at the Faculty.

Our book contains many pictures obtained through scanning electron microscopy. Every one of them has required many work phases. We thank the Institute of Biotechnology of the Helsinki University. Its staff handled our parasite samples with expertise and kindly allowed us to use their equipment.

Colleagues Dr. Antti Lavikainen and Professor Antti Oksanen have helped us with many parasitological challenges and Dr. Sami Junnikkala has done the same with immunology. We are grateful for their cooperation.

Jouko Koppinen and Pamela White have done a huge job in translating the book from Finnish to English. Our editing and finalizing was much easier after your work. Thank you both!

Linda Versteeg-Buschman, Carlos Rodriguez, Punithavathy Govindaradjane, and others in the Elsevier editorial team have kindly answered our countless questions, considered our last-minute ideas, and guided us through the publishing process. Thank you for your patience with us.

We would like to express our warmest thanks to the following colleagues who provided us their superb photographic or parasite material: Finnish veterinarians and scientists (Annette Brockmann, Heikki Henttonen, Marina Hultholm, Mirja Kaimio, Veera Karkamo, Antti Oksanen, Lotta Pänkälä, Leena Saijonmaa-Koulumies, Kirsti Schild, Hanna-Kaisa Sihvo, Thomas Spillmann, Pentti Tapio, Marika Tenhunen), their assistants (Sofie Alakoski, Erja Juvakka and Merja Ranta), dog owners (Marja Lehtiö, Erik Lindholm and Christel Sivula) and graphic/photographic experts (Sami Karjalainen, Olli Immonen and Tom Björklund), and colleagues abroad (Yazmin Alcala-Canto, Walter Basso, Svetlana Belova, Emanuele Brianti, Jitender P. Dubey, Bengt Ekberg, Heidi Enemark, Juan Antonio Figueroa Castillo, Jennifer Gerner, Katarzyna Goździk, Lotta Gunnarsson, Anja Heckeroth, Kristel Kegler, Dawie Kok, Klaus Earl Loft, Guadalupe Miró, Daniel Młocicki, Tapio Nikkilä, Maria Pennisi, Arlett Perez, Rusłan Sałamatin, Alexandr Stekolnikov, Mousa Tavassoli, Roberta di Terlizzi, Rebecca Traub and her research group, and Jennifer Vander Kooi). The following companies and institutes have provided us with photographs or samples: Bayer Animal Health, ClinVet, Centers for Disease Control and Prevention (CDC), Elanco Animal Health, Finnish Food Safety Authority Evira, IDEXX Laboratories, Medical University of Warsaw, MSD Animal Health, Novartis Animal Health National Veterinary Institute of Sweden (SVA), University of Helsinki and Witold Stefanski Institute of Parasitology. The support is greatly appreciated. In addition some of the photos were purchased from the commercial stock photo libraries.

For understanding my long days and nights at the computer, I'd (SS) like to thank my dear and supportive wife, Tuija, and my sons, Sebastian and Oliver.

Seppo Saari
Anu Näreaho
Sven Nikander

Abbreviations

AHR	anthelmintic resistance	**IFAT**	immunofluorescence antibody test
BAL	broncho-alveolar lavage	**L1, L3**	1st larval stage, 3rd larval stage in Nematodes
BID	two times a day (medication dose)	**MAC**	membrane attack complex
CAPC	Companion Animal Parasite Council	**NBL**	newborn larva
CLM	cutaneous larva migrans	**OLM**	ocular larva migrans
DIC	disseminated intravascular coagulation	**opg**	oocysts per gram
ELISA	enzyme-linked immunosorbent assay	**p.o.**	per os, orally
epg	eggs per gram	**PCR**	polymerase chain reaction
ESCCAP	European Scientific Counsel Companion Animal Parasites	**SAF**	sodium acetate formalin
FECRT	fecal egg-count reduction test	**TLR**	toll-like receptor
HE	hematoxylin and eosin stain	**VLM**	visceral larva migrans
HPO	hypertrophic pulmonary osteoarthropathy	**Z-N-stain**	Ziehl-Neelsen stain

Chapter 1

Introduction

Parasites are eukaryotic pathogenic organisms belonging to protozoa (unicellular organisms) or metazoa (multicellular animals). Parasitism is a subtype of symbiosis, in which one of the symbionts (parasite) benefits from the coexistence and the other one (host) is adversely affected. The disservice to the host, however, is debatable in many parasitic infections. Typically, it does not benefit the parasite if the host becomes unwell or even dies. On the other hand, it is often more beneficial for the host to tolerate a moderate number of parasites that do little harm than to strive after a parasite-free state, which would demand a disproportional immunological effort. Many dog owners believe that a single parasite can adversely affect the dog's welfare and thus cannot be tolerated. This is part of the reason that parasite diagnostics and antiparasitic treatments have a significant role in everyday animal care. Some canine parasite infections, even with no or minor effect on the dog itself, are zoonotic. With these infections too, medical interference is in place to protect the humans in the household.

An adult dog often tolerates a moderate parasitic burden well without getting clinical signs or disease. Because the acquired immunity of the host is important in the management of parasitic diseases, parasites cause more severe problems to young animals. Canine immunity, protecting dogs from excess parasitic infections, is unexpectedly an important cause of clinical disease. Ectoparasite infestations often cause a hypersensitivity reaction, manifesting as pruritus and scratching, which leads to trauma and secondary cutaneous bacterial infection. Many clinical parasitic diseases are therefore primarily the result of the reaction of the host against the parasite rather than damage caused by the parasite itself.

A parasite's life is described as a life cycle. The definitive host is the host animal species in which the sexual reproduction of the parasite takes place. The result of this is offspring in the form of eggs, cysts, oocysts, or larvae. If the next definitive host can be infected directly from the end-results of the reproduction, the life cycle is called direct. Nematodes usually have a direct life cycle. In an indirect life cycle, one or several intermediate host species are required for maturation and asexual reproduction of the parasite. The definitive host can be infected only after these necessary phases. The animal is usually infected when it eats an intermediate host and the infective parasite forms the host carries. Cestodes and trematodes typically have an indirect life cycle.

The complex life cycles of parasites, developed in evolution, may appear bizarre and even impractical. Why does a larva of a canine roundworm have to embark on a dangerous odyssey in the body of the puppy before it can mature into an adult in the gut? Why do certain flatworms have to have two intermediate hosts before they can infect the definitive host? The parasite always has a reason for its life cycle. For example, stages in intermediate hosts facilitate the asexual increase of the parasite population and may offer a safe haven during periods when unfavorable conditions endanger the rest of the life cycle. The parasite stages in the environment, in the intermediate hosts, and in vectors make the life cycle difficult to break and infection hard to control.

Dogs' parasites can be classified by their location to endo- and ectoparasites (Fig. 1.1). Endoparasites are usually helminths or protozoans. Most of the ectoparasites are arthropods: insects or acari. Some parasites are obligatory, and constantly need their host for survival. Others are facultative parasites that perform part of their life cycle outside the host and only, for example, suck blood from the host animal or convert to parasitism when the living conditions become unfavorable. Some organisms are considered as normal fauna, but in exceptional conditions they may cause clinical signs and act as parasites. In addition to these parasite behavioral classifications, taxonomy based on the (genetic) systematics is used for precise classification of the parasite species.

In parasite diagnostics, classical fairly inexpensive methods are still in routine use, but newer methods have been shown to be a useful addition to these traditional diagnostics. The aim should always be to base the treatment on a correct diagnosis.

The guidelines for canine anthelmintic treatments vary geographically because of the difference in the prevalence of parasites. They also vary by time, as more knowledge and research data becomes available. For example, data on anthelmintic resistance may have an influence on the recommendations. Different drugs are in use around the world due to countries' different regulations.

Canine Parasites and Parasitic Diseases. https://doi.org/10.1016/B978-0-12-814112-0.00001-5

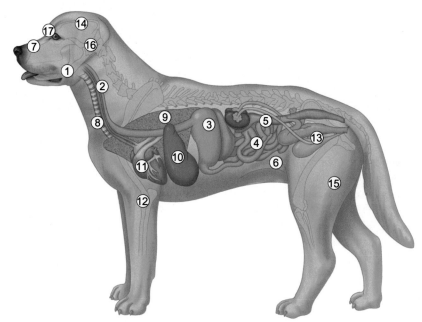

FIG. 1.1 Canine parasites by their most common anatomical location.

(1) **Mouth and pharynx—Protozoa:** *Tetratrichomonas canistomae, Trichomonas tenax.*

(2) **Esophagus—Nematoda:** *Spirocerca lupi.*

(3) **Stomach—Nematoda:** *Physaloptera* species.

(4) **Small intestine—Protozoa:** *Isospora canis, Isospora ohioensis complex, Cryptosporidium canis, Neospora caninum, Sarcocystis* species, *Giardia canis;* **Cestoda:** *Dipylidium caninum, Diphyllobothrium latum, Hymenolepis* species, *Mesocestoides* species, *Spirometra* species, *Taenia* species, *Echinococcus granulosus* complex, *Echinococcus multilocularis;* **Trematoda:** *Alaria alata, Mesostephanus* species, *Apophallus donicum, Heterophyes, Dicrocoelium dendriticum, Nanophyetus salmincola;* and **Nematoda:** *Toxocara canis, Toxascaris leonina, Baylisascaris procyonis, Strongyloides stercoralis, Uncinaria stenocephala, Ancylostoma caninum, Ancylostoma braziliense, Trichinella* species, **Acantocephala:** *Macracanthohynchus* species, *Oncicola canis.*

(5) **Large intestine—Protozoa:** *Entamoeba histolytica* and **Nematoda:** *Trichuris vulpis.*

(6) **Peritoneum and the abdominal cavity—Cestoda:** *Mesocestoides* species, *Spirometra* species and **Nematoda:** *Acantocheilonema dracunculoides.*

(7) **Nose and the nasal cavities—Nematoda:** *Eucoleus boehmi* and **Arthropoda:** *Pneumonyssoides caninum, Linguatula serrata.*

(8) **Trachea and bronchus—Nematoda:** *Oslerus osleri, Eucoleus aerophilus.*

(9) **Lower respiratory tract—Protozoa:** *Toxoplasma gondii;* **Nematoda:** *Toxoacara canis (larval stages), Oslerus osleri, Filaroides hirthi, Filaroides milksi, Crenosoma vulpis;* and **Trematoda:** *Alaria alata* (larval stages), *Paragonimus kellicotti.*

(10) **Liver—Protozoa:** *Toxoplasma gondii, Leishmania* species; **Trematoda:** *Clonorchis sinensis, Dicrocoelium dendriticum, Heterobilharzia americana, Metorchis* species; and **Nematoda:** *Capillaria hepatica.*

(11) **Blood and circulation—Protozoa:** *Toxoplasma gondii, Babesia* species, *Hepatozoon canis, Leishmania* species; **Trematoda:** *Heterobilharzia americana;* and **Nematoda:** *Angiostrongylus vasorum, Dirofilaria immitis, Dirofilaria repens* (microfilaria), *Acantocheilonema reconditum* (microfilaria), *Acantocheilonema dracunculoides* (microfilaria), *Microfilaria* species (microfilaria).

(12) **Locomotion organs and connective tissue—Protozoa:** *Leishmania* species, *Toxoplasma gondii, Neospora caninum;* **Cestoda:** *Spirometra* species; and **Nematoda:** *Trichinella* species

(13) **Urogenital organs—Protozoa:** *Leishmania* species and **Nematoda:** *Capillaria plica, Dioctophyma renale.*

(14) **Brain and nervous system—Protozoa:** *Toxoplasma gondii, Neospora caninum* and **Nematoda:** *Toxocara canis* (larval stages), *Baylisascaris procyonis* (larval stages).

(15) **Skin, subcutis, fur—Protozoa:** *Leishmania* species, *Sarcocystis* species; **Nematoda:** *Strongyloides stercoralis* (larval stages), *Pelodera strongyloides* (larval stages), *Uncinaria stenocephala* (larval stages), *Ancylostoma caninum* (larval stages*), Ancylostoma braziliense* (larval stages), *Dracunculus insignis, Dirofilaria repens, Acantocheilonema reconditum, Cercopithifilaria* species; **Annelida:** leaches; and **Arthropoda:** *Linognathus setosus, Trichodectes canis, Heterodoxus spiniger, Cimex lectularius, Ctenocephalides* species and other fleas, Tabanidae, Muscidae, and Fanniidae, Oestridae, Calliphoridae, Culicidae, Simulidae, *Culicoides* species, *Hippobosca longipennis, Lipoptena cervi, Ixodes ricinus, Dermacentor reticulatus, Rhipicephalus sanguineus,* Other Ixodidae-ticks. *Ornithodoros moubata,* avian and rodent mites, *Cheyletiella yasguri, Demodex canis, Demodex injai, Demodex cornei,* Trombiculidae and Leeuwenhoekiidae *mites, Sarcoptes scabiei.*

(16) **Ear—Arthropoda:** *Otodectes cynotis, Otobius megnini, Demodex canis.*

(17) **Ocular region—Protozoa:** *Toxoplasma gondii* and **Nematoda:** *Toxocara canis* (larval stages), *Thelazia callipaeda, Thelazia californiensis, Onchocerca lupi.*

Increased travel and importation of the dogs, and gradually also climate change, will lead to a greater variety of canine parasites in countries where canine parasites have not previously been an issue. In contrast, the use of efficient and long-acting antiparasitic drugs will diminish the spectrum of canine parasites and may even endanger some parasite species.

PARASITOLOGICAL CONCEPTS

Life cycle describes the stages of the parasite's life span: what kinds of host species the parasite needs, in what forms it parasitizes in each host and in what organs it visits or colonizes in the host. The direct life cycle involves no intermediate hosts, while the indirect life cycle involves at least one intermediate host species.

The *definitive, final, or primary host* is the host in which the parasite reproduces sexually.

The *intermediate host* is a host species that is obligatory for the life cycle of certain parasites. The development to the stage infectious to the next host takes place in the intermediate host, and occasionally also asexual reproduction—for instance, by cell division. If the life cycle includes an intermediate host, direct transmission between definitive hosts is not possible, apart from a few exceptions.

The *paratenic host* refers to a species that is accidentally infected, but the parasite will not undergo any development while staying infectious. Thus, the paratenic host may act as a source of infection for the definitive hosts. In some cases, paratenic hosts may have an important epidemiologic role as parasite storage.

The *dead-end host* is a host where the parasite's life cycle ends. Humans are dead-end hosts for many parasitic infections, because human flesh is not used for animal feed, thus stopping the life cycle. Human parasitic infections are also treated effectively, which reduces the significance of this host for parasitic life cycles.

The *prepatent period* is the time starting from the infection up to the time when the parasite starts to reproduce recognizably in its definitive host, or the infection can otherwise be diagnosed. Thus, the prepatent period is a diagnostically and therapeutically a problematic stage: a dog may already be infected but the infection cannot be diagnosed. Antiparasitic medicines may be ineffective against some parasites during the prepatent period. Different parasites have distinct prepatent periods.

The *patent period* refers to the time that the parasite lives in the host, reproduces, and can be diagnosed.

Hypobiosis is the adaptive developmental stage of nematode worms. It is a rest period, during which the life cycle stops—for instance, due to unfavorable conditions—but continues later, when the conditions allow.

For more terms, see the glossary at the end of this book.

Chapter 2

Protozoa

Protozoa are eukaryotic unicellular organisms, which together with single-cell algae and slime molds belong to the Protista kingdom. They possess a simpler and more primitive structure than the members of the animal kingdom. The protozoans contain a membrane-surrounded nucleus and cellular organs. Most protozoa have, at least in some stage of their life, structures such as flagella or cilia that enable them to move and, for some species, to obtain nutrients. The traditional classification of protozoa is based on their structures of movement (e.g., flagellates, ciliates). Most protozoa are microscopical. They live in moist conditions and only a few are parasites. Protozoans usually multiply asexually by binary or multiple fission. Some are capable of sexual reproduction.

Eucoccidiorida-order protozoans are called coccidians and they cause the disease coccidiosis. In dogs, coccidians are *Isospora* type and they reproduce sexually in the dog's intestine. After cycles of asexual reproduction, merogony (also known as schizogony) and gametogony take place, producing oocysts to be spread to the environment. Depending on the coccidian, the oocysts are directly infective to the next host or they require a certain period of time in the oxygen-rich environment to sporulate into the infective form. Sporulated *Isospora*-type oocysts have two spocysts inside, with four sporozoites within them. In Eimeria-type oocysts, which are shed by herbivorous animals, there are four or more sporocysts with two sporozoites within them.

Some protozoans infect dogs with the aid of arthropod vectors. Piroplasmida-order (*Babesia*) protozoans spread by tick bites and spend their life cycle in a dog as intraerythrocyte forms. *Trypanosoma*, which lives in the cytoplasm of white blood cells, spreads to dogs through ingestion of an arthropod vector.

Flagellate protozoans in Diplomonadida and Trichomonadida orders have characteristic flagellae in their trophozoite forms. Some genera, such as *Giardia*, also produce resistant cysts for better survival in their environment. They infect the dog directly, without any vectors.

As treatment, antibiotics such as benzimidazoles or toltrazuril are used for intestinal protozoans. These protozoans affect puppies in particular, and require good hygiene for the prevention of the disease. For systemic protozoan infections, there are both unspecific and specific medications.

The vector-borne protozoans may harm adult dogs too, and for prevention the arthropod exposure should be controlled.

ISOSPORA (CYSTOISOPORA) CANIS, ISOSPORA OHIOENSIS-Complex

- Coccidian parasites of small intestine.
- Infects especially puppies with oocysts from their living environment.
- Causes diarrhea in puppies; stress is usually a predisposing factor for clinical disease.
- Diagnosis by detecting *Isospora*-type oocysts from fecal sample.
- Treatment with toltrazuril or sulfonamides.

Identification

Isospora species are coccidian protozoans that multiply sexually in the small intestine of the dog and secrete into feces oval oocysts lacking a micropyle, which is a small opening and a lid-like structure in the surface of the oocyst. The size of *Isospora canis* oocysts is $37 \times 30\,\mu m$, while *Isospora ohioensis*-complex oocysts are smaller, about $25 \times 20\,\mu m$. The species of *I. ohioensis*-complex parasites cannot be identified morphologically. In fresh feces, the oocysts are in unsporulated and in noninfective form, but they, after 1–4 days, become infectious through sporulation. A sporulated *Isospora*-type oocyst contains two sporocysts with four sporozoites inside each sporocyst (Fig. 2.1).

Life Cycle

Puppies are usually infected by ingesting sporulated *Isospora* oocysts from their living environment. If sporulated oocysts end up orally in dogs' food, the freed sporozoites remain infectious and the dog may be infected by eating this paratenic host. The prepatent period of *I. canis* is 8–12 days and that of *I. ohioensis* complex parasites 4–9 days. The shell of the oocyst is broken down and the sporozoites are released in the intestinal tract. The sporozoites invade the epithelial cells of the small intestine as a kick-off of

Canine Parasites and Parasitic Diseases. https://doi.org/10.1016/B978-0-12-814112-0.00002-7

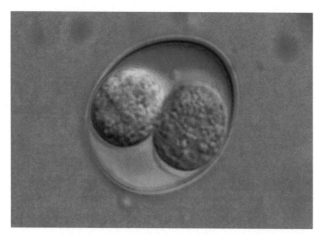

FIG. 2.1 A partially sporulated oocyst belonging to *Isospora ohioensis*-complex. The size of the cyst is $23 \times 20 \mu m$.

the asexual reproduction merogonia (also known as schizogonia), which takes place in several repeated cycles. Asexual cycles are followed by the phase of sexual reproduction: gametogonia. The end-result of the cycle is an oocyst, which is voided in the feces. These oocysts may number up to 200,000 in a gram of feces. In the environment, the oocysts sporulate in a few days, depending on conditions (e.g., in $+20^{\circ}C$ this takes 48 h) and subsequently become

infective for their next hosts. The oocysts are viable and remain infectious for months. The lifecycle of *Isospora* spp. is illustrated in Fig. 2.2.

Distribution

Four *Isospora* species parasitize dogs: *I. canis*, *I. ohioensis*, *I. burrowsi*, and *I. neorivolta*. The three latter ones are often classified as so-called *I. ohioensis*-complex, because they cannot be distinguished from each other on the basis of oocyst morphology. *Isospora* infections, often referred as coccidiosis, are common in dogs, especially in puppies, around the world. Dense dog populations, such as kennel conditions, are conducive for transmission. Coccidian oocysts found in the feces of adult dogs can usually be traced to the stools of herbivore animals, such as sheep or hares, which have been eaten by the dog. Those belong to the Eimeria genus and are not infective to dogs; they are only passing by the intestinal tract.

Importance to Canine Health

The clinical signs are due to destruction of the intestinal epithelial cells. The damage of the epithelium results in the diminution of the absorptive surface of the gut or

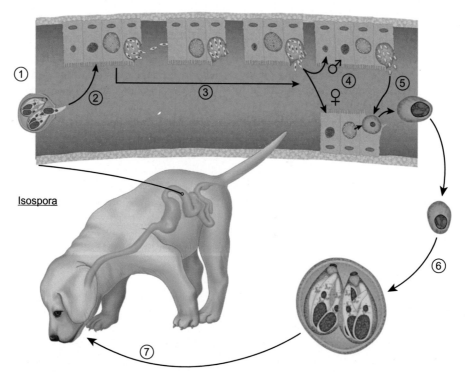

FIG. 2.2 Life cycle of *Isospora canis*: (1) the dog is infected when sporulated oocysts of *Isospora* enter its gut; (2) the shell of the oocyst breaks down and releases parasitic sporozoites, which penetrate intestinal epithelial cells; (3) the asexual reproduction of the parasite (merogony/schizogony) begins in the epithelial cells of the small intestine, is repeated during several cycles, and leads to the infection of new epithelial cells; (4) the next state is sexual reproduction, or gametogonia, producing both male microgametes and female macrogametocytes; (5) the sexual cycle results in the fertilized zygote, which develops into an oocyst that exits the canine host in feces; and (6) the oocysts sporulate in the environment in a few days and become infectious to new dogs.

full-thickness epithelial damage extending to the underlying connective tissue of the mucosa. This may be accompanied by hemorrhage into the lumen of the intestine and inflammation. The most important sign is watery or bloody, yet often self-limiting diarrhea, lasting sometimes for weeks. There may be vomiting and abdominal pain. Clinical signs manifest typically in puppies under 4 months of age. The growth and development of the puppy may be affected even in subclinical cases. Coccidia are opportunistic pathogens; if pathogenic, their virulence may be influenced by various stressors such as changes in living conditions or feeding (e.g., when solid foods are introduced to puppies). Coinfections with viruses, bacteria, and other parasites are common in dogs displaying clinical signs.

Diagnosis

The fecal oocysts are detected with flotation methods. As diarrhea may start before the secretion of oocysts, it may be necessary to analyze several fecal samples. When oocysts are found in feces, it is recommended to sporulate the cysts to ascertain that they really are of the *Isospora*-type (two sporocysts in each oocyst). Sporulation takes place in moist and oxygen-rich conditions, for instance, on a petri dish, and it can be enhanced with potassium dichromate. Dogs often practice coprophagia, and it is very common to find *Eimeria* coccidia (with four sporocysts in a sporulated oocyst) of hares or ruminants, for example, in canine feces. They do not infect dogs, cause no adverse effects in dogs, and do not require intervention.

Treatment and Prevention

All puppies that have been in contact with dogs with coccidiosis should be treated (the whole litter). Early treatment minimizes the epithelial damage in the gut. Common medicinal treatments are sulfonamides or toltrazuril. For supportive therapy, rehydration and antimicrobial treatment can be used, if secondary bacterial infection is suspected.

Avoiding stress and maintaining good hygiene in the environment of puppies is important for prophylaxis. Stools should be removed without delay and the surfaces allowed to dry after washing. Disinfection with steam or chemicals such as 10% ammonia may increase the efficacy of cleaning, but oocysts are generally very resistant to common disinfectants, which emphasizes the significance of mechanical cleaning. Heat and dryness help to kill and control environmental oocysts. The personnel handling infected puppies must maintain good hygiene to prevent the transfer of the infection between dogs and kennel facilities.

NEOSPORA CANINUM

- Coccidian with canines as definitive hosts and herbivores, especially cattle, as intermediate hosts.
- Infection orally from oocysts or tissue cysts; puppies may acquire the infection transplacentally from the dam.
- Clinically progressive paralysis of the hind limbs, encephalitis, meningitis, and other signs.
- In cattle an important cause of abortions.
- Diagnosis serologically or from oocysts in the feces.

Identification

Neospora is a coccidian protozoa. The size of its tachyzoite is $6 \times 2\,\mu m$ (Fig. 2.3). The wall of the tissue cyst filled with bradyzoites (Fig. 2.4) is about $4\,\mu m$ thick, and the size of the cyst may be over $100\,\mu m$ (Fig. 2.5). The diameter of the oocysts is about $10\,\mu m$, and having sporulated in the environment, two sporocysts form inside them, each containing four sporozoites.

Life Cycle

Canids are the definitive hosts of *Neospora* and many herbivorous animals are its intermediate hosts. *Neospora* does not infect humans. The dog is infected by the feco-oral route by infective oocysts or by ingesting the tissues of an infected intermediate host. The unborn puppies may be infected by the transplacental route. The motile and rapidly dividing tachyzoites are released from the oocyst or from tissues in the intestinal tract and they begin multiplying first asexually and then sexually in the dog's intestinal epithelium. As the result of sexual gametogony, oocysts are released into the environment in the feces. They are in unsporulated form in fresh feces. In a few days, the oocysts

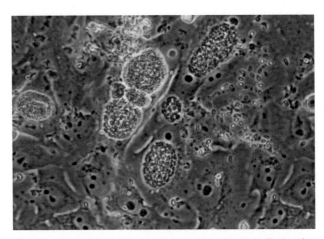

FIG. 2.3 Tachyzoites of *Neospora caninum* in cell culture. Tachyzoites can be seen as small, bluish organisms, both free and as intracellular cystic groups. *(Reproduced with permission from Katarzyna Goździk.)*

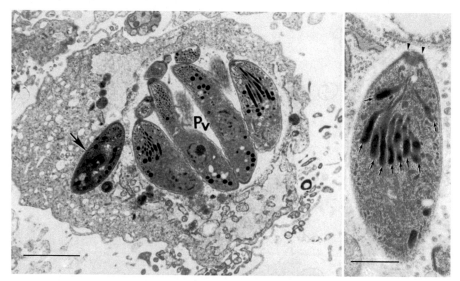

FIG. 2.4 TEM of *Neospora caninum* tachyzoites in cell culture (on the *left*). A group of tachyzoites can be seen in a parasitophorous vacuole (Pv). One tachyzoite (*arrow*) is located in the host cell cytoplasm without any visible surrounding parasitophorous vacuole; scale bar = 2 μm. On the *right*, TEM of a tachyzoite of *N. caninum*. Apical end showing a conoid (*arrowheads*) and nine rhoptries (the arrows pointing to blind ends of rhoptries) with electron-dense contents; scale bar = 1 μm. *(Reproduced with permission from The TEM micrographs from Dubey JP, Barr BC, Barta JR, Bjerkås I, Björkman C, Blagburn L, Bowman D., et al. Redescription of* Neospora caninum *and its differentiation from related coccidian, Int J Parasitol 3:929–946, 2002.)*

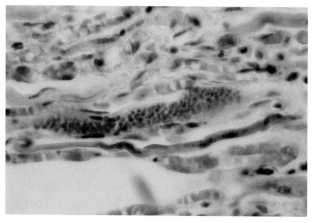

FIG. 2.5 Light microscope micrograph of a tissue section taken from a dog suffering from neosporosis. Myositis and the light-blue tissue cyst filled with bradyzoites are present.

become infective through sporulation. Animals at pasture, typically cattle, serve as an intermediate host, and ingest oocysts while grazing. In the ruminant's intestine the oocyst breaks down and the released sporozoites disseminate throughout the body. In response to the intermediate host's immune response, the oocysts differentiate into bradyzoites, which form cysts in muscle and tissue. Tachyzoites are able to invade the fetus through the placenta. Bradyzoites multiply slowly in the tissues of both definitive and intermediate hosts, and form tissue cysts. Recent studies have broadened the list of known intermediate hosts to include birds. The life cycle of *Neospora caninum* is illustrated in Fig. 2.6.

Distribution

Canine as well as bovine *Neospora* infections are ubiquitous around the world. Sheep, goats, and horses—even birds—may also be infected and act as intermediate hosts. The sexual reproduction of the parasite, however, only occurs in canids. *Neospora* infections originating from dogs are a significant cause of bovine abortions and production losses.

Importance to Canine Health

Tissue cysts that grow in the host may lead to many types of clinical signs. The cysts are most common in nervous tissue and muscle, but all organs may become infected. In dogs, typically in puppies under 6 months of age, the most obvious sign of *Neospora* infection is generally a progressive paralysis that starts from the hind limbs. It is caused by myositis and neuritis (polyraculoneuritis-myositis syndrome), which are results of the immune response against the tissue cysts. Gradually the hind limbs often overextend and the dog cannot stand anymore. Instead, it sits with its legs stiffly pointing forward (Fig. 2.7). Encephalitis and meningitis and the infection and inflammation of diverse parts of the central nervous system cause fainting, loss of balance, ataxia, and paralytic signs. Myocarditis, hepatitis, dermatitis, pulmonary and splenic infection and ocular lesions have also been associated with neosporosis. A dog over 6 months is assumed in most cases to display clinical signs due to a reemergence of an earlier infection. In these cases, central nervous signs are usually dominant. In experimental infections involving

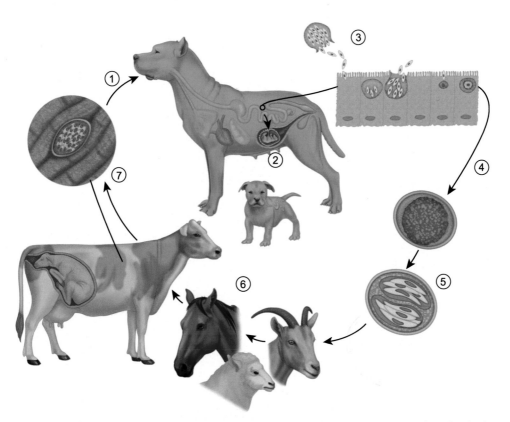

FIG. 2.6 Life cycle of *Neospora caninum*: (1) the dog is infected by the feco-oral route by infective oocysts or by ingesting the tissues of an infected intermediate host; (2) the unborn puppies may be infected by the transplacental route; (3) the motile and rapidly dividing tachyzoites are released from the oocyst or from tissues in the intestinal tract and they begin multiplying first asexually and then sexually in the dog's intestinal epithelium; (4) as the result of sexual gametogony, oocysts are released in the environment in the feces; (5) in a few days, the oocysts become infective through sporulation; (6) animals at pasture, typically cattle, but also horses, goats, and sheep, for example, serve as intermediate hosts. Even birds may serve as an intermediate hosts. The oocyst breaks down in the intermediate host's intestine and the released sporozoites disseminate throughout the body; in response to the intermediate host's immune response, the sporozoites differentiate into bradyzoites, which form cysts in muscle and tissue; and (7) tachyzoites are able to invade the fetus through the placenta. Bradyzoites multiply slowly and form tissue cysts.

pregnant bitches, *Neospora* has caused abortions and the birth of weak puppies.

In cattle, the infection causes abortions and subsequently great production losses worldwide. The calf may be born

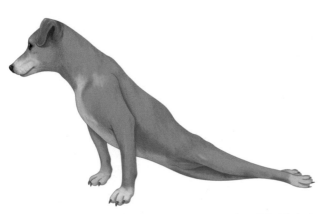

FIG. 2.7 A hind limb paresis with rigid hyperexpension of hind limbs is considered a classical sign of polyradiculoneuritis-myositis syndrome associated with *N. caninum* infection in puppies.

infected and, when pregnant later, transfer the infection to its own offspring. Carriers of *Neospora* infection often have to be culled.

Diagnosis

Commercial serological indirect fluorescent antibody test (IFAT) and enzyme-linked immunosorbent assay (ELISA) assays are available. The serological diagnosis in puppies is difficult, because the maternally derived antibodies may cause a false positive result up to the age of 32 days. The result of the serological test is inconclusive at the time of oocyst release in terms of the infectivity of the dog. While the small-sized oocysts may be seen in routine fecal tests based on flotation, their number is low and secretion intermittent. Consequently, the risk of false negative results is high. The dog is not the definitive host of the feline *Toxoplasma*, but it may eat feline feces. Thus, oocysts of *Toxoplasma* can be found in canine feces after coprophagy. The oocysts of *Neospora*, *Toxoplasma*, and *Hammondia* are all small, and cannot be morphologically differentiated reliably. The finding can be identified as *Neospora* with PCR analysis. A dog may secrete a small number of *Neospora* oocysts variably after infection during a long period. Thus, an infected dog should always be considered a *Neospora* risk on cattle farms. The parasite can be identified with PCR from tissue samples or the cerebrospinal fluid. A negative result does not guarantee noninfection, as cysts are scarce and unevenly distributed in the tissues. Suspicious cysts found in tissues samples can also be confirmed as *Neospora* cysts with immunohistochemical staining methods.

Treatment and Prevention

Clindamycin, trimethoprim, sulfadiazine, and pyrimethamine, alone or in combinations, are recommended for the treatment of neosporosis. The use of corticosteroids is contraindicated, since they may worsen the clinical signs. If one puppy in a litter has a confirmed *Neospora* infection, the whole litter should be treated. Prognosis depends on the promptness of the treatment. If the disease has proceeded to the overextension of hind limbs, the prognosis is poor, because irreversible tissue damage has already occurred.

Dogs should not be allowed to eat aborted fetuses or fetal membranes of pastured animals or deer. The meat of these animals should be cooked or thoroughly frozen before given to dogs. Dog or wild canids should not be allowed to contaminate bovine feed or drinking fountains with their feces. If dogs are used for herding cattle, their access to the feeding areas, including pastures, should be minimized and limited to work. Leisure time should be spent elsewhere. If dogs defecate into cattle's feeding area, the stools should be discarded before possible oocysts turn infective.

TOXOPLASMA GONDII

- Felines as definitive hosts; dogs get infected as intermediate hosts and do not spread oocysts.
- Infection from oocysts from the environment or tissue cysts from under-cooked meat.
- Usually subclinical, but central nervous system signs or abortions may occur.
- Diagnosis with immunological tests or PCR.
- No registered treatment, but clindamycin, trimethoprim, sulfadiazine, and pyrimethamine have been used.

Identification

Toxoplasma is a coccidian protozoa belonging in the family Sarcocystidae. Three different genotypes (I–III) of different virulence are known, together with atypical strains. The size of sickle-shaped tachyzoites is $6 \times 2\,\mu m$. The diameter of the early tissue cyst containing a few bradyzoites is only $5\,\mu m$, but it may grow to a cyst of up to $100\,\mu m$, containing thousands of bradyzoites. The shape of tissue cysts in muscle are more longitudinal than, for instance, those in the brain. The size of the oocyst is $10 \times 12\,\mu m$. In sporulation, two sporocysts develop inside the oocyst, each containing four sporozoites.

Life Cycle

Felids are the definitive hosts of *Toxoplasma*, and the sexual reproduction and the production of oocysts take place only in them. Many other animals, including dogs, are intermediate hosts of *Toxoplasma*. The infection may pass also between the intermediate hosts, without sexual reproduction. The dog is typically infected after having eaten infective meat. The infection may happen transplacentally from the bitch to puppies, or after the ingestion of sporulated oocysts in feline stools. The parasites are freed from the oocyst or the tissue cyst in the intestinal tract, distributed to the dog's tissues, then start multiplying asexually and form tissue cysts.

Distribution

Toxoplasma is considered the most widely distributed parasite in the world, both geographically as well as in regard of the number of host species. Almost all warm-blooded animals can serve as intermediate hosts. Different genotypes and atypical strains have geographically distinct, albeit partly overlapping areas of distribution. *Toxoplasma* is common in cats, and cystic forms of the parasite are frequently found in the muscle samples of different species. It is therefore probable that many dogs get the infection during their lives.

Importance to Canine Health

The *Toxoplasma* infection of an adult and healthy dog is usually subclinical. Tissue cysts are typically found in skeletal muscles, heart, or brain, but other organs may be infected and the dog may start showing clinical signs. The infection of brain, meninges, and the central nervous system causes seizures, ataxia, shaking, circling, changes in consciousness, and behavioral abnormalities. In eyes, manifestations of toxoplasmosis may vary from slight photophobia to blindness. A pregnant bitch may abort or give birth to dead puppies. Thus, the clinical manifestations of toxoplasmosis vary greatly.

Diagnosis

Commercial serological tests based on agglutination, IFAT, or ELISA are available. However, the seropositivity confirms only the infection, not the association of *Toxoplasma* and the clinical findings and disease. The parasite can also be detected in tissue samples or cerebrospinal fluid with PCR; however, the absence of parasites in tissue samples does not guarantee noninfection, because tissue cysts are scarce and they are unevenly distributed. *Toxoplasma* can be confirmed with immunohistochemical staining of tissue cysts. Since the dog is not the definitive host of *Toxoplasma*, the diagnosis cannot be made through coprological examination.

Treatment and Prevention

Clindamycin, trimethoprim, sulfadiazine, and pyrimethamine, alone or in combinations, are recommended for treatment, although these substances are not registered for toxoplasmosis therapy in dogs. Meat and organs should be cooked in +67°C or frozen thoroughly before being given to dogs. Canine *Toxoplasma* infection does not pose a risk to humans in countries where dogs are not eaten. However, the dog has been proven to serve as a mechanical vehicle of oocysts from the environment to the vicinity to humans, when the dog has been rolling in feline feces or ingested them.

HAMMONDIA SPECIES

- Close relative to *Neospora* and *Toxoplasma*.
- Infection by eating tissue cysts, not oocysts.
- Usually no clinical signs.
- Diagnosis by finding oocysts in fecal sample; differentiation from *Toxoplasma* and *Neospora* requires PCR.
- Treatment is rarely required, but clindamysin may be used if necessary.

Identification

Hammondia is a close relative of *Neospora* and *Toxoplasma*, and its oocysts are morphologically indistinguishable from them. Species that are known to infect dogs are *Hammondia hammondi* and *Hammondia heydorni*. The oocyst size is about 12 × 11 μm, and the shape is round. They sporulate as *Isospora*-type oocysts: two sporocysts, with four sporozoites within them.

Life Cycle

Carnivores are the definitive hosts for *Hammondia*, and sexual reproduction and oocyst production happen in them after the prepatent period of 5–13 days (*H. hammondi*) or 7–17 days (*H. heydorni*). Herbivores and rodents act as intermediate hosts. Unlike in the case of *Toxoplasma*,

the oocysts are only infective to the intermediate hosts, and the definitive hosts become infected only after eating tissue cysts.

Distribution

Hammondia species are distributed worldwide, but because the differentiation from *Neospora* and *Toxoplasma* requires PCR, the true prevalence is often not known.

Importance to Canine Health

Most often the infection is subclinical, and the oocysts are an accidental finding in feces. If signs appear (e.g., in immuno-compromised dogs), they are gastrointestinal and later in the course of infection, they may vary according to the organs involved. Neurological signs have been reported, for example.

Diagnosis

Hammondia oocysts can be found in fecal examination with routine methods, such as flotation techniques. These oocysts are morphologically similar to small *Neospora* and *Toxoplasma* oocysts.

Treatment and Prevention

Usually treatment is not needed; however, if there are clinical signs, clindamycin for 2–4 weeks is the drug of choice. Puppies may need supportive therapy to recover. If neurological signs are involved, the prognosis is guarded as irreversible tissue damage might have already occurred.

SARCOCYSTIS SPECIES

- Coccidians with carnivorous definitive host and herbivorous intermediate host.
- Dog becomes infected by eating tissue cysts from the intermediate host.
- Dogs usually have no clinical signs of infection, mild diarrhea may occur.
- Diagnosis from fecal sample, where the oocysts are present in already sporulated and infective forms.
- Treatment is rarely required.

Identification

Sarcocystis species belong to coccidian protozoa. The oocysts sporulate in the definitive host and are thus sporulated while voided in the feces of the dog. The sporulated oocyst is elliptical and about 20 μm in diameter. It contains two sporocysts, each holding four sporozoites. The wall of the oocyst is fragile and breaks down readily, releasing the sporocysts in the feces of the definitive host. Depending on the species, the size of the sporocyst is about $15 \times 10\,\mu m$. The cystic tissue form of this parasite is called a sarcocyst (or sarcosporid) and contains bradyzoites; it is located in the muscle of the intermediate hosts, rarely in a dog (Figs. 2.8–2.10). Sarcocysts can be large enough to be seen by the naked eye, or may be microscopical, depending on the host species.

Life Cycle

Sarcocystis protozoa have typically a carnivorous definitive host and a herbivorous intermediate host. The species are named after the hosts. For instance, *Sarcocystis bovicanis*, also known as *S. cruzi*, is named after the intermediate host cattle and the definitive host dog. The dog is infected by eating bradyzoites of the parasitic cysts with bovine meat. In the intestinal tract, the liberated zoites penetrate the gut epithelium and multiply sexually by gametogonia. Oocysts sporulate before being secreted and are consequently infectious when they end up in the environment in the dog's feces. They remain infective in the environment for months, even years, depending on the conditions. The prepatent period from infection through sexual reproduction to secretion of the oocyst of new generation is 1–4 weeks, and the patent period is several months. The intermediate host eats feed contaminated with oocysts and the asexual reproduction starts in the intestinal tract and mesenteric veins by merogony. The merozoites end up in the host's muscles and multiply there slowly by division as bradyzoites, forming tissue cysts. In the host's organism, the asexual reproduction happens via endopolygonia, in which the internal splicing produces several new organisms within the parent organism.

Distribution

There are many *Sarcocystis* species, with dogs as their definitive hosts. At least 21 species have been identified in the canine feces. The geographical distribution depends on the local spectrum of intermediate hosts. During the meat inspection or histopathology, cysts of *Sarcocystis* are a common incidental finding when analyzing the muscle tissue of herbivorous intermediate host species.

Importance to Canine Health

Sarcocystis does not usually cause clinical signs to the dog, but mild diarrhea is sometimes associated with the infection. The infection is self-limiting. In isolated cases, an extraintestinal or even generalized form of the disease has been described in dogs. Its characteristic is that the infection spreads from the intestine elsewhere in the body. Necrotic lesions in the liver and infection of muscle or nerve

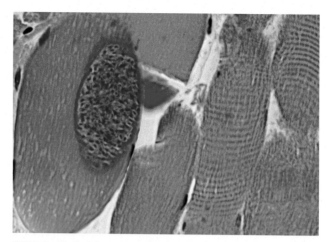

FIG. 2.8 Typical tissue cyst with bradyzoites of *Sarcocystis* in the canine striated muscle. *(Reproduced with permission from Antti Sukura.)*

tissues may be seen. The signs may then be severe: fever, pain, elevated liver or muscle enzyme activity, weakness, and inappetence. Purulent and ulcerative skin lesions have been described in association with extraintestinal sarcocystosis, especially in Rottweilers. *Sarcocystis neurona* is found in horses and in rare cases it can be carried by opossums to dogs, which act as intermediate hosts and can develop neurological signs. Canine *Sarcocystis* infections are not transmitted to humans.

Diagnosis

Sporulated *Sarcocystis* oocysts or freed sporocysts can be detected in a canine stool sample, for instance, with flotation methods. If the rare canine muscular sarcocystosis (sarcosporidiosis) is suspected, organisms may be made visible in a muscle biopsy or in cytological samples (Figs. 2.8–2.11), and sometimes even in peripheral blood (Fig. 2.12). If needed, immunohistochemical methods (Fig. 2.13) and PCR may provide confirmation of the diagnosis. PCR is used to define the *Sarcocystis* species.

Treatment and Prevention

Since the infection does not usually cause clinical signs to the dog and is self-limiting, no treatment has described against the parasite. In cases of diarrhea, supportive treatment is indicated. To interrupt the parasite's life cycle, the canine feces should not be allowed to contaminate food or drinking water given to domestic animals. Giving raw infected meat to dogs should be avoided. Thorough cooking of meat at 70°C or freezing (−20°C for 4 days) destroys *Sarcocystis*.

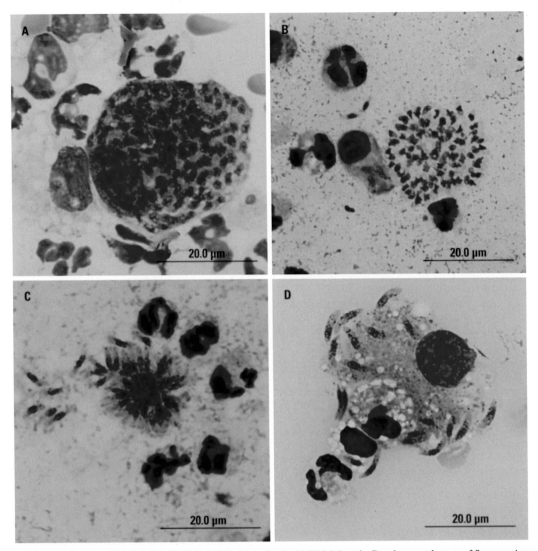

FIG. 2.9 Cytological findings from the dog with a draining skin lesion stained with Wright's stain. Developmental stages of *Sarcocystis neurona* can be observed. During division, the parasite nucleus became highly lobulated (A) and merozoites are budded from the periphery (B), sometimes leaving a centrally located residual body (C). Individual merozoites vary in shape and size (D). Most merozoites seen here are slender, but stubby merozoites are also present (D). *(Reproduced with permission from Roberta di Terlizzi.)*

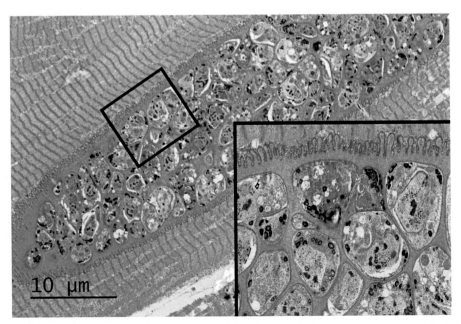

FIG. 2.10 Transmission electron microscopy of a tissue cyst of *Sarcocystis* in striated muscle tissue. Bradyzoites are seen in the detail. *(Reproduced with permission from Antti Sukura.)*

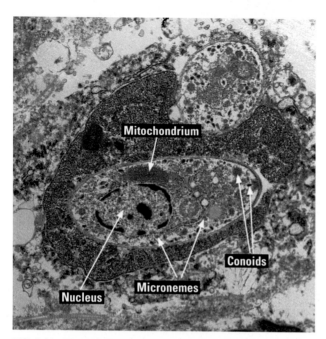

FIG. 2.11 Transmission electron microscopy (TEM) of an intracellular merozoite of *Sarcocystis neurona*. The organism is located directly in the host cell cytoplasm, without any apparent parasitophorous vacuole. Note the presence of conoids (C), micronemes (Mi) distributed throughout the parasite, a nucleus (N), a mitochondrium (Mc), and absence of rhoptries. The latter feature distinguishes *Sarcocystis* merozoites from other Apicomplexa tachyzoites. *(Reproduced with permission from Roberta di Terlizzi.)*

CRYPTOSPORIDIUM CANIS

- Recently reclassified as a gregarine instead of coccidian.
- Infection orally from oocysts; the infection dose is very low.
- Clinically, diarrhea is the primary sign.
- Diagnosis from fecal sample with Ziehl-Nielsen stain or immunological tests.
- No specific treatment available.

Identification

The *Cryptosporidium* genus has been recently classified as gregarine (phylum Apicomplexa, class Gregarinomorphea, subclass Cryptogregaria) instead of belonging to Coccidia, as it was previously classified. Gregarines are capable of completing their lifecycle even without a host. The oocyst of *Cryptosporidium* is small, only about 5 μm in diameter (about the size of a red blood cell). The oocyst contains four sporozoites but no sporocysts. Oocysts are secreted in feces in a sporulated form with an immediate infective effect.

Low Zoonosis Risk Associated With Canine Cryptosporidiosis

Cryptosporidium canis has been isolated in human samples in rare cases involving immunocompromised patients or young children. Even in at-risk groups (young children, organ transfer patients, cancer patients, or people receiving immunosuppressive glucocorticoid medication or having other immunosuppressive conditions), the transfer of cryptosporidia from dog to human is very rare, considering the close coexistence of these two species. Human cryptosporidiosis is often transferred via water, and this method of contagion cannot be ruled out in canine infections either.

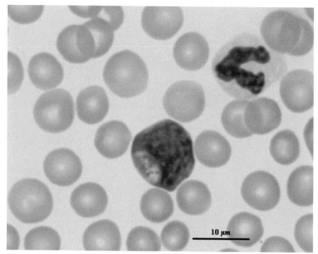

FIG. 2.12 Peripheral blood of a dog, Wright's stain. A reactive lymphocyte contains a *Sarcocystis neurona* merozoite. *(Reproduced with permission from Roberta di Terlizzi.)*

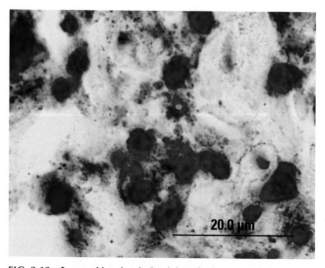

FIG. 2.13 Immunohistochemical staining of a tissue sample from a dog. Strong positive reaction for *Sarcocystis neurona* can be observed with anti *S. neurona* polyclonal antibodies. *(Reproduced with permission from Roberta di Terlizzi.)*

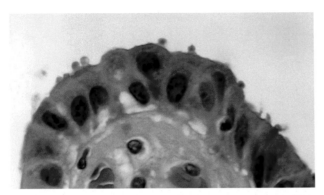

FIG. 2.14 *Cryptosporidium* protozoa seen as spherical structures within microvillus surface of epithelium. *(Courtesy of Dr. Edwin P. Ewing, Jr./ CDC.)*

Life Cycle

The dog receives the infection orally from *Cryptosporidium* oocysts. The infectious dose is very small and the prepatent period varies from days to weeks. Sporozoites that are released from the oocyst penetrate the gut epithelial cells and multiply through asexual (merogony/schizogony) (Figs. 2.14 and 2.15) and sexual cycles (gametogony), resulting in oocysts that sporulate inside the host and are readily infectious when they reach the environment. This early sporulation also enables autoinfection. An infected dog secretes large amounts of oocysts in the feces. An illustrated life cycle of *Cryptosporidium* is presented in Fig. 2.16.

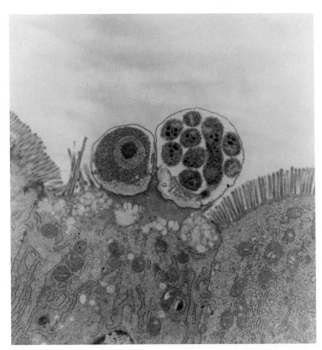

FIG. 2.15 Transmission electron microscopy showing *Cryptosporidium* protozoa in the intestinal microvillus surface of epithelium. Two developmental stages can be seen: a trophozoite (left) and meront (right). *(Reproduced with permission from Science Source Images. Photo by Biophoto Associates.)*

Distribution

Cryptosporidium infections are ubiquitous in humans as well as in animals. Many host species have their specific *Cryptosporidium* species. *C. canis* is specific to dogs. It is common especially in kennels with high dog density. It is also known that dogs frequently visiting dog parks are at greater risk of infection than other dogs.

Importance to Canine Health

The pathogenesis of canine cryptosporidiosis is poorly known, but it is assumed that the canine cryptosporidia behave in the same way as those infecting mice, cattle, and humans, which are better known and studied.

The penetration of cryptosporidia into the intestinal epithelium is limited. Yet they do affect the surface membrane of epithelial cells, which facilitates their access inside the cells. Clinical signs may be caused either by cryptosporidia themselves or by the dog's immune response activated by the infection. Signs may be triggered, for instance, by the inflammation mediators, the shortening of the microvilli covering the epithelial cells of the intestine, or the increased permeability of the gut epithelial lining. The cryptosporidia may loosen the intercellular adhesion between the epithelial cells, which may in turn weaken the epithelial defense barrier. This leads to increased epithelial cell death and the activation of mucosal associated immune-defense. There is little published information on the clinical importance of cryptosporidia to dogs. It appears that *C. canis* is well adjusted to coexistence with dogs, and consequently subclinical infections are common. The infection may manifest in especially young dogs as diarrhea of small-intestine origin, and immunocompromised dogs or dogs with concomitant diseases may have chronic signs, such as weight loss and signs associated with nutrient malabsorption.

Diagnosis

Oocysts in fecal sample are colored bright red in modified Ziehl-Nielsen stain (Fig. 2.17). Several commercial ELISA or immunofluorescence assays have been developed for Crytosporidium diagnosis (Fig. 2.17). The species is defined with PCR.

Therapy and Prevention

There is no specific medical therapy for canine cryptosporidiosis. The treatment is symptomatic and supportive. Sick animals should be isolated from the healthy, if possible, and the environment should be cleaned and good hygiene maintained. *Cryptosporidium* oocysts are resistant to disinfectants but sensitive to heat and drought.

Thorough mechanical cleaning of surfaces is important. Exposure to 3% hydrogen peroxide for 20 min reduces the number of infective oocysts. The cleaned surfaces must be totally dry before dogs are allowed in the space.

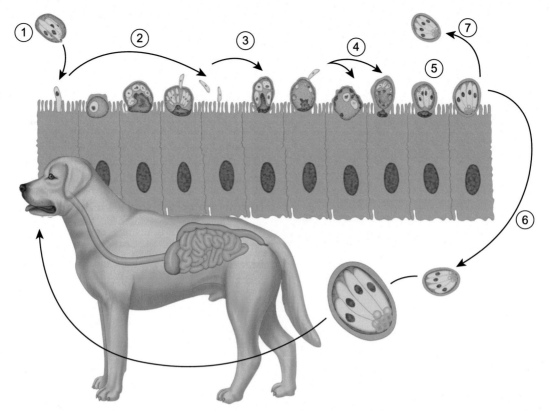

FIG. 2.16 Life cycle of *Cryptosporidium* spp.: (1) the dog gets the infection orally from *Cryptosporidium* oocysts. The infectious dose required is very low and the prepatent period varies from days to weeks. Sporozoites released from the oocyst penetrate the gut epithelial cells; (2) cryptosporia multiply first by merogonia resulting in type I meront, followed by another asexual cycle, type II meront as an end-result (3); (4) type II meronts, or rather the gamonts inside them, serve as a source for sexual cycle called gametogony, producing microgamonts (male) and macrogamonts (female); (5) microgametes fertilize the macrogamont, resulting in the oocyst, which sporulates in the infected host. Oocysts are infective upon excretion, thus permitting direct and immediate fecal-oral transmission as well as auto-infection. There are thick-walled oocysts, which are commonly excreted from the host (6); and thin-walled oocysts, which enable the autoinfection (7). An infected dog secretes large amounts of oocysts in feces.

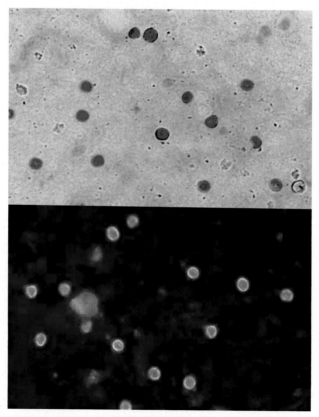

FIG. 2.17 Cryptosporidia in a fecal sample. The small-sized cryptosporidia have been made to stand out and stained red with modified Ziehl-Nielsen staining. A strong specific immunofluorescence reaction can be seen in the immunofluorescence assay (micrograph below). *(Reproduced with permission from Heidi Enemark.)*

BABESIA SPECIES

- Protozoans within the red blood cells.
- Tick-borne parasitic infection.
- Clinical signs resulting from hemolysis.
- Diagnosis from blood smear or immunological tests.
- Treatment depends on *Babesia* species; tick control is an important preventive measure.

Identification

Babesia are protozoans found within red blood cells and belong to the order Piroplasmida. The so-called large canine piroplasms, *B. canis*, *B. rossi*, and *B. vogeli*, are drop-shaped, about 4–5 μm in diameter, and commonly found in pairs (Fig. 2.18). Small canine piroplasms, *B. gibsoni*, *B. annae* (also known as *B. microti*-like and *Theileria annae*), and *B. conradae*, are round or oval, less than 2 μm in diameter, and are usually found singly (Fig. 2.19).

Life Cycle

Babesiosis is a tick-borne disease. When the tick sucks blood, infective sporozoites of *Babesia* are transferred to the dog's blood circulation and penetrate red blood cells. During the repeated asexual cycles (merogony), erythrocytes are broken

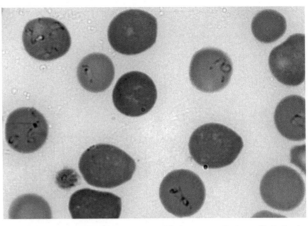

FIG. 2.19 *Babesia gibsoni* is classified as so-called small *Babesia*. Typical forms are seen in several erythrocytes. Blood smear stained with Giemsa.

down and merozoites are liberated to infect yet more red blood cells. Another tick ingests *Babesia* during the blood meal. In the tick, *Babesia* reproduces through sexual cycles and invades the organs of the tick including ovaries, thus enabling also the infection of the future tick generation. In dogs, the prepatent time varies according to the species. Usually it is 2–3 weeks. For instance, the prepatent time of *B. canis* infection is 10–21 days and that of *B. gibsoni* 14–28 days. The life cycle of *Babesia canis* is presented in Fig. 2.20.

Distribution

The distribution of *Babesia* species depends on which tick species are endemic in the area. *B. canis* is transmitted by *Dermacentor reticulatus*, which is endemic in southern and central Europe. The vector of *B. rossi* is *Haemaphysalis leachi*, endemic in South Africa. *Babesia vogeli* is carried by the brown dog tick *Rhipicephalus sanguineus*, which is found in Asia, Africa, the Americas, Australia, and Europe. *Babesia gibsoni* is endemic in Asia, North Africa, and occasionally North America and Europe. Its vectors are *Haemaphysalis bispinosa*, *Haemaphysalis longicornis*, and, according to some sources, *R. sanguineus*. Evidently, *B. gibsoni* could be spread by dog bite or intraplacentally without vector involvement. This is supported by the relatively high prevalence in fighting dogs compared to other dogs. It has been suspected that the vector of *B. annae*, endemic in southern Europe, is *Ixodes hexagonus*. Infections caused by canine *Babesia* have not been diagnosed in humans. Traveling dogs also import *Babesia* cases into nonendemic areas, but the emergence of these cases depends on tick species present in new areas.

Importance to Canine Health

The clinical signs of babesiosis may vary and involve many organs. The seriousness depends on the *Babesia* species and

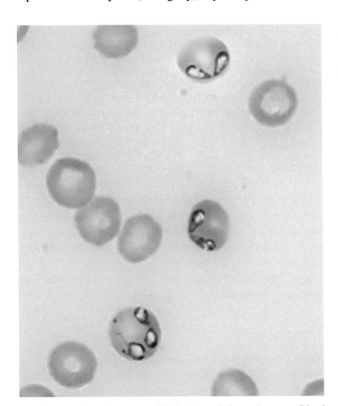

FIG. 2.18 Merozoite stages of *Babesia canis* in erythrocytes. Blood smear stained with Giemsa.

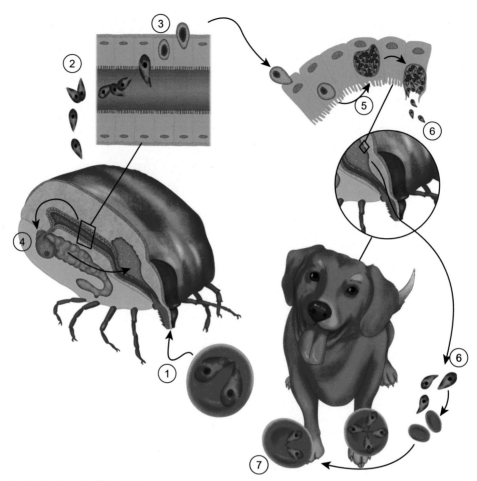

FIG. 2.20 Life cycle of *Babesia canis*: (1) the tick ingests *Babesia* merozoites while sucking blood. Merozoites liberated from disintegrated erythrocytes change their form, developing spiky and filamentous appendages; (2) two *Babesia* with appendages, or so-called ray bodies, join forming a zygote and followed by a stage called kinete; (3) kinetes migrate from the intestine to other parts of the tick and infect different cell types, including muscle cells, cells of Malpighian tubules, ovary cells, and gonads; (4) *Babesia* may pass into the offspring of the female tick in the gametes. Intracellular kinetes change their form and go through several division cycles. The result is the development of new kinetes. These also penetrate the salivary gland epithelium; (5) when the tick sucks blood from a dog in its next developmental stage, the parasites in the salivary gland activate and start dividing, resulting in a large number of sporozoites; (6) sporozoites invade though the salivary ducts into the dog when blood is being sucked. The transfer usually takes place about two days after the attachment of the tick; and (7) in the dog, the sporozoites infect erythrocytes and multiply in them asexually. These new *Babesia* infect more red blood cells.

strain, other infections, the dog's age, and immune defense. Babesiosis cases may be divided into uncomplicated and complicated forms on the basis of the clinical signs. In an uncomplicated case of babesiosis, the signs are usually limited to anemia, while the complicated form affects several organ systems. Both types manifest as a result of the host's inflammatory response. When the erythrocytes undergo lysis, hemolytic anemia develops, causing lethargy, weakness, enlargement of the spleen and liver, and possibly disturbances in the function of several organs. Fever, poor appetite, and pale mucous membranes or jaundice may be the initial observed signs. Tachycardia, hemoglobinuria, uremia, mucous membrane petechiae, low blood pressure, ischemia, coma, and ultimately death may follow. Central nervous system signs are possible. The signs associated with especially *B. rossi* infection can be peracute. The infection caused by *B. vogeli* is the least severe in adult

dogs, but can cause severe signs in puppies, whereas *B. gibsoni* infection is characterized by chronic signs and transient fever. Because the elimination of red blood cells damaged by protozoa takes place in the spleen, splenectomized dogs tend to have more severe clinical signs. Dogs with compromised immunity or those on immunosuppressive medication may become seriously ill. In these dogs, chronic babesiosis may become active and start showing clinical signs.

Diagnosis

Babesia organisms may be seen in a stained blood smear. The sensitivity of the smear may be enhanced by puncturing a peripheral capillary vein (e.g., the tip of pinna or tail), in order to yield a maximum number of protozoa-carrying erythrocytes. Infected red blood cells are often found in the edges of the smear. In a Giemsa-stained blood smear, the parasites are visible inside erythrocytes and the morphological evaluation may reveal whether the *Babesia* is of a small or large type (Figs. 2.18 and 2.19). Several commercial immunological assays are available. The *Babesia* species is determined with PCR methods and also with ELISA tests. It is therapeutically important to distinguish large and small *Babesia*, as they are sensitive to different drugs.

Other hematological findings in babesiosis reflect the hemolytic anemia caused by the infection. Thrombocytopenia is a common finding in babesiosis regardless of the protozoa species, and it often precedes anemia and circulatory parasitemia.

Treatment and Prevention

In the endemic areas of vector ticks, dogs should be protected with continuous preventative medication for the duration of the tick season. Attached ticks must be removed without delay, because the transmission of the tick-borne disease takes place for a few days, and in the case of *B. canis* at least 48 h. *Babesia* vaccines are available in some countries. They do not stop the infection, but do prevent the development of severe signs. The efficacy of the vaccine depends on the *Babesia* species.

Whenever dogs are given a blood transfusion, the *Babesia* status of the donor should be checked to prevent iatrogenic infection.

The disease caused by large *Babesia* is treated with imidocarb given twice at a 2-week interval. Small *Babesia* are more difficult to manage. There are varying therapy recommendations, including treatment with atovaquone combined with azitromycin daily for 10 days. Symptomatic treatment is also necessary. The prognosis of a treated dog is good, but naturally depends on the therapy and the *Babesia* species. It is important to remember that an infected dog is considered a carrier of *Babesia* even after it has been cured of the disease.

HEPATOZOON CANIS

- A tick-borne protozoan, but the infection comes from eating the tick, not from the bite.
- Usually subclinical, but unspecific signs of lethargy, fever, anemia, etc. may appear.
- Parasitic gamonts can be seen inside the neutrophilic granulocytes in a blood smear.
- Treatment with imidocarb; prevention by acarisidic substances.

Identification

Of the currently recognized 300 *Hepatozoon* protozoa, two, *H. canis* and *H. americanum*, are known to infect dogs. Of the life cycle stages of Hepatozoon, gamonts

are the most likely to be detected in the laboratory. In a stained blood smear, they are visible in the cytoplasm of white blood cells (neutrophilic granulocytes, rarely also in monocytes) Gamonts are elongated, ellipsoidal, and surrounded by a membrane, with an eccentrically located nucleus (Fig. 2.21). The nucleus of *H. canis* is elongated and sometimes shaped like a horseshoe. Its gamont is about 8–12 µm long and 3–6 µm wide.

Another form found in the dog is the meront (also known as the schizont). It can be seen in histological sections or cytological samples taken from lymph nodes, spleen, or bone marrow. Meront is a round or oval tissue cyst and is capsulated in the tissue. At an early stage, the meront contains only amorphic material, but with the development of the cyst, a nucleus develops, which divides into elongated merozoites. The size of a typical meront of *H. canis* is about 30×30 µm. Within the meront, there are two or four macromerozoites, or over 20 micromerozoites. Micromerozoites are often in a cartwheel pattern around the central core of the meront (Fig. 2.22).

Life Cycle

Hepatozoonosis is a tick-borne disease. Unlike in many other tick-borne infections, the dog is infected orally and not during the tick's blood meal. Infection takes place when the dog ingests a hepatozoon-carrying tick from its fur or from a prey animal that has ticks on its skin. The scene of sexual reproduction and hence the definitive host in the life cycle of *H. canis* is the brown dog tick, *R. sanguineus*. The infection is passed transtadially from one stage of the tick development to another. The dog is usually infected by an adult tick, which has been infected during the larval or nymphal stage. Both male and female ticks can infect the dog.

After the dog has eaten the tick carrying *H. canis*, the sporozoites penetrate the gut wall. They infect circulatory monocytes and macrophages, which transfer the sporozoites primarily to lymph nodes, bone marrow, and spleen.

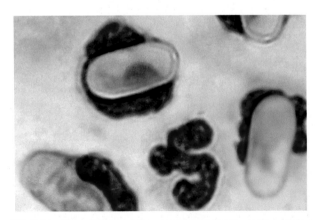

FIG. 2.21 Gamont forms of *Hepatozoon canis* inside granulocytes in a Giemsa-stained blood smear. Since they struggle to fit into the cytoplasm of the neutrophil, they distort its morphology.

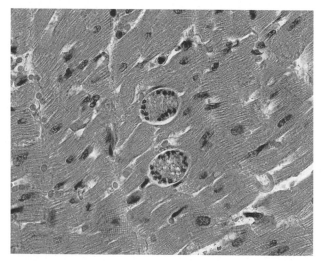

FIG. 2.22 A tissue stage, meront, of *Hepatozoon* showing characteristic cartwheel pattern seen in histological section. The sample is from a cat. *(Reproduced with permission from Kristel Kegler.)*

They can also end up in the liver, kidney, and lungs, for instance. Hepatozoon may pass from the bitch to puppies through the transplacental route.

Parasitic cysts, or meronts, are developed in the tissues of the dog. The parasite multiplies asexually in a process called merogony. Mature merozoites are released from the meront and infect neutrophilic granulocytes and monocytes. Before they infect the white blood cells, the parasite may repeat the cycle of asexual reproduction developing new meronts. The tick is infected when sucking blood from an infected dog. The disintegrating white blood cells release male and female gamonts in the tick's intestine. A stage of sexual reproduction called gametogony now takes place in the tick. At the end of the cycle, male and female gametes are developed. After conception, they form the fertilized egg cell, the zygote. The zygote divides, finally resulting as oocysts in the body cavity of the tick. The oocyst of *H. canis* is a large and round parasite store that can contain hundreds of membrane-confined sporocysts, containing sporozoites, infectious to the dog. The life cycle of *H. canis* is illustrated in Fig. 2.23.

Distribution

Hepatozoonosis is a widely spread vector-borne disease and endemic wherever the brown dog tick is found, especially in the Mediterranean area. Apart from *H. canis*, dog can be infected with *H. americanum*. It is endemic in North America and its tick vector is *Amblyomma maculatum*.

Importance to Canine Health

H. canis infection is usually subclinical or the signs are mild. Clinical signs are commonly seen in the summer, when the ticks are most active. These signs may include

somnolence, fever, poor appetite, weight loss, anemia, and enlarged lymph nodes. *Hepatozoon americanum* causes a more severe disease than its European cousin, often leading to death. The signs are fever, severe weight loss, lethargy, myositis and muscle atrophy, purulent eye discharge, and anemia. The pathogenesis of hepatozoonosis is insufficiently understood.

Diagnosis

The diagnosis is often based on the microscopical findings of a stained (Diff Quick or Giemsa) blood smear. Parasitic gamonts can be seen in neutrophilic granulocytes. They are oval with straight sides, and often situated in the center of the neutrophil, pressing the nucleus toward the edges. Since they do not seem to fit into the cytoplasm, they distort the cell's morphology (Fig. 2.20). The best way to find the organisms is to prepare the blood smear of the buffy coat layer that is between the plasma and the erythrocytes in the centrifuged blood sample. The parasites are typically seen in about 5% of the neutrophils of a dog without signs or with mild signs. Gamonts are sparse in *H. americanum* infection. Typical laboratory findings include neutrophilia, eosionophilia, lymphocytosis, and monocytosis. Meronts may be found in cytological samples. Modern diagnosis of hepatozoonosis include PCR methods and the analysis of antibodies.

Treatment and Prevention

Hepatozoonosis is most commonly treated with imidocarb. The prevention is based on tick control.

LEISHMANIA SPP.

- Infection from a sandfly bite, or from dog bites, from dam to puppy, in mating from male to female, blood transfusions and possibly through blood-sucking ectoparasites.
- Zoonosis; dogs are an important reservoir of human infections.
- Clinical status varies from no signs to lethal generalized disease.
- Diagnosis with immunological tests or PCR-based methods.
- Treatment takes months, and possibly continues for the rest of the dog's life.

Identification

Leishmania is a parasitic protozoa belonging to the family Trypanosomatidae. There are over 50 species and at least 12 of them are reported to infect dogs. The most significant species is *Leishmania infantum*. In the cytoplasm of mammal cells, *Leishmania* is present as a nonflagellated amastigote form (Figs. 2.24 and 2.25). It is roundish and

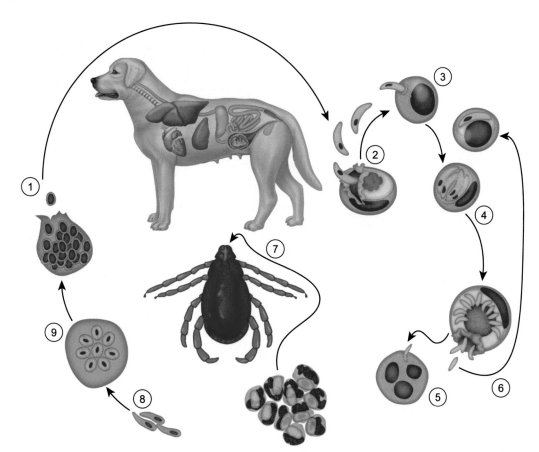

FIG. 2.23 Life cycle of *Hepatozoon canis*: (1) infection takes place when the dog ingests a hepatozoon-carrying tick or a prey animal that has ticks on its skin. Both male and female ticks can infect the dog; (2) after the dog has eaten the tick carrying *H. canis*, the sporozoites are released in the gastrointestinal tract and penetrate the gut wall; (3) they infect monocytes and macrophages, which transfer the sporozoites primarily to lymph nodes, bone marrow, and spleen. They may also end up in the liver, kidney, and lungs, for example. Hepatozoon may pass from the bitch to puppies through the transplacental route; (4) parasitic cysts, or meronts, are developed in the tissues of the dog. The parasite multiplies asexually in a process called merogony (also known as schizogony); (5) mature merozoites are released from the meront and infect neutrophilic granulocytes and monocytes; (6) before they infect the white blood cells, the parasites may repeat the cycle of asexual reproduction, developing new meronts; (7) the tick is infected when sucking blood from an infected dog; (8) the disintegrating white blood cells release male and female gamonts in the tick's intestine. A stage of sexual reproduction called gametogony now takes place in the tick. At the end of the cycle, male and female gametes are developed; and (9) after conception, they form the fertilized egg cell, the zygote. This divides, resulting as oocysts in the body cavity of the tick. The oocyst of *H. canis* is a large and round parasite store that can contain hundreds of membrane-confined sporocysts, containing sporozoites, which are infectious to the dog.

about 2–6 μm in diameter. The nucleus, consisting of the short flagellum that is embedded in the anterior end without projecting out and a tiny but intensively stained rod-like kinetoplast, associated with flagella, can be seen even with a light microscope. In its Anthropod vector, the sandfly (Fig. 2.26), *Leishmania* is present as an extracellular promastigote. A promastigote is elongated and in the anterior end it has a flagellum for active movement. The promastigote is 15–30 μm long and about 5 μm thick.

Life Cycle

Apart from reproduction in mammals, the vector insects, genera *Phlebotomus* and *Lutzomyia*, have an important role in the distribution and multiplication of *Leishmania*. While sandflies use the blood pooling at the skin bite for nutrition, they get the parasite in the infected cells present in the skin. *Leishmania* parasitizes the vector as a highly motile promastigote form and it multiplies in the central alimentary tract of sandflies by longitudinal division. Initially the promastigotes are located in the posterior part of the central gut, but while the infection matures, over 1–2 weeks, they move toward the anterior part of the central gut and prepare to infect the following host. The gelatinous secretion of the promastigotes, together with the parasites themselves, forms a plug in the gut of the sandfly, preventing the fly from satisfying its thirst for blood. The insect that usually stops feeding on blood for days after a meal continues to attempt feeding. This enhances the spread of the infection to new hosts. Inside the mammal host, the macrophages ingest the alien parasitic material and transfer it further to tissues. The sandfly saliva contains substances that interfere with the host immune defense and block the action of many molecules that participate in this defense, preventing the

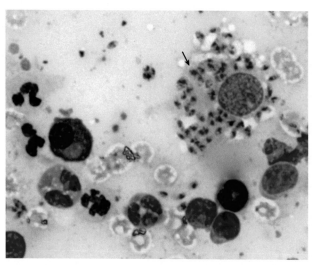

FIG. 2.24 Giemsa-stained cytological sample of the skin of a dog suffering from leishmaniosis. A macrophage, with many *Leishmania* amastigotes in the cytoplasm, is indicated with an arrow. There are also many inflammatory cells, mostly neutrophilic granulocytes and a single plasma cell.

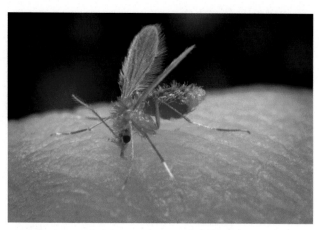

FIG. 2.26 Phlebotomine sandfly is the most important vector insect of *Leishmania*. The name reflects the sandy-brown color of the insect. *(Reproduced with permission from Science Source Images. Photo by James Gathany/CDC.)*

macrophages from presenting *Leishmania* antigens to T-lymphocytes. Without the insect saliva, the host's immune defense could easily eliminate the *Leishmania*. The promastigote turns into the nonflagellated amastigote in 1–5 days. The amastigotes start to divide inside the cell and when the cells undergo lysis, yet more cells are infected with the liberated amastigotes. Apart from the sandfly, other bloodsucking arthropods such as fleas and the brown dog tick are reportedly able to act as vectors for *Leishmania*. Furthermore, the dog can be infected via blood transfusion,

via semen at breeding from the male to female or vertically from the bitch to the puppy. Infection via bite in dog fights is also possible. The illustrated life cycle of *Leishmania* is presented in Fig. 2.27.

Distribution

In addition to dogs, *Leishmania* can infect humans and other mammals. The dog is the most significant source of human *Leishmania*, and it is the species that maintains the parasitic infection. The disease is endemic in several countries in the Mediterranean, Near East, Far East, Africa, and Central and South America. The vectors of *Leishmania* have moved north along with climate change. Thanks to its long incubation

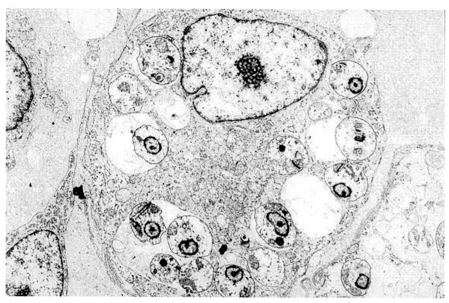

FIG. 2.25 A *Leishmania*-infected macrophage in a transmission electron microscope image. The visible parasite forms are amastigotes. The nuclei of the amastigotes and occasionally also kinetoplasts can be seen. *(From Saari S, Rasi J, Anttila M: Leishmaniosis mimicking oral neoplasm in a dog: an unusual manifestation of an unusual disease in Finland, Acta Vet Scand 41:101–104, 2000.)*

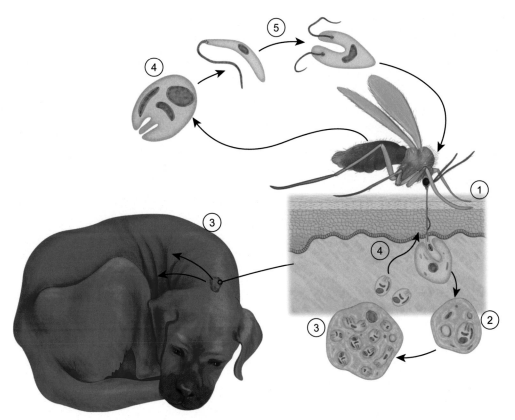

FIG. 2.27 Life cycle of *Leishmania infantum*: (1) dog gets infected when the sandfly, while sucking blood, inoculates promastigotes of *Leishmania* into the skin; (2) the promastigote forms lose their flagellas, developing into amastigotes. They infect macrophages that are attracted into the area by the dog's immune response. If the macrophages succeed in killing the parasites in phagocytosis, the infection dies out. *Leishmania*, however, has many methods of avoiding the canine immune response, allowing the amastigotes to multiply inside the macrophages and then infect new macrophages; (3) depending on the canine immune response, the infection is eliminated, it is contained in the skin, or macrophages transfer it elsewhere in the organism, and it can develop into a condition called visceral leishmaniosis; (4) the sandfly obtains parasitic amastigotes while sucking blood; and (5) amastigotes develop into promastigotes, multiplying by division, in the gut of the sandfly.

period, leishmaniosis is frequently diagnosed in nonendemic countries in dogs imported from endemic areas, although the dogs had been clinically healthy at the time of importation. In nonendemic areas, the infection have passed from dog to dog, for instance, at breeding, without vector involvement.

Leishmaniosis Is a Zoonosis

Leishmania infantum is an important pathogenic organism for humans. In endemic areas, dogs act as reservoirs for the disease, but humans become infected via sandflies. Visceral leishmaniosis caused by *Leishmania infantum* is most common in small children. The symptoms of visceral leishmaniosis are similar to those of canine leishmaniosis. Splenomegaly is a common clinical finding. *Leishmania* has recently become an important pathogen in immunocompromised humans. The combined infection of HIV and *Leishmania* is well known. HIV infection reduces the ability of the immune defense to control intracellular pathogens. A person infected with HIV has an increased risk of getting the *Leishmania* infection and manifesting clinical symptoms, and of reactivation of a latent, earlier infection.

Importance to Canine Health

The incubation period of leishmaniosis is long, lasting up to several years. The infection may also stay latent and activate if the host's immune defense undergoes a change that is favorable for the *Leishmania*. The clinical manifestations of leishmaniosis vary from subclinical carrier status to cutaneous leishmaniosis involving the skin and further to fatal, generalized visceral leishmaniosis. The host immune defense plays a major role in the infection. In some dogs, the immune defense quickly eliminates the pathogen. In some, the infection establishes itself but it is limited to a local lesion by the immune defense. The most serious disease type in a dog develops when the pathogens are able to spread all over the organism. Skin lesions are often first noted (Figs. 2.28–2.30). They usually manifest as flaky, dry, and hairless skin in the pinnae, nose, around the eyes and elsewhere on the head, elbows, and hocks. The dermatitis may be associated with ulcers and papules. Abnormalities in paws and nails are common. Systemic signs include weakness, weight loss, lack of appetite, fatigue, enlarged lymph nodes, fever, and pale mucous membranes. The liver and spleen are

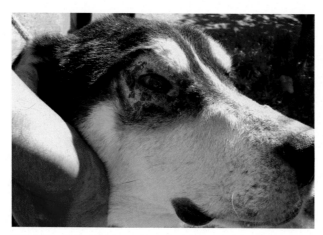

FIG. 2.28 Periorbital dermatitis typical to leishmaniosis. *(Reproduced with permission from Maria Pennisi.)*

often enlarged, and kidney function is impaired. Proteinuria is common. Some dogs display lameness and ocular signs as well as epistaxis. Prognosis is guarded and an untreated visceral leishmaniosis is usually fatal. Boxers, Cocker Spaniels, Rottweilers, and German Shepherds appear to have an increased sensitivity to leishmaniosis, whereas many breeds typical for the endemic *Leishmania* areas, such as Podencos, rarely manifest the disease.

Diagnosis

When *Leishmania* infection is suspected in nonendemic areas, it is important to record the history of the dog's travels and possible contacts with dogs that have visited endemic areas. If an infection is considered possible, antibodies

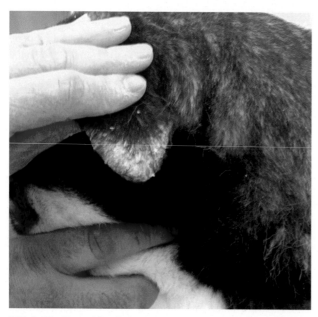

FIG. 2.29 Dermatitis of pinna associated with leishmaniosis. *(Reproduced with permission from Maria Pennisi.)*

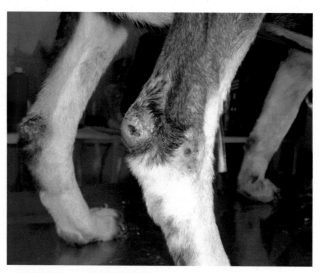

FIG. 2.30 Deep pyogranulomatous dermatitis with ulceration, typical to leishmaniosis. *(Reproduced with permission from Maria Pennisi.)*

against *Leishmania* are assayed serologically. There are several commercial tests available. The most commonly used are ELISA, IFAT, indirect hemagglutination assay (IHA), and direct agglutination test (DAT). PCR analysis of the blood and tissues is also possible. The histological analysis of tissue samples can be complemented with immunohistochemistry, to highlight amastigotes that stain typically and the inflammatory reaction associated with in the infection. *Leishmania* diagnosis can also be made with a cytological sample, since protozoa are clearly visible in the cytoplasm of macrophages taken, for instance, from a skin lesion, lymph node, or bone marrow (Fig. 2.24). *Leishmania* can be cultured in a research laboratory; however, the method is not feasible for routine diagnosis, because it is slow and laborious. Dogs originating from endemic areas are often seropositive for *Leishmania* antigens and positive in a PCR test. It proves that the dog has got the infection, but it is not a confirmation of leishmaniosis disease.

Treatment and Prevention

Meglumine antimoniate or miltefosine are used for the medical treatment of leishmaniosis, often combined with allopurinol. The condition of the patient improves after the onset of therapy, but the cure can take months. It is common that the patient undergoes a relapse of the disease after the medical treatment. After the initiation of therapy, there are fairly poor chances to visualize amastigotes in histopathology or cytology anymore. Vaccines have been developed against canine leishmaniosis, but their efficacy is not perfect. Nevertheless, vaccination will probably be the future solution for *Leishmania* control. The use of insect repellents to protect dogs in endemic areas is indicated. Infections may also be prevented by confining dogs inside at dusk and dark times of day, when sandflies are active. When dogs are sleeping outside, it is important to cover them with an insect net. Dogs imported from endemic areas pose a risk for other dogs. Although *Leishmania* lacks a sandfly vector outside endemic regions, breeding and bites can transmit the disease between dogs. Conducting the *Leishmania* assay is recommended for imported dogs to control the transmission risk. Since blood-sucking arthropods other than the sandfly can also act as a vector, ectoparasites should be controlled. The risk of *Leishmania* should be considered when operating a canine blood bank.

TRYPANOSOMA SPP.

- Hemoprotozoans with arthropod vectors.
- Infection via vector bite or blood or mucous membrane contact with arthropod feces.
- Unspecific clinical signs with involvement of several organ systems.
- Diagnosis from a blood smear or with immunological or PCR tests.
- Prevention by controlling the vector population.

Clinical Staging of Canine Leishmaniosis Based on Serological Status, Clinical Signs, Laboratory Findings, and Type of Therapy and Prognosis for Each Stage

Clinical Stages	Serology[a]	Clinical Signs	Laboratory Findings	Therapy	Prognosis
Stage I. Mild disease	Negative to low positive antibody levels	Dogs with mild clinical signs such as peripheral lymphadenomegaly, or papular dermatitis	Usually no clinicopathological abnormalities observed Normal renal profile: creatinine < 1.4 mg/dL; nonproteinuric: UPC < 0.5	Scientific neglect/ allopurinol or meglumine antimoniate or miltefosine/ allopurinol + meglumine antimoniate or allopurinol + miltefosine[b]	Good
Stage II. Moderate disease	Low to high positive antibody levels	Dogs, which apart from the signs listed in stage I, may present: diffuse or symmetrical cutaneous lesions such as exfoliative dermatitis/onychogryphosis, ulcerations (planum nasale, footpads, bony prominences, mucocutaneous junctions), anorexia, weight loss, fever, and epistaxis	Clinicopathological abnormalities such as mild nonregenerative anemia, hyperglobulinemia, hypoalbuminemia, serum hyperviscosity syndrome *Substages* (a) Normal renal profile: creatinine < 1.4 mg/dL; nonproteinuric: UPC < 0.5 (b) Creatinine < 1.4 mg/dL; UPC = 0.5–1	Allopurinol + meglumine antimoniate or allopurinol + miltefosine	Good to guarded
Stage III. Severe disease	Medium to high positive antibody levels	Dogs, which apart from the signs listed in stages I and II, may present signs originating from immune-complex lesions: vasculitis, arthritis, uveitis and glomerulonephritis	Clinicopathological abnormalities listed in stage II Chronic kidney disease (CKD) IRIS stage I with UPC > 1 or stage II (creatinine 1.4–2 mg/dL)	Allopurinol + meglumine antimoniate or allopurinol + miltefosine Follow IRIS guidelines for CKD	Guarded to poor
Stage IV. Very severe disease	Medium to high positive antibody levels	Dogs with clinical signs listed in stage III. Pulmonary thromboembolism, or nephrotic syndrome and end stage renal disease	Clinicopathological abnormalities listed in stage II CKD IRIS stage III (creatinine 2–5 mg/dL) and stage IV (creatinine > 5 mg/dL). Nephrotic syndrome: marked proteinuria UPC > 5	Allopurinol (alone) Follow IRIS guidelines for CKD	Poor

[a]*Dogs with negative to medium positive antibody levels should be confirmed as infected by other diagnostic techniques such as cytology, histology, immunohistochemistry or PCR. High levels of antibodies, defined as a three- to fourfold elevation above the cut off level of a well-established reference laboratory, are conclusive of a diagnosis of CanL.*

[b]*Dogs in stage I (mild disease) are likely to require less prolonged treatment with one or two combined drugs or alternatively monitoring with no treatment. However, there is limited information on dogs in this stage and, therefore, treatment options remain to be defined.*

(Data from Laia Solano-Gallego, Guadalupe Miró, Alek Koutinas, Luis Cardoso, Maria Grazia Pennisi, Luis Ferrer, Patrick Bourdeau, Gaetano Oliva and Gad Baneth: LeishVet guidelines for the practical management of canine leishmaniosis, Parasites & Vectors 2011 4:86.)

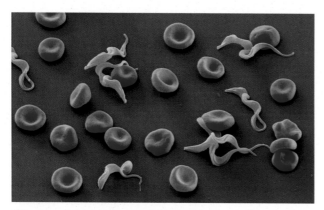

FIG. 2.31 Trypanosomes and red blood cells in colored scanning electron micrograph (SEM). *(Reproduced with permission from Eye of Science/Science Photo Library.)*

Identification

Trypanosomas (Fig. 2.31) are hemoprotozoans that can infect a variety of vertebrate hosts. The morphological forms of order Trypanosomatida can be differentiated by the presence or absence of undulating membrane and flagella, and the kinetoplast's location in relation to the nucleus. *Trypanosoma* species are divided into categories salivaria and stercoraria; these are morphologically based on the shape of the posterior end of the organism, which is blunt in salivaria and pointed in stercoraria.

Life Cycle

Trypanosoma species usually need an insect vector in their life cycle. The vertebrate host becomes infected when the insects infected saliva or contaminated mouthparts are in contact with it during blood meal. In Africa, biting flies (tsetse flies from genus *Glossina*) and in Americas hemipteran triatomine species (kissing bugs) act as vectors for canine trypanosomiasis. In addition, nonvector borne infections have been demonstrated in dogs from eating infected meat, organs, or blood. A triatomine bug defecates during the blood meal and passes trypomastigotes within its feces. Trypomastigotes enter the body of the dog through bite wounds or mucous membranes. In a dog, trypomastigotes may infect various types of cells and transform into intracellular amastigotes. Amastigotes multiply by binary fission in infected tissues. Amastigotes transform again into trypomastigotes and burst out of the cell and enter the blood stream. Trypomastigotes may infect cells from a variety of tissues and transform into intracellular amastigotes in new infection sites. The tsetse fly or triatomine bug receives the infection by ingesting trypomastigotes during the blood meal. The entire life cycle of African trypanosomes is represented by extracellular stages, and they lack intracellular stages with amastigotes. In circulation, African trypanosomes are present in two forms: slender and stumpy. Evidently, nonreplicating stumpy trypanosomes are needed for the continuation of the life cycle in tsetse fly. In the insect vector's midgut, the parasite multiplies by binary fission. In the tsetse fly, the parasites have to reach the fly's salivary glands, enabling transmission to new hosts. Fig. 2.32 illustrates the life cycle of *Trypanosoma cruzi*.

Distribution

In dogs, certain *T. brucei* species appear in Africa and Asia, and *T. cruzi* in the USA and South America. There is one case report of *Trypanosoma pestanai* in dogs in Europe. In endemic areas, over half of the dog population may be seropositive.

Importance to Canine Health

Dogs have two types of trypanosomiasis: African (Surra) and American (Chagas), which are both zoonotic. Other *Trypanosoma* species may infect dogs too, but they are nonpathogenic to dogs with normal immunological status. In trypanosomiasis, the clinical picture depends on the parasite strain, host's age and immunological status, and other factors. Clinical signs appear about 1 week to 2 months after the infection, with fever, weakness, edema, and anemia being the most common signs. For example, *T. brucei evansi* has been reported to cause a rapid course of disease in dogs, leading to death in a week or weeks. Lower body parts' edema and petechial hemorrhages and paralysis or paresis may occur in addition to the general signs. *Trypanosoma cruzi* involves especially young dogs about 6 months of age, and heart and respiratory symptoms are typical. Deaths from heart failure, caused by parasite-induced cell damage, occur. Acute phase takes about 2 months, and after that, if the dog survives, the chronic phase with arrhythmias, myocardial dilatation, and right-side cardiac insufficiency follows.

Diagnosis

The clinical signs of trypanosomiasis are common with several other systemic diseases and may involve several organs. For definite diagnosis, a blood smear (preferably Giemsa stained) should be drawn to visualize the trypomastigote forms of *Trypanosoma*. Unfortunately, this method is insensitive due to the low number of parasites in the blood. Serological methods detecting antibodies or antigens have been designed for more sensitive diagnostics of trypanosomiasis. These, however, lack specificity, due to cross-reactions between different *Trypanosoma* species and even with *Leishmania*. PCR methods are also in use, especially for the confirmation of the diagnostics and

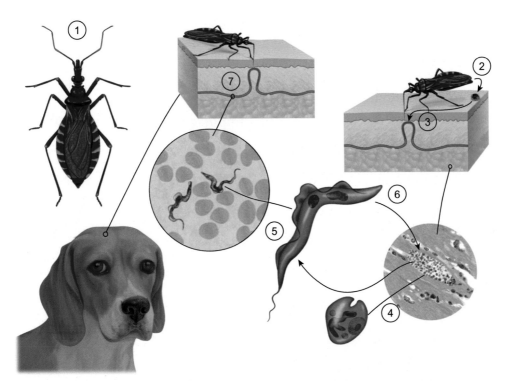

FIG. 2.32   Life cycle of *Trypanosoma cruzi*: (1) hemipteran triatomine bugs (kissing bugs) act as vectors for *T. cruzi* infection; (2) triatomine bug defecates during the blood meal and passes trypomastigotes of *Trypanosoma* within its feces; (3) trypomastigotes enter the body of the dog through bite wound or mucous membranes; (4) in a dog, trypomastigotes may infect various types of cells and transform into intracellular amastigotes. Amastigotes multiply by binary fission in infected tissues; (5) amastigotes transform again into trypomastigotes and burst out of the cell and enter the blood stream; (6) trypomastigotes may infect cells from a variety of tissues and transform into intracellular amastigotes in new infection sites; and (7) the triatomine bug gets the infection by ingesting trypomastigotes during the blood meal. In the insect vector's midgut, the parasite multiplies by binary fission.

Trypanosoma species identification. Biological methods involve the infection of laboratory animals or blood/cell cultures.

Treatment and Prevention

Diminazene aceturate has been shown to be an effective treatment for *T. evansi* in dogs, with a subcutaneous dose of 7 mg/kg on the first day and 3.5 mg/kg on the following day. The problem with the treatment is that the disease tends to recur and the treatment then has to be repeated or prolonged. In rats, for example, the drug has been administered for five consecutive days. Other drugs have been tested in dogs too, but the side-effects have been too serious.

In general, the disease can be contained by controlling the vector population. For prophylaxis, several kinds of insecticides can be used. Drugs in the isoxazoline group have been shown to be effective in killing triatomine vectors. Dogs should also be prevented from eating possible infected material. Vaccine trials have been made with dogs with promising results; however, to date, no commercial vaccine is available. Motivation to vaccinate dogs is usually based on their reservoir role in human trypanosomiasis.

ENTAMOEBA HISTOLYTICA

- Cause of amebiasis of humans and other primates, zoonosis.
- Dog may get infected feco-orally from contaminated food or water.
- Clinical signs vary from asymptomatic to prolonged diarrhea. Extra-intestinal signs may also appear.
- Diagnosis from cysts or trophozoites from fecal sample.
- Treatment with metronidazole; prevention with good hygiene.

Identification

Entamoeba histolytica causes human amebiasis and diarrhea, which can sometimes also infect dogs. The size of trophozoites (Fig. 2.33) increasing in the organism is usually 15–20 µm, and they may contain erythrocytes that have been ingested. The diameter of cysts (Fig. 2.34) that are released in the environment is 10–14 µm. A fully developed cyst contains four nuclei. Cigar-shaped chromatoidal bodies can be seen inside the cyst.

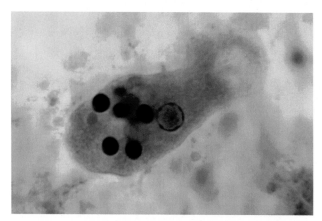

FIG. 2.33 A micrograph depicting *Entamoeba histolytica* trophozoite in a specimen stained with trichrome. Ingested erythrocytes can be seen as dark inclusions. *(Courtesy of Dr. Mae Melvin and Dr. Green/CDC.)*

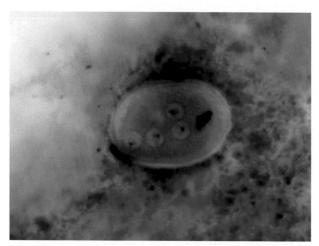

FIG. 2.34 A micrograph depicting a chlorazol black-stained specimen, with a cyst of the *Entamoeba*. A fully developed cyst contains four nuclei and a chromatoidal body. *(Courtesy of Dr. George R. Healy/CDC.)*

Distribution

E. histolytica is endemic in the tropics and subtropics as the protozoa of humans and other primates. Dogs and other mammals can become infected transiently. The parasite has been found more often in domestic dogs with disease signs than with stray dogs, possibly thanks to the former's closer contact with humans. Dog breeds also seem to play a role in prevalence.

Life Cycle

The dog receives a feco-oral infection from food or water contaminated with human feces and containing cystic stages of the protozoa. The cysts are broken down in the stomach and the intestine and the released trophozoites colonize the large intestine. They multiply by binary fission and produce robust cysts ready to be secreted to the external environment. It was previously thought that dogs do not often secrete cysts of *Entamoeba* and they therefore do not have any role in the epidemiology of the disease. This has been proved wrong; dog stools can contain cysts.

Importance to Canine Health

The clinical signs of amebiasis vary. Cases without any symptoms are found in humans as well as in dogs. Sometimes the signs are limited spontaneously without intervention, and sometimes the infection becomes chronic. The disease is occasionally fatal in humans. The *Entamoeba* that penetrate the intestinal wall may cause inflammation, ulceration and bleeding of the epithelium, resulting in acute or long-lasting diarrhea. If the disease is prolonged, the appetite is affected and the patient loses weight. Sometimes the *Entamoeba* can infect the viscera outside the intestine, such as the liver, kidneys, lungs, and brain, causing abscesses.

Diagnosis

Both cysts as well as trophozoites may be searched in a fecal sample. It should be noted that trophozoites cannot withstand the hypertonicity of flotation solutions, and they are found most readily in direct microscopy of the stools. Distinguishing *Entamoeba* from nonpathogenic amoebas with similar morphology is, however, done with immunological or PCR methods. Parts of the human diagnostic methods are also suitable for the diagnosis of canine amebiasis. Diagnosis can additionally be reached with the endoscopy of the large intestine and the analysis of tissue biopsies taken.

Cases of Extraintestinal Entamoebiasis also occur in Dogs

While *Entamoeba* are known primarily as the causative organism of intestinal infections, the group includes other types of rare canine pathogens. They live freely in the environment but are capable of pathogenicity. Protozoa of the genus *Acanthamoeba* live in freshwater as well as salt water. They cause diseases primarily in humans, but canine infections have also been described. The infection affects eyes and, in the case of immunocompromised individuals, may also spread into other organs. In dogs, the signs may resemble those of distemper: ocular and nasal discharge, poor appetite, and fever. The signs of a systemic infection have similarities with distemper: pulmonary infection and central nervous system signs. A member of the genus *Hartmannella*, a close relative, may cause ocular infections too. *Balamuthia mandrillaris* and its relatives *Naegleria* and *Sappinia* may cause a generalized canine infection. They are known primarily as rare causative organisms of meningitis.

Treatment and Prevention

The dog's food and water must be uncontaminated. If amebiasis is diagnosed in a family, it is advisable to examine also the dog, especially if it has any signs of disease. Good hand hygiene is important in infection outbreaks. Humans are treated with metronidazole, and this is also suitable for canine therapy.

TETRATRICHOMONAS CANISTOMAE (SYN. *TRICHOMONAS CANISTOMAE*)

- Commensal of oral mucous membranes.
- Not important in canine medicine.

Identification

Tetratrichomonas canistomae is a small drop or pear-shaped protozoan flagellate. It is 7–12 μm long and its maximum width is 3–4 μm. Typical morphological features (Fig. 2.35) are four anterior flagella, which are approximately as long as the body, and a longer, posteriorly pointing flagellum. It is attached to the body with an undulating membrane and continues as a free flagellum further posteriorly. The length of the free flagellum is about half of the body's length. The organism is supported by an axostylum, a thread-like structure that gives the body rigidity and sticks out from the posterior end.

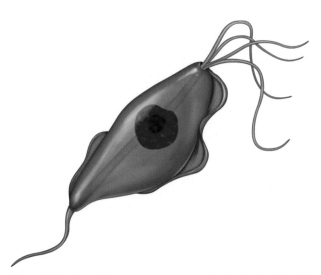

FIG. 2.35 *Tetratrichomonas canistomae*. Typical morphological features of this parasite are the four flagella of the anterior end, the longer, posteriorly pointed thread-like flagella with the undulating membrane attached to it and posteriorly pointed axostyle.

Life Cycle

The parasite only has a flagellar trophozoite form, living on oral mucous membranes as a commensal organism. It generally cannot survive the passage through the alimentary tract and is thus transferred from dog to dog in saliva, when dogs lick each other, or when they eat or drink from same bowls. Reproduction is by longitudinal binary fission.

Distribution

The distribution of *T. canistomae* is not known.

Importance to Canine Health

T. canistomae is considered a harmless commensal without veterinary significance. *Trichomonas tenax*, another protozoon living in the oral cavity, may cause periodontitis.

Diagnosis

T. canistomae can primarily be sought from the mucous membrane folds of the oral cavity. The initial identification can be based on the jerky rolling movement of the parasite in a fresh sample. Morphological features can be seen in a stained cytological smear taken from the mouth. Culture media used for growing Trichomonas in laboratories are suitable for culturing *Tetratrichomonas*.

GIARDIA CANIS, GIARDIA DUODENALIS Strains C and D

- A very common flagellate protozoan among dogs.
- Infection from the cyst forms from the environment.
- Mostly subclinical in adults; in puppies may cause severe diarrhea.
- Diagnosis from fecal sample detecting stained cysts or finding antigen in immunological tests or with PCR.
- Cure results are better if treatment is combined with hygiene measures.

Identification

Giardia is a flagellated protozoan parasite. The active stages, trophozoites (Fig. 2.36), are drop shaped, and are 9–21 μm long and 5–15 μm wide. There are four pairs of flagella. Light microscopy reveals that the trophozoites have two nuclei and an adhesive disc. The cysts (Fig. 2.37) are oval, sized 8–15 × 7–10 μm, and have four nuclei. The cyst wall consists of two layers, which makes it tough and robust.

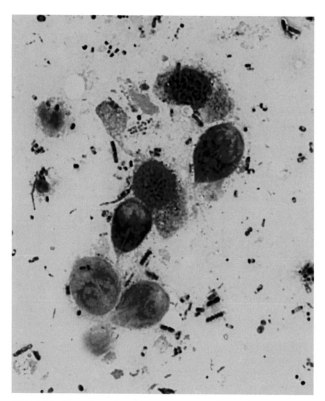

FIG. 2.36 Four drop-shaped *Giardia* trophozoites in a Giemsa-stained cytological sample taken from the intestinal epithelium. Bacteria and two epithelial cells are visible.

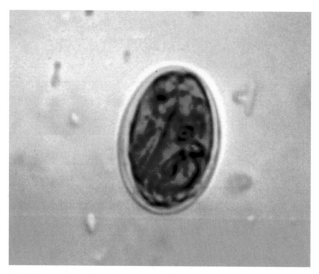

FIG. 2.37 A *Giardia* cyst. *(Courtesy of CDC.)*

Life Cycle

The trophozoites of *Giardia* multiply asexually by binary replication on the small intestine mucous membrane, to which they are attached with the adhesive disc. The life cycle involves the periodic secretion of *Giardia* cysts into feces as cysts form that withstand environmental conditions well. A cyst is developed to envelop the trophozoite, as it travels caudally in the gut. The prepatent period is short: 4–16 days. The cysts are infective to the new host immediately and the dose required for infection is small. A few cysts are sufficient. The dog is infected by getting cysts in its alimentary tract. The cyst cell is digested and the two trophozoites freed to multiply. Fig. 2.38 illustrates the life cycle of *Giardia*.

Distribution

Giardia are ubiquitous in the world. *Giardia* is the most common endoparasite of puppies in many areas, according to prevalence studies. There are several strains and assemblages of *Giardia duodenalis*. Some are host-specific while others are capable of infecting several types of host species. Dogs and other canids are typically colonized by their own *Giardia* types (*Giardia canis* or *G. duodenalis* strains C and D), which are not zoonotic, but zoonotic strains have also been found in dogs' fecal samples.

Importance to Canine Health

Subclinical infections are common, especially in adult dogs. Puppies are more prone to develop clinical signs and puppy infections are common. The pathogenesis of giardiasis signs is poorly known. *Giardia* lives on the surface of the intestinal villi. It is assumed that a severe *Giardia* infection involves a layer of trophozoites that covers the gut wall and interferes with the absorption of nutrients (Fig. 2.39). The unabsorbed carbon hydrates and other nutrients may support an overgrowth of intraluminal bacteria, leading to diarrhea. Villus flattening, caused by *Giardia* infection, leads to similar signs. The adhesion between brush border endothelial cells loosens. The result is increased intestinal permeability and the leakage of tissue fluids and protein into the intestine. In addition, the proteins of the food and many of its antigens escape in between the loosened epithelial cells into the body and become needlessly presented to the immune defense. For instance, in humans a *Giardia* infection is associated with the risk of developing lactose intolerance—either a permanent condition or one lasting for some months. In normal circumstances, the renewal of the intestinal epithelial cells happens through apoptosis, the programmed death of epithelial cells, making space for new cells. In giardiasis, apoptosis is enhanced. The associated diarrhea may be acute or chronic and periodical. Mucus may be secreted. Bloody diarrhea is not common. Other signs may include anorexia, vomiting, lethargy, and weight loss. Fever is rare. The diarrhea is self-limiting if the immune defense of the dog functions normally. The acquired immunity may prevent future disease signs, but not necessarily a new infection.

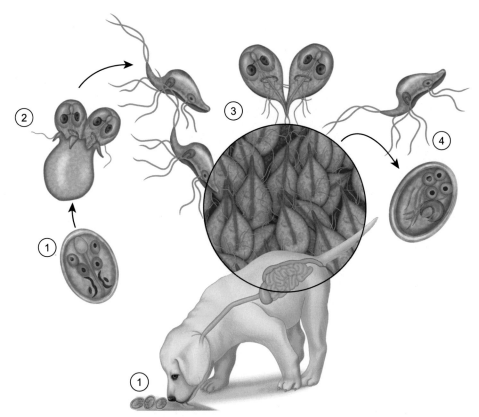

FIG. 2.38 Life cycle of *Giardia*: (1) a dog gets the infection from the environment when it ingests *Giardia* cysts; (2) in the gastrointestinal tract, the cyst capsule breaks down and each cyst releases two actively moving trophozoite stages; (3) the trophozoites attach to the intestinal epithelium and multiply by binary division; and (4) finally they start to secrete cyst-forming protein and transform into cysts, which are transferred in feces into the external environment and are readily infectious for other dogs.

Diagnosis

Testing dogs without signs of disease for *Giardia* is infeasible. It may be beneficial to take fecal samples from dogs with clinical signs over several days to look for cysts, since the cyst secretion is intermittent. Samples taken over three consecutive days provide sufficient sensitivity. Veterinary clinics often use quick *Giardia* tests, which are supportive for a rapid diagnosis of diarrhea signs. However, these quick tests should be used with caution in monitoring the efficacy of treatment. Since these tests detect antigens, they do not inform clinicians about the vitality of the infection, but instead only reveal if traces of the antigenic structure are present in the sample. For most tests, this is the cyst-forming protein. Antigens may be secreted in the feces for weeks after the treatment. It may be advisable not to test after the treatment, if the dog is clinically cured. In laboratory conditions, the test can be conducted with an antigen ELISA. Its limitations are the same as those of the quick test. To learn if the infection is at the cyst-producing stage, the best method is to show the cysts with immunofluorescence. *Giardia* cysts can also be visualized with routine sedimentation or flotation methods, combined with direct microscopy, especially if the sample has been stained with Lugol (iodine) solution. This method is not very sensitive and requires expertise of microscopy, because many common fecal particles may resemble cysts. In addition, saturated salt or sugar solutions may distort the shape of the cyst. In direct microscopy of the stool sample, trophozoites have a

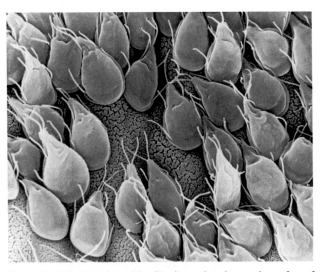

FIG. 2.39 The layer formed by *Giardia* trophozoites on the surface of the small intestine, scanning electron microscopy. *(Reproduced with permission from Ami Images/Science Photo Library.)*

characteristic "falling leaf" movement pattern. *Giardia* trophozoites can also been detected in histological biopsies and scraping samples of the intestinal epithelium, as well as more rarely conducted cytological analysis of feces. The PCR method is feasible especially when the *Giardia* strain needs to be detected. It is seldom used in routine diagnostics.

Treatment and Prevention

Fenbendazole and metronidazole are the most common medicines used to treat *Giardia* infections. Ronidazole as well as a single dose of nitazoxanide has been recently tested in dogs with success. The duration of the therapy varies in the literature. Fenbendazole is often given longer (e.g., 5 days) than when treating nematode infections. Many medicinal products combine several active substances and often include febantel, which is turned into fenbendazole by metabolism. Thus, products containing febantel are efficacious, if the treatment lasts long enough. Combining medical treatment with chlorhexidine shampooing of the dog increases the efficacy. It is beneficial to dry the dog, especially its rear end, with a hair dryer, since moisture favors the survival of *Giardia* cysts that may have attached to the hair. The therapeutic goal is not to achieve a negative test result. Instead, clinical cure of diarrhea is desired. Therefore, repetition of *Giardia* assays is not needed if the dog has no more signs of disease. If a repeat sample after the treatment is analyzed, the test should be based not on antigen detection, but on visualization of the cysts.

The interior spaces are carefully cleaned of feces contamination and the dirty surfaces are washed with a solution of sodium hypochlorite or quaternary ammonium compounds) during the drug treatment. *Giardia* maintains its virulence in room temperature for about a week, and moisture is beneficial for it. Subzero temperatures are lethal for most cysts, but some can survive. In water, *Giardia* can survive for weeks or even months, depending on the temperature. Raw or insufficiently purified drinking water is considered the most important source of giardiosis in humans.

Dog stools are removed from the environment, including the kennel and the yard, and discarded with household waste. Clean drinking water is provided for dogs. If the dog has

shampoo. All unnecessary bedding and toys of the dogs should be discarded. Textiles still in good condition should be washed at 60°C and with detergent, and allowed to dry thoroughly. Bowls and dishes should be washed with hot water daily. The spaces occupied by dogs should be cleaned with a solution containing sodium hypochlorite or quaternary ammonium compounds, which is then allowed to function preferably for 5–20 min before rinsing and careful drying. Elevating the temperature in the cleansed kennel over 26°C for 24 h is reported to enhance the effect. Dogs should be allowed in only after the space is totally dry. Dog keepers must apply strict hygiene to prevent the infection from spreading to other spaces—for instance, with contaminated footwear.

Typical sources of reinfection are outside yard or pens, where the infected dog has defecated stools containing large numbers of *Giardia* cysts. The kennel structures can be washed with the same disinfectants as the inside spaces, but several washes may be needed to remove layers of dirt and to allow the disinfectants to take effect. The only efficient method to clean the ground is to remove and replace the surface layer. This is unfortunately seldom practical, explaining why the *Giardia* test often returns to positive despite medication and meticulous cleaning. The most important preventative measure against soil contamination is the diligent and timely removal of stools from the premises.

If soil removal is embarked upon, it should be arranged to occur when the dogs are being medically treated. This helps to prevent immediate recontamination with cysts. The top soil should be scraped off and replaced. It may be feasible to replace the soil with a more permeable material, such as rough gravel. Vegetation, while enjoyable for dogs, provides shelter for *Giardia* and helps to retain moisture, which is important for *Giardia* survival. The contours and the runoff of the ground give hints as to where *Giardia* cysts tend to aggregate and where they remain in moist conditions. It is advisable to prevent puddles from forming on the ground in a dog pen.

Giardia Control in a Kennel

Giardia infections are difficult to manage in kennel circumstances with puppies that readily show disease signs. Managing the infection demands planning in cooperation with a veterinarian, and perseverance and commitment from the breeder.

The dogs should be treated along with the instructions given by the veterinarian and washed with chlorhexidine

---

diarrhea and *Giardia* infection has been diagnosed, swimming and contact with other dogs should be minimized until the signs have passed. For humans, it is recommended that a *Giardia* patient avoids swimming for 2 weeks after the symptoms have stopped. Although canine *Giardia* strains do not typically infect humans, dog keepers should maintain good hand hygiene. The risk is greatest for immunocompromised individuals and small children.

FURTHER READING

Alam M, Maqbool A, Nazir M, Lateef M, Khan M, Lindsay D: Entamoeba infections in different populations of dogs in an endemic area of Lahore, Pakistan, *Vet Parasitol* 207:216–219, 2015.

Alcolea P, Alonso A, Gómez M, et al: Temperature increase prevails over acidification in gene expression modulation of amastigote differentiation in *Leishmania infantum*, *BMC Genomics* 11:31, 2010.

Allen K, Johnson E, Little S: Hepatozoon spp. infection in the United States, *Vet Clin North Am Small Anim Pract* 41:1221–1238, 2011.

Altreuther G, Gasda N, Schroeder I, et al: Efficacy of emodepside plus tol-trazuril suspension (Procox® oral suspension for dogs) against pre-patent and patent infection with *Isospora canis* and *Isospora ohioensis*-complex in dogs, *Parasitol Res* 109:9–20, 2011.

Baneth G: Perspectives on canine and feline hepatozoonosis, *Vet Parasitol* 181:3–11, 2011.

Baneth G, Mathew JS, Shkap V, Macintire DK, Barta JR, Ewing SA: Canine hepatozoonosis: two disease syndromes caused by separate Hepatozoon spp., *Trends Parasitol* 19:27–31, 2003.

Baneth G, Samish M, Shkap V: Life cycle of hepatozoon canis (apicom-plexa: adeleorina: hepatozoidae) in the tick *Rhipicephalus sanguineus* and domestic dog (Canis familiaris), *J Parasitol* 93:283–299, 2007.

Bates P: Transmission of Leishmania metacyclic promastigotes by phlebo-tomine sand flies, *Int J Parasitol* 37:1097–1106, 2007.

Birkenheuer A, Correa M, Levy M: Geographic distribution of babesiosis among clogs in the United States and association with dog bites. 150 cases (2000–2003), *J Am Vet Med Assoc* 227:23–27, 2005.

Blagburn B, Lindsay D, Swango L, Pidgeon G, Braund K: Further charac-terization of the biology of *Hammondia heydorni*, *Vet Parasitol* 27:193–198, 1988.

Bowman D, Lucio-Forster A: Cryptosporidiosis and giardiasis in dogs and cats: veterinary and public health importance, *Exp Parasitol* 124:121–127, 2010.

Bresciani K, Costa A, Toniollo G, et al: Experimental toxoplasmosis in pregnant bitches, *Vet Parasitol* 86:143–145, 1999.

Cicco M, Downey M, Beeler E, et al: Re-emerge of *Babesia conradae* and effective treatment of infected dogs with atovaquone and azithro-mycin, *Vet Parasitol* 187:23–27, 2012.

Corza V, Lappin M: Chapter 8, cryptosporidiosis and cyclosporidiasis. In Greene, editor: *Infectious diseases of the dog and cat*, 4 ed., 2012, Elsevier, pp 840–851.

Darwich L, Cabezón O, Echeverria I, et al: Presence of *Toxoplasma gondii* and *Neospora caninum* DNA in the brain of wild birds, *Vet Parasitol* 183:377–381, 2012.

de Brito A, de Souza L, da Silva A, Langoni H: Epidemiological and sero-logical aspects in canine toxoplasmosis in animals with nervous symptoms, *Mem Inst Oswaldo Cruz* 97:31–35, 2002.

Dubey J: The evolution of the knowledge of cat and dog coccidia, *Para-sitology* 136:1469–1475, 2009.

Dubey JP, Barr BC, Barta JR, et al: Redescription of *Neospora caninum* and its differentiation from related coccidian, *Int J Parasitol* 3:929–946, 2002.

Dubey J, Lindsay D, Lappin M: Toxoplasmosis and other intestinal coc-cidial infections in cats and dogs, *Vet Clin North Am Small Anim Pract* 39:1009–1034, 2009.

Dyachenko V, Steinmann M, Bangoura B, et al: Case report: co-infection of Trypanosoma pestanai and Anaplasma phagocytophilum in a dog from Germany, *Vet Parasitol Reg Stud Reports* 9:110–114, 2017.

Eloy L, Lucheis S: Canine trypanosomiasis: etiology of infection and implications for public health, *J Venom Anim Toxins Incl Trop Dis* 15:4, 2009.

Eloy L, Lucheis S: Hemoculture and polymerase chain reaction using primers TCZ1/TCZ2 for the diagnosis of canine and feline trypanoso-miasis, *ISRN Vet Sci* 2012:419378, 2012.

European Scientific Counsel Companion Animal Parasites (ESCCAP): *Control of intestinal protozoa in dogs and cats. Guideline 6, 2018:* ed 1, https://www.esccap.org/uploads/docs/2l5qc8kt_0701_ESCCAP_Guideline_GL6_v5.pdf. (Accessed January 2018).

Fiechter R, Deplazes P, Schnyder M: Control of Giardia infections with ronidazole and intensive hygiene management in a dog kennel, *Vet Parasit* 187:93–98, 2012.

Gjerde B, Dahlgren S: Hammondia triffittae n. comb. of foxes (Vulpes spp.): biological and molecular characteristics and differentiation from Hammondia heydorni of dogs, *Parasitology* 138:303–321, 2011.

Gondim L, Abe-Sandes K, Rosângela S, et al: *Toxoplasma gondii* and *Neospora caninum* in sparrows (Passer domesticus) in the Northeast of Brazil, *Vet Parasitol* 168:121–124, 2010.

Gunn A, Pitt S: *Parasitology: an integrated approach,* West Sussex, 2012, Wiley-Blackwell, 442 p.

Holman P, Snowden K: Canine hepatozoonosis and babesiosis, and feline cytauxzoonosis, *Vet Clin North Am Small Anim* 39:1035–1053, 2009.

Imre M, Farkas R, Ilie M, Imre K, Dărăbuş G: Survey of babesiosis in symptomatic dogs from Romania: occurrence of *Babesia gibsoni* asso-ciated with breed, *Ticks Tick Borne Dis* 4:500–502, 2013.

Irwin P: Canine babesiosis, *Vet Clin North Am Small Anim Pract* 40:1141–1156, 2010.

Itoh N, Oohashi Y, Ichikawa-Seki M, et al: Molecular detection and char-acterization of *Cryptosporidium* species in household dogs, pet shop puppies, and dogs kept in a school of veterinary nursing in Japan, *Vet Parasitol* 200:284–288, 2014.

Jordan H: Amebiasis (*Entamoeba histolytica*) in the dog, *Vet Med Small Anim Clin* 62:61–64, 1967.

Karkamo V, Kaistinen A, Näreaho A, et al: The first report of autoch-thonous non-vector-borne transmission of canine leishmaniosis in the Nordic countries, *Acta Vet Scand* 56:84, 2014.

Lindsay D, Dubey J, Butler J, Blagburn B: Mechanical transmission of Toxoplasma gondii oocysts by dogs, *Vet Parasitol* 73:27–33, 1997.

Little S, Allen K, Johnson E, Panciera R, Reichard M, Ewing S: New devel-opments in canine hepatozoonosis in North America: a review, *Parasit Vectors* 2:5, 2009.

Louhelainen M, Spillmann T: Case report: *Babesia canis* -infektio koiralla, *Suomen Eläinlääkäril* 115:143–148, 2009 (in Finnish).

Loza A, Talaga A, Herbas G, et al: Systemic insecticide treatment of the canine reservoir of Trypanosoma cruzi induces high levels of lethality in Triatoma infestans, a principal vector of Chagas disease, *Parasit Vectors* 10:344, 2017.

Meneses D, Schares G, Rezende-Gondim M, Galvão G, Gondim L: Ham-mondia heydorni: oocyst shedding by dogs fed in vitro generated tissue cysts, and evaluation of cross-immunity between *H. heydorni* and *Neospora caninum* in mice, *Vet Parasitol* 244:54–58, 2017.

Mitchell S, Zajac A, Charles S, Duncan R, Lindsay D: Cystoisospora canis neméseri, 1959 (syn. *Isospora canis*), infections in dogs: clinical signs, pathogenesis, and reproducible clinical disease in beagle dogs fed oocysts, *J Parasitol* 93:345–352, 2007.

Moron-Soto M, Gutierrez L, Sumano H, Tapia G, Alcala-Canto Y: Efficacy of nitazoxanide to treat natural *Giardia* infections in dogs, *Parasit Vectors* 10:52, 2017.

Northway R: *Entamoeba histolytica* in a dog, *Vet Med Small Anim Clin* 70:306, 1975.

Olson M: Coccidiosis caused by *Isospora ohioensis*-like organisms in three dogs, *Can Vet J* 26:112–114, 1985.

Rimhanen-Finne R, Enemark HL, Kolehmainen J, Toropainen P, Hänninen ML: Evaluation of immunofluorescence microscopy and enzyme-linked immunosorbent assay in detection of *Cryptosporidium* and *Giardia* infections in asymptomatic dogs, *Vet Parasitol* 145:345–348, 2007.

Ryan U, Paparini A, Monis P, Hijjawi N: It's official—Cryptosporidium is a gregarine: what are the implications for the water industry? *Water Res* 15:305–313, 2016.

Saari S, Rasi J, Anttila M: Leishmaniosis mimicking oral neoplasm in a dog: an unusual manifestation of an unusual disease in Finland, *Acta Vet Scand* 41:101–104, 2000.

Saleh M, Gilley A, Byrnes M, Zajac A: Development and evaluation of a protocol of *Giardia duodenalis* in a colony of group-housed dogs at a veterinary medical college, *J Am Vet Med Assoc* 249:644–649, 2016.

Santín M: Clinical and subclinical infections with Cryptosporidium in animals, *N Z Vet J* 61:1–10, 2013.

Schares G, Heydorn A, Cüppers A, Conraths F, Mehlhorn H: Hammondia heydorni-like oocysts shed by a naturally infected dog and *Neospora caninum* NC-1 cannot be distinguished, *Parasitol Res* 87:808–816, 2001.

Schares G, Pantchev N, Barutzki D, Heydorn A, Bauer C, Conraths F: Oocysts of *Neospora caninum*, *Hammondia heydorni*, *Toxoplasma gondii* and *Hammondia hammondi* in faeces collected from dogs in Germany, *Int J Parasitol* 35:1525–1537, 2005.

Schetters T: Vaccination against canine babesiosis, *Trends Parasitol* 21:179–184, 2005.

Schetters T, Moubri K, Cooke B: Comparison of *Babesia rossi* and *Babesia canis* isolates with emphasis on effects of vaccination with soluble parasite antigens: a review, *J S Afr Vet Assoc* 80:75–78, 2009.

Schoeman J: Canine babesiosis, *Onderstepoort J Vet Res* 76:59–66, 2009.

Slapeta J, Koudela B, Votýpka J, Modrý D, Horejs R, Lukes J: Coprodiagnosis of Hammondia heydorni in dogs by PCR based amplification of ITS 1 rRNA: differentiation from morphologically indistinguishable oocysts of *Neospora caninum*, *Vet J* 163:147–154, 2002.

Solano-Gallego L, Miró G, Koutinas A, et al: Vet guidelines for the practical management of canine leishmaniosis, *Parasit Vectors* 4:86, 2011.

Sykes J, Dubey J, Lindsay L, et al: Severe myositis associated with *Sarcocystis* spp. infection in 2 dogs, *J Vet Intern Med* 25:1277–1283, 2011.

Tangtrongsup S, Scorza V: Update on the diagnosis and management of *Giardia* spp. infections in dogs and cats, *Topics Comp Anim Med* 25:155–162, 2010.

The Center for Food Security and Public Health, *Giardiasis*, 2018, Iowa State University. http://www.cfsph.iastate.edu/Factsheets/pdfs/giardiasis.pdf. (Accessed 25 January 2018).

Thomas W: Inflammatory diseases of the central nervous system in dogs, *Clin Tech Small Anim Pract* 13:167–178, 1998.

Uehlinger F, Greenwood S, McClure J, Conboy G, O'Handley R, Barkema H: Zoonotic potential of *Giardia duodenalis* and *Cryptosporidium* spp. and prevalence of intestinal parasites in young dogs from different populations on Prince Edward Island, Canada, *Vet Parasitol* 196:509–514, 2013.

Visvesvara G, Martinez A, Schuster F, et al: Leptomyxid ameba, a new agent of amebic meningoencephalitis in humans and animals, *J Clin Microbiol* 28:2750–2756, 1990.

Wang A, Ruch-Gallie R, Scorza V, Lin P, Lappin M: Prevalence of *Giardia* and *Cryptosporidium* species in dog park attending dogs compared to non-dog park attending dogs in one region of Colorado, *Vet Parasitol* 184:335–340, 2012.

Chapter 3

Trematoda (Flukes)

Parasitic worms of the dog are classified as flatworms (Platyhelminthes), roundworms (Nematoda), thorny headed worms (Acantocephala) and ringed worms (Annelida). Flatworms are further separated into tapeworms (Cestoda) and flukes (Trematoda). Trematodes or flukes are soft, usually flat worms without segments. They generally reside in the alimentary canal or the organs associated with it. In addition to the intestine, depending on fluke species, they can be found in the liver, bile duct, gall bladder, and pancreatic ducts, but also in the lungs and bladder.

There is a lot of variation in size, shape, and internal anatomy in trematodes. A typical trematode has two suckers: a well-developed oral sucker and a ventral sucker or acetabulum. The position and the shape of these suckers are used to aid the morphological diagnosis of flukes. Some species (e.g., *Alaria* spp.) have an additional organ of attachment or acetabulum located behind the ventral sucker. Morphology of a typical trematode is presented in Fig. 3.1.

Trematodes have an intestinal tract with a mouth and an intestine branching from the esophagus. Some trematodes have an intestine comprising two pouches (ceca). In some, they diverge further into smaller subbranches. The trematode intestinal track is incomplete, because there is no anus. Small molecules can be absorbed through the tegument.

Most of the parasitic trematodes are hermaphroditic, with the exception of blood flukes. The reproductive organs vary in different species and their morphology and position are key features in identification. There are usually two testes, but there are also species with one testis or several testes. The male copulatory organ is referred to as a cirrus, and is usually vaginated in a pouch-like structure. There is usually a single ovary connected to a short oviduct. In addition, there are follicular vitelline glands, which are arranged in two lateral clusters. Again, there is a lot of variation in the shape of the uterus, which can be short and straight or fairly long and coiled. In many species, the egg-containing uterus fills most of the parasite. Both self- and cross-fertilization are possible. The species-level identification of trematodes is based primarily on the localization and structure of suckers, the intestinal tract, and the genitals.

Trematodes have a complex and indirect life cycle, which may involve several intermediate hosts, depending on the parasite species. There is one common denominator: the first intermediate host is usually a gastropod. A "classical" life cycle is as follows. Adult worms are producing eggs voided in the feces. A free-swimming larva or miracidium hatches from the egg and penetrates the first intermediate host, usually a gastropod. In a gastropod, a larva develops into a sporocyst stage. In the sporocyst, the worm reproduces asexually as number of embryos develops within them. These embryos will develop to become rediae. The asexual reproduction continues within the rediae with new embryos becoming cercariae. These will leave the intermediate host. Cercariae usually possess a tail for a swimming aid and many trematodes need further development to the cystic stage called metacercaria, which is infective for the definitive host. There is species-specific variation of the life cycle: sporocyst or redia stages may be lacking in some species, and in some species cercaria without metacercarial stage is a source of infection for a definitive host. Dogs are definitive hosts for many species, as are several mammals and birds. They get the infection from metacercaria-larvae from the intermediate (usually the second) host.

Trematode eggs can be found in the feces of the definitive host by routine sedimentation/flotation methods. The possible clinical signs caused to dogs depend on the anatomical location of the fluke species. In mild infections, there are no signs at all. Praziquantel and fenbendazole have been mentioned as medical treatments for dogs. As a control measure, dogs should be prevented from eating undercooked fish or other sources of infection. Several species may infect dogs, because trematodes are not too specific about their definitive hosts.

ALARIA SPP.

- A genus residing in the small intestine of the carnivorous definitive host, such as a dog.
- Indirect life cycle; dog becomes infected by ingestion of the metacercarial larval stage in the tissues of second intermediate hosts or paratenic hosts.
- The first intermediate hosts are snails, the second tadpoles and frogs.
- Adults 5 mm long and scoop-shaped.
- Canine infections are rarely associated with clinical signs.
- Diagnosis is based on the detection of operculated eggs in the fecal sample.

Canine Parasites and Parasitic Diseases. https://doi.org/10.1016/B978-0-12-814112-0.00003-9

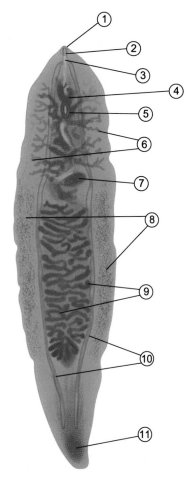

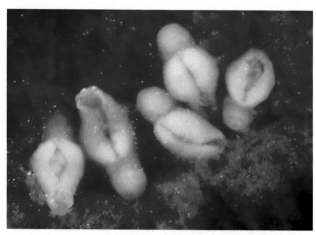

FIG. 3.2 *Alaria alata* trematodes on the intestinal mucosa.

FIG. 3.1 Morphology of a typical fluke, with *Clonorchis sinensis* as an example: (1) oral opening and oral sucker, (2) pharynx, (3) esophagus, (4) genital opening (gonophore), (5) ventral sucker or acetabulum, (6) uterus, (7) ovary, (8) vitellinic grands (vitellaria), (9) testes, (10) intestinal caeci, and (11) excretory bladder.

Identification

Alaria is a genus of trematode intestinal parasites found in carnivores (Fig. 3.2). The adults are about 5 mm long and resemble a short-handle scoop (Figs. 3.2 and 3.3). They produce moderately sized (110–140 × 65–80 μm) eggs with a clearly defined operculum.

Alariosis is a Zoonosis

Humans can be infected by *Alaria*, but this is very rare. A case has been described in the literature of a man who was trekking and ate poorly cooked frog's legs. After a few days, he got flu-like symptoms lasting a few days, descended into a coma, and perished. This was due to a large number of mesocercaria that had invaded his body. Respiratory and cutaneous symptoms have also been described, as well as neuroretinitis and anaphylactic reactions. Recently, knowing the zoonotic potential of *Alaria alata*, food hygienists have raised concerns about finding metacercariae in wild boar during meat inspections. The mesocercariae of *A. alata* are very robust: freezing for 5 days in −18°C is not sufficient to kill them in meat.

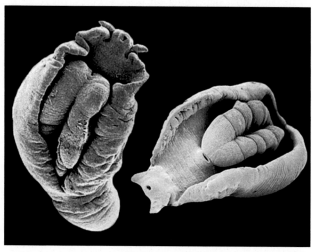

FIG. 3.3 *A. alata* trematodes in scanning electron microscopy. The cylindrical tail of the worm and the curling hem-like protrusions of the lateral edge create an image of a scoop. The figure shows clearly the oral sucker and the somewhat bigger ventral sucker, or acetabulum, of the trematode. The large, slit-like tribocytic organ for grasping is located immediately posteriorly to the ventral sucker. It guarantees the tight attachment of the worm to the intestinal mucosa.

Life Cycle

Alaria have a complex life cycle comprising stages in several intermediate hosts. The eggs of these hermaphrodite trematodes, living in the intestine, are transferred to the external environment in feces. The requirement for the continuity of the life cycle is that the eggs reach freshwater. After the development, which lasts about 2 weeks, the egg hatches to release an actively swimming larva, or miracidium. It penetrates the first intermediate host, the gastropod (several species are suitable intermediate hosts: Planorbis, Heliosoma, Lymnea, and Anisus). The parasite reproduces asexually in the snail, forming first sporocysts and then further daughter sporocysts. This enables the development of one miracidium into a large number of trematode larvae, which at the end of the cycle develop into cercaria stages, and exit the gastropod host. The cercaria swim with their forked tails to the surface, where they sink and then swim to the surface again, and thus attract the second intermediate host, an amphibian. The cercaria penetrate through the skin of the frog or tadpole, and develop in a few weeks into mesocercaria, a developmental stage between cercaria and metacercaria, which are infective for the definitive host. Carnivores are infected with *Alaria* by eating a tadpole or adult frog. If the frog is eaten by a snake or a bird, the parasite retains its infectivity and the definitive host may be infected by eating this paratenic, parasite-carrying host. In the alimentary tract of the definitive host, the larvae travel through the diaphragm and the pleura to the lungs, where the development of larvae into the diplostomulae of the metacercaria stage takes place. The diplostomulae penetrate into the respiratory tract, further with the sputum to the pharynx and, after swallowing, to the alimentary tract, where the worm matures. The prepatent period is about 3 weeks. In a suckling bitch, the diplostomulae may travel into the mammary gland and further to the puppies. The life cycle of *A. alata* is illustrated in Fig. 3.4.

Distribution

Distribution is worldwide, but the *Alaria* species vary. *A. alata* is common in wild carnivores in Europe, having local hot-spots in prevalence.

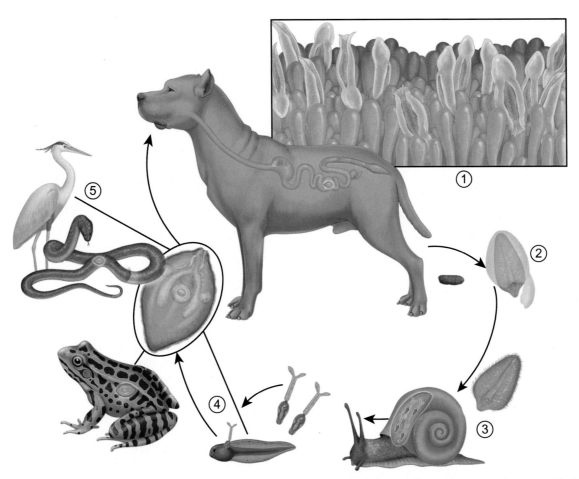

FIG. 3.4 Life cycle of *A. alata*: (1) *A. alata* have a complex life cycle requiring stages in several intermediate hosts. The adults live burrowed in the folds of the intestinal mucosa. The eggs are transferred into the environment in feces; (2) a swimming miracidium hatches from the egg in water; (3) the miracidium penetrates into the first intermediate host, Helisoma gastropod. The asexual reproduction of the parasite takes place in the gastropod, forming first sporocysts and then daughter sporocysts. As a result of the cycle in the gastropod, a large number of trematode larvae are developed, which at the end stages of the cycle develop into mesocercaria stages that exit the gastropod host; (4) the second intermediate host of the *A. alata* is the tadpole. The cercariae penetrate its skin. The larvae develop in the frog to mesocercaria stages, infectious to the definitive host; (5) if the frog is eaten by, e.g., a bird or snake, the parasite remains infectious in the new host; and (6) the dog is infected by eating the tadpole, the mature frog, or the infection-carrying paratenic host. In the alimentary tract of the definitive host, the larvae penetrate the gut wall into the abdominal cavity or the liver. They travel through the diaphragm into the thoracic cavity, where their development into the diplostomulae takes place. The diplostomulae penetrate the respiratory tract and further with the sputum to the pharynx, and are then swallowed to the alimentary tract, where they mature. The prepatent period is about 3 weeks.

Importance to Canine Health

Several *Alaria* species apparently have the capability to infect dogs. Infections, however, are rather rare in owned dogs compared to wild canids. The infection is usually subclinical. The most common clinical signs are respiratory or systemic signs during the migration of the larvae. A severe patent trematode infection may manifest as enteritis.

Diagnosis

Diagnosis is based on the presence of large operculated eggs in the feces. Sedimentation methods are best for finding *Alaria* eggs. A much less sensitive method is centrifugation flotation. The flotation solution should be, for instance, sugar or magnesium sulfate solution, which have high specific gravity.

Treatment and Prevention

The registered drugs for treatment or prevention of canine trematosis are scarce. Praziquantel, epsiprantel or fenbendazole are most often used for treatment. The dog is not infected unless it is allowed to eat infected intermediate or paratenic hosts.

Morphology of *A. alata*

The front of *A. alata* is dorso-ventrally flat. It has a clearly visible small oral sucker. Lateralle at both edges, there are ear-like tentacles (Fig. 3.5). The curled hem-like wings (alata means equipped with wings) of the lateral edge create an image of a spoon (Fig. 3.3) The lateral hems may cover a large area of the worm's ventral surface, which has a ventral sucker, slightly larger than the oral sucker. A large tribocytic organ is located immediately posterior from the ventral sucker. It ensures a tight attachment of the parasite to the intestinal mucosa (Fig. 3.3). Typical of trematodes, the outer surface of *Alaria* is covered with clusters consisting of small spines (Fig. 3.6). The posterior end of the worm is cylindrical. The genitalia of the hermaphrodite worm are situated in the posterior end, except for the vitellar glands. The genital pore is close to the worm's front end, slightly dorsally, and the secretory pore is posterior to it. The alimentary tract begins at the oral sucker. It consists of a well-developed pharynx and a branched caecum. The branches pass the tribocytic organ latero-dorsally and blind-end at the posterior end of the worm. There are two testes. They are located in the mid part of the rear end slightly dorsally. The anterior testis is smaller and the posterior is shaped like a horseshoe. The oval ovary is located at the junction of the anterior and posterior parts of the worm. The vitellary glands are at the front part and are evenly distributed. The general morphology and internal organs of *A. alata* are presented in Fig. 3.7.

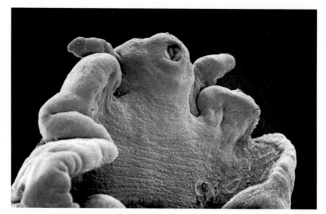

FIG. 3.5 The front end of *A. alata* trematode in electron microscopy. The oral sucker and the ear-like tentacles of the head's lateral edges can be clearly seen.

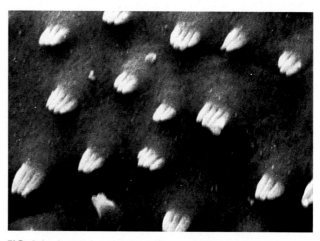

FIG. 3.6 A scanning electron microscopy image of the spine clusters present on the tegument of an *A. alata* trematode.

CLONORCHIS SINENSIS

Identification

The adult worm (Fig. 3.1) is leaf-shaped and 1–2.5 cm long. Branched testes are located posteriorly. The oval egg is about $15 \times 30\,\mu m$ and has an operculum with a visible rim and a knob in the other end.

Life Cycle

The fluke lives in the liver, bile ducts, and gall bladder. It produces eggs, which are carried with bile to the gut contents and finally with fecal material to the environment. The eggs have to reach water where they are eaten by snails. It is noticeable that unlike most other trematodes, the miracidium larval stage hatches from the egg inside the snail, not in the water. After asexual multiplication within the snail, the cercariae are released. They do not swim, but float and sink in turns. The cercariae are not able to feed, so their

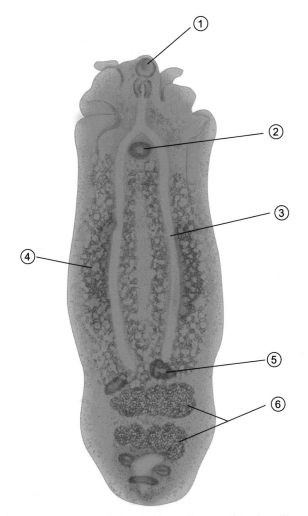

FIG. 3.7 General morphology and internal organs of *A. alata*. (1) oral sucker, (2) ventral sucker, (3) intestine (caecum branches), (4) vitellaria (5) ovary (6) testes.

life span is limited to only couple of days and finding the second intermediate host, fish, has to happen quickly. When a fish swims by, the cercaria attaches to its scales and penetrates the skin to the muscles, where it forms a hard cyst cover for protection and develops into the metacercaria phase. There are tens of freshwater fish species (mainly cyprinids) known to be suitable as hosts. Definitive hosts are several fish-eating species including humans and dogs. In their intestines, the metacercariae are released from the protective cyst and larvae penetrate the intestinal mucosa and migrate to the bile ducts to mature. The prepatent period is about a month.

Distribution

Clonorchis is one of the most prevalent flukes humans in the world. It is endemic in the Far East and eastern Russia, where dogs are also at high risk. The prevalence in dogs has been shown to be extremely high in certain areas.

Importance to Canine Health

Most of the cases are asymptomatic, but obstruction of bile ducts causes acute pain, nausea, and diarrhea. The chronic inflammation may cause diarrhea, anorexia, fatigue, and jaundice, and even trigger a neoplastic process which leads to cholangiosarcoma. Heavy infection has been reported to cause signs in several organs and to lead to dog's death.

Diagnosis

The eggs can be found in feces, but species identification according to egg morphology alone is discouraged, because several trematode eggs are very similar. In human diagnostics, ELISA and PCR methods are also used nowadays, but in endemic areas it should be remembered that serology does not differentiate between old and patent infections.

Treatment and Prevention

Dogs should be prevented from eating uncooked freshwater fish in endemic areas. In diagnosed cases, praziquantel can be used. In different human and canine trematode infections, the dose varies from a single high dose (up to 100 mg/kg) to a few days lower dose.

MESOSTEPHANUS SPP.

- A parasite of fish-eating birds, but infects other fish-eaters, such as dogs, as definitive hosts as well.
- Indirect life cycle, which is not yet clarified in detail.
- The life cycle involves mollusks and fish.
- Couple of mm long; operculated eggs.
- Canine infections are rarely associated with clinical signs.
- Diagnosis is based on the detection of operculated eggs in the fecal sample.

Identification

Mesostephanus species (Fig. 3.8) are trematode parasites occurring especially in fish-eating birds. Many are poorly host-specific and also infect other animals that eat fish, such as marine mammals, reptiles, dogs, and cats. The most common canine parasite of this group is *Mesostephanus milvi*. It can be up to 2 mm long, and the width is about half of this. The oral and the ventral sucker, or acetabulum, are small. The acetabulum is located in the middle part of the worm, and the circular tribocytic organ is posterior to it. Its length is about one-third of the whole length of the worm. The genitals are located posteriorly from the acetabulum and the tail end of the worm gets clearly thinner

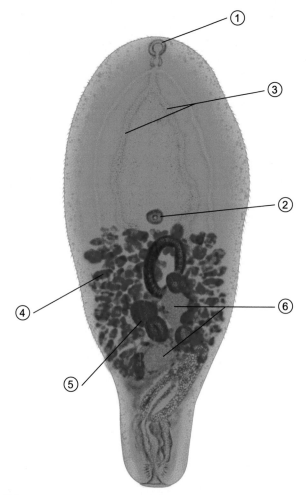

FIG. 3.8 General morphology and internal organs of *Mesostephanus* sp. (1) oral sucker, (2) ventral sucker, (3) intestine (caecum branches), (4) vitellaria (5) ovary (6) testes.

while forming an extension. The size of eggs is about 100–120 × 60–80 μm. They are yellowish brown and with dissimilar poles.

Life Cycle

The life cycle of *Mesostephanus* trematodes is not known in detail, but it includes stages at least in mollusks and fish.

Distribution

Mesostephanus trematodes have been identified in dogs and cats in Africa, India, Japan, and Europe.

Importance to Canine Health

Mesostephanus is not expected to cause clinical signs of disease for dogs.

Diagnosis

The diagnosis is based on the presence of large opeculated eggs in the feces. Sedimentation methods are best for finding *Mesostephanus* eggs. Centrifugation-flotation is much less sensitive and the flotation solution should be high in specific gravity—for instance, saturated magnesium sulfate solution.

Treatment and Prevention

There is no information on treatments against *Mesostephanus* infections.

Praziquantel is probably efficient. The infection is prevented by preventing the dogs from eating raw fish.

Apophallus donicus

- A parasite of fish-eating mammals, such as dogs, as its definitive hosts.
- Indirect life cycle involving mollusks and fish as intermediate hosts.
- About 1 mm long.
- Canine infections are rarely associated with clinical signs.
- Diagnosis is based on the detection of eggs in the fecal sample.

Identification

A. donicus (Fig. 3.9) is an intestinal trematode infecting fish-eating mammals. It is small, with a length of 0.5–1.15 mm. The width of the worm is 0.2–0.4 mm. The ventral sucker is small. The testes are large and located in the posterior part of the worm partly overlapping with each other. The vitellaria extend only to the level of the ventral sucker. The size of eggs is 35–39 × 22–24 μm.

Life Cycle

The worm lays embryonated eggs that contain fully developed miracidium larva, and they are excreted into the environment. Once a mollusk has eaten them, they hatch and the miracidium penetrates the gut wall of the mollusk. Redia and cercaria stages of the parasites have been found in Flumencola mollusks that live in streams. Mollusk-eating fish serve as the second intermediate hosts. Metacercaria, the stage infectious for mammals, develop in them. Known intermediate host species include the European perch (redfin) and sander of the perch group, and the common

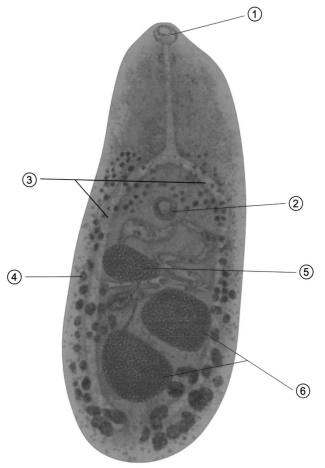

FIG. 3.9 General morphology and internal organs of *Apophallus donicus*. (1) oral sucker, (2) ventral sucker, (3) intestine (caecum branches), (4) vitellaria (5) ovary (6) testes.

rudd, a bentho-pelagic freshwater fish. The definitive host is infected by eating raw, insufficiently cooked, or poorly salted fish. The prepatent period is a few days.

Distribution

In addition to dogs, *Apophallus* is a small-intestine parasite of at least cats, seals, foxes, and, in rare cases, humans. It is endemic at least in Central and Eastern Europe.

Importance to Canine Health

The infection is usually subclinical. The worms are small and live deeply embedded in the mucosa. They may cause lesions in the site of attachment, which may manifest as enteritis.

Diagnosis

The infection is diagnosed by detecting eggs in a fecal sample.

Treatment and Prevention

There are no registered drugs for the treatment of canines. Praziquantel, epsiprantel, or fenbendazole are most often used for treatment of canine trematosis. Dogs are not infected unless they are allowed to eat infected intermediate or paratenic hosts.

HETEROPHYES HETEROPHYES

- A parasite of fish-eating mammals, such as dogs, as its definitive hosts.
- Indirect life cycle involving mollusks and fish as intermediate hosts.
- About 1 mm long; eggs have opercula.
- Canine infections rarely associated with clinical signs.
- Diagnosis based on the detection of eggs in the fecal sample.

Identification

H. heterophyes (Fig. 3.10) is an intestinal trematode parasite of fish-eating mammals. It is small, less than 2 mm long. The size of *Hetrophyes* eggs is about 20–30 × 15 μm and they have a distinctive lid (operculum).

Life Cycle

Like other trematodes, *Heterophyes* needs intermediate hosts for its life cycle. The worm lays embryonated eggs that contain fully developed miracidium larvae, and they are excreted into the environment. Once they have been eaten by a mollusk, they hatch and the miracidium penetrates the mollusk's gut wall. The asexual reproduction of the parasite takes place. After the sporocyst and redia stages, cercariae are developed. They are transferred to the second intermediate host, the fish. Many fish species living in fresh or brackish water can act as intermediate hosts. Flathead mullet, *Mugil cephalus*, is considered the most important of these. The stage infectious to the definitive host, metacercaria, grows in fish tissues. The definitive host is infected by eating raw, poorly cooked, or poorly salted fish.

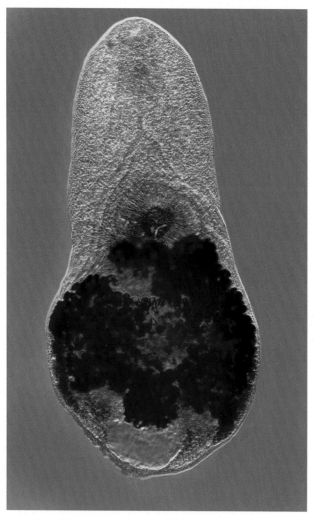

FIG. 3.10 *Heterophyes heterophyes* is a small trematode, under 2 mm long, of fish-eating mammals.

Morphology of *Heterophyes heterophyes*

All *Heterophyes* species are small trematodes, under 2 mm long. Their outer surface is covered by tiny spikes. The pharynx is long and well developed. The caecae of the intestine extend to the tail end of the worm. The genital pore is surrounded by a sucker with spiky structures. The identification of *Heterophyes* is commonly based on the number of these spikes. The sucker of the genital pore is close and posterio-lateral to the well-developed ventral sucker (acetabulum). The testes are side by side, close to the distal parts of the intestinal caecae. The ovary is located medially. The vitellar glands are located at the anterior side of the testes and grouped symmetrically. The general morphology and internal organs of *H. heterophyes* are presented in Fig. 3.11.

Distribution

Several *Heterophyes* species are capable of infecting dogs. Trematodes of this genus are endemic in dogs, especially in African, Middle Eastern, and Asian countries.

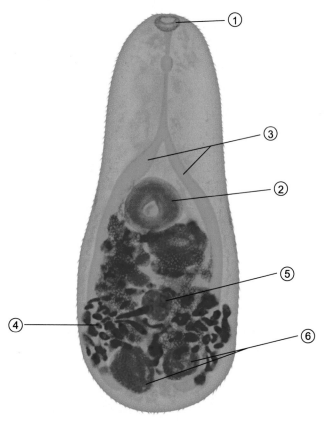

FIG. 3.11 General morphology and internal organs of *H. heterophyes*. (1) oral sucker, (2) ventral sucker, (3) intestine (caecum branches), (4) vitellaria (5) ovary (6) testes.

Importance to Canine Health

The infection is usually subclinical. A severe intestinal infection caused by adult trematodes may manifest as enteritis. *H. heterophyes* is a zoonotic parasite, but the dog is not the source of human infection.

Diagnosis

The diagnosis is based on finding eggs with operculum in the fecal sample. Immunological assays have been developed for diagnostics, but they are not known to be commercially available.

Treatment and Prevention

There are no registered drugs for the treatment of canine trematosis. Praziquantel is the treatment most often used. The dog is safe from the infection if it has no access to infected intermediate or paratenic hosts.

DICROCOELIUM DENDRITICUM, Lancet Liver Fluke

- A parasite of grazing animals as definitive hosts.
- Indirect life cycle involving a land snail and an ant as intermediate hosts. Dog is an accidental host after ingesting ants.
- Adults live in bile ducts and are 6–10 mm long; eggs are small and with operculum.
- Canine infections and clinical signs are rare.
- Diagnosis based on the detection of eggs in the fecal sample.

Identification

The lancet liver fluke (Fig. 3.12) is a flat, transparent, elliptical, and leaf-shaped trematode. Its length is 6–10 mm and its width is 1.5–2.5 mm. The egg is small, 45 × 30 μm, thick-shelled, dark brown, and equipped with an obscure operculum. It is flatter on one side. The miracidium larva with visible "eye spots" occupies the egg entirely (Fig. 3.13).

Life Cycle

Adult *D. dendriticum* trematodes live in the bile ducts of the liver. The hermaphrodite worms copulate and the eggs are voided in bile into the intestine and further into the environment within the fecal mass. Terrestrial mollusks act as the first intermediate hosts. They are infected while ingesting egg-contaminated dung. In the snail, the hatched miracidium larva penetrates the intestinal wall and asexually develops into the sporocyst, creating daughter sporocysts. The snail secretes slime containing these daughter sporocysts and, inside them, cercariae infectious to the next intermediate host. An ant acting as a second intermediate host is necessary for the next developmental stage of the lancet liver fluke. The ant eats the slime and cercariae secreted by the snail. A major part of the cercariae penetrates into the ant's body cavity, where they develop into metacercariae, the form infectious to the definitive host. A single cercaria penetrates the neural center of the ant, the subesophageal ganglion. The cercaria alters the behavior of the ant. When the ambient temperature gets cooler in the evening, the ant, manipulated by the cercariae, climbs high on the shaft of a grass, grasps the shaft with its jaws, and remains immobile during the night. The morning sun frees the ant into its daily activities, but the same action repeats night after night until the ant is eaten by an animal foraging early in the morning. In the alimentary tract of the host animal, the ant is digested and the liver fluke penetrates the bile ducts. The prepatent period is about 10–12 weeks.

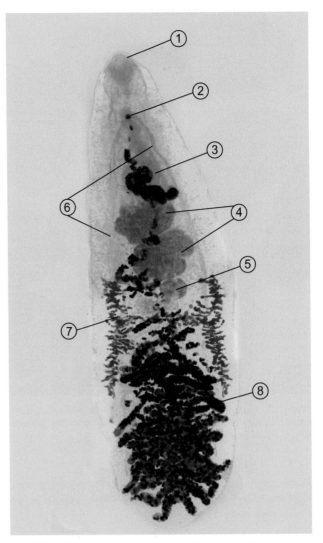

FIG. 3.12 *Dicrocoelium dendriticum*, the lancet liver fluke stained to enhance the morphological details in light microscopy: (1) oral sucker, (2) genital pore, (3) ventral sucker, (4) testis, (5) ovary, (6) caecum branch, (7) vitellaria, and (8) egg-filled uterus.

Distribution

The lancet liver fluke is common especially in Europe and in most parts of North America.

Importance to Canine Health

The lancet liver fluke parasitizes primarily in herbivorous animals. It is nonhost-specific but the ants, acting as intermediate hosts and carrying infective forms, are the most probable prey for foraging animals. Dogs are infected only in exceptional circumstances. The infection is passed similarly to with other animals: by eating grass. The significance of the lancet liver fluke to a dog's health is poorly known. The infection is generally subclinical. Nonspecific

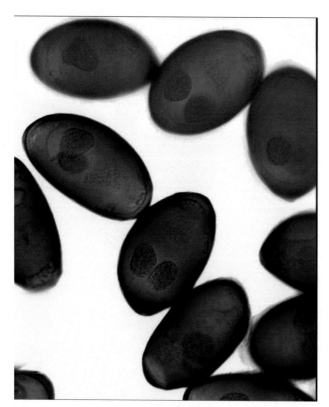

FIG. 3.13 Eggs of *D. dendriticum*. They are quite small, 45 × 30 μm, *brown*, flat on one side, and the "eye spots" of the miracidium larva can be seen inside them.

NANOPHYETUS SALMINCOLA

- A parasite of fish-eating birds and mammals, such as dogs, as its definitive hosts.
- Indirect life cycle involving a fresh water snail and a (salmonid) fish as intermediate hosts.
- Adults are couple of mm long; eggs have opercula.
- The clinical signs are usually the result of a microbe *Neorickettsia helminthoeca*, a symbiont of the trematode and the cause of salmon poisoning.
- The trematode diagnosis is based on the detection of eggs in the fecal sample; salmon poisoning is suspected if the signs and history fit.

alimentary tract signs, such as diarrhea and vomiting, have been described in the literature. Declining condition has reported in some dogs.

Diagnosis

If eggs of lancet liver fluke are found in a dog's fecal sample, the primary suspicion is that the eggs are passing though the intestine after having been eaten together with ruminant or lagomorph feces by the dog. The infection can be confirmed by preventing the dog from moving freely in the nature and continuing to analyze fecal samples for parasite eggs. If the infection is authentic, eggs will also turn up in the subsequent tests. The diagnosis is hampered by the fact that eggs are infrequently secreted in feces also in real infections.

Treatment and Prevention

Infections of the lancet liver fluke in other animals are most commonly treated with drugs belonging to the benzimidazole group, so that could also be the drug of choice in canine infection.

Identification

N. salmincola (Fig. 3.14) is an intestinal trematode found in fish-eating mammals and in some fish-eating birds. The *Nanophyetus* are small, 0.8–2.5 mm long, and about 0.3–0.5 mm wide. The size of eggs is 87–97 × 38 μm and they have a distinct lid (operculum) and a vaguely visible blunt bump at the other end.

Life Cycle

Typical of trematodes, *N. salmincola* needs intermediate hosts in its life cycle. The adult flukes live in the small intestine, mostly buried between the intestinal villi. The eggs are transferred in feces into the environment, where they must reach fresh or brackish water. The eggs develop slowly, about 3 months in room-temperature water, while in a natural environment, development often takes more than 6 months. *Oxytrema silicula*, a freshwater snail living in streams, acts as an intermediate host. The asexual reproduction of the parasite takes place in the snail. After the sporocyst and redia stages (while it is not certain that sporocysts belong to the life cycle of this parasite), the cercaria that develop in the snail attach to the second intermediate host, fish, as they swim past.

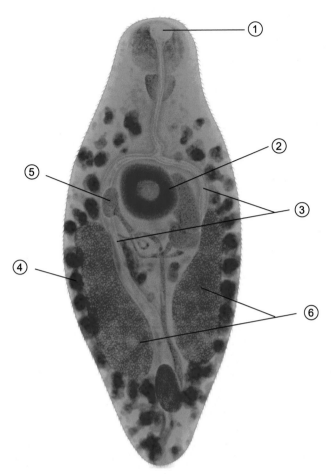

FIG. 3.14 General morphology of *Nanophyetus salmincola*. (1) oral sucker, (2) ventral sucker, (3) intestine (caecum branches), (4) vitellaria (5) ovary (6) testes.

Salmonids in particular act as second intermediate hosts. Metacercaria, the stage infectious to the definitive host, develops in the fish tissues. The definitive host is infected by eating raw, poorly cooked, or poorly salted fish. Fig. 3.15 presents the life cycle of *N. salmincola*.

Distribution

N. salmincola is endemic especially on the west coast of North America.

Importance to Canine Health

The infection is usually subclinical. This trematode is best known for acting as a vector species for *N. helminthoeca* infection. The trematodes carry in their system rickettsia microbes and transfer them to the intestinal epithelial cells. The microbes take over the lymphatic tissue of the intestinal mucosa, lymph nodes, and spleen. After the incubation period of 2–14 days, a dog gets salmon poisoning, a serious gastrointestinal infection, manifesting with fever, anorexia, and lethargy. Lymphadenopathy is an additional sign.

Without treatment, salmon poisoning is often fatal within 10–14 days of the onset of the disease.

Diagnosis

Trematode diagnosis is based on finding eggs with opercula in the fecal sample. The eggs are heavy and best detected with sedimentation methods.

Treatment and Prevention

Praziquantel, epsiprantel, and fenbedazole are reported to be effective against *Nanophyetus* trematodes. Tetracycline is used to treat neorickettsiosis. Dogs have been immunized in high-risk areas by being fed raw fish and treated with tetracycline immediately when signs of neorickettsiosis have manifested.

> **Morphology of *Nanophyetus salmincola***
> *N. salmincola* is 0.8–2.5 mm long and 0.3–0.5 mm wide. Its shape varies from spherical to rod-shaped. The oral sucker is slightly bigger than the ventral one. The ovary is located at the right side of the ventral sucker. The genital pore is behind the posterior edge of the ventral sucker. In young individuals, the uterus is U-shaped, and, when filled with eggs, W-shaped. There are usually 5–16 eggs. The vitellarias are grouped into rather large follicles that are irregularly scattered mostly in the dorsal parts of the parasite, also partly extending to the ventral parts. Large, elongated testes are in the posterior third of the fluke lateral from the branches of the intestine. They are surrounded by the tightly packed vitellary follicles, except medially. The general morphology and internal organs of *N. salmincola* are presented in Fig. 3.14.

PARAGONIMUS KELLICOTTI

- A pulmonary parasite of crayfish-eating animals, such as dogs, as its definitive hosts.
- Indirect life cycle involving aquatic gastropod and crayfish as intermediate hosts.
- Adults are 1 cm long; eggs have on operculum.
- The most common clinical signs are cough, intolerance to exercise, and dyspnea (difficulty breathing).
- Sudden deaths have been reported.
- The diagnosis is based on the detection of eggs in the fecal sample.

Identification

P. kellicotti (Fig. 3.16) is a trematode and a pulmonary parasite. It is 1 cm long, dorso-ventrally flat, oval, reddish-brown, and roughly resembles a coffee bean. It has distinctive

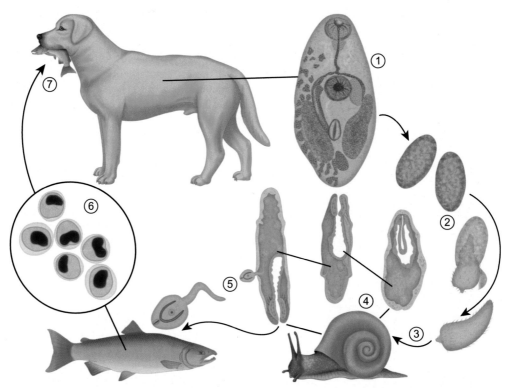

FIG. 3.15 Life cycle of *N. salmincola*: (1) the adult flukes live in the small intestine mostly buried between the intestinal villi. The eggs are transferred in feces into the environment, where they must reach fresh or brackish water; (2) the eggs develop slowly and an actively swimming miracidium hatches from the egg in water; (3) the miracidium penetrates into the first intermediate host: *O. silicula*, a freshwater snail living in streams; (4) the asexual reproduction of the parasite takes place in the snail; (5) after the sporocyst and redia stages (while it is not certain that sporocysts belong to the life cycle of this parasite), the cercaria that developed in the snail attach and penetrate to the second intermediate host, fish, as they swim past. Salmonids in particular act as second intermediate hosts; (6) metacercaria, the stage infectious to the definitive host, develops in the fish tissues; and (7) the definitive host is infected by eating raw, poorly cooked, or poorly salted fish.

oral and ventral suckers of similar size. The genus *Paragonimus* also includes other species, some of which can also parasitize dogs. The species identification is often based on the recognition of small scales covering the skin of the fluke and their shape, and in the differences in the morphology of the metacercaria larvae. *Paragonimus* eggs are oval, yellow-brown, and 75–118 × 42–67 μm in size. While in the canine feces, they are still monocellular and they have a distinguishable lid (operculum).

Paragonimios is a Zoonosis

Humans can also be infected with *P. kellicotti*. The source of infection is usually raw or partially cooked crustaceans. Since the fluke requires two intermediate hosts for its life cycle, the dog cannot infect a human. The pulmonary symptoms of human paragonimiosis are similar to those in dogs. Humans can experience symptoms also in the beginning of the infection, when the larvae penetrate the gut wall and start their migration. The abdominal pain and fever associated with this stage are, however, nonspecific signs.

Life Cycle

Adult parasites live encapsulated in the lung tissue. In exceptional cases, stray larvae can also be found elsewhere in the organism. The flukes usually live in communities of two or more individuals in the fluke cysts or granulomas formed in the lungs. The diameter of cysts varies from 2 to 5 cm, and they are covered in a capsule of connective tissue, up to several millimeters thick. There is a connection from the cysts to bronchioli. The fluke eggs migrate within sputum to the pharynx, and are swallowed and transferred in feces into the external environment. The parasite has an indirect life cycle that necessitates intermediate hosts. *Paragonimus* eggs must get to fresh water. The development of the larva stage inside the egg capsule usually takes several weeks. The miracidium larva, hatching from the egg, needs to find the first intermediate host, aquatic gastropods of Pleuroceridae or Thiaridae family. These snails occupy often rapidly streaming rivers, which makes finding a suitable intermediate host challenging for the miracidium. The following development stages, with asexual reproduction, take place in the snail. These asexual cycle stages facilitate the survival of the fluke, although

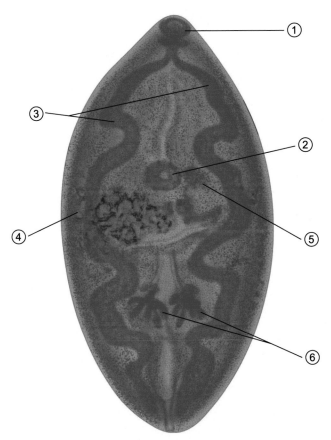

FIG. 3.16 General morphology of *P. kellicotti*, which is a pulmonary trematode. (1) oral sucker, (2) ventral sucker, (3) intestine (caecum branches), (4) vitellaria (5) ovary (6) testes.

only a small minority of miracidium larvae are able to find a gastropod for an intermediate host. The miracidium first develops into a sporocyst, in which rediae and further great quantities of cercariae develop. The cercariae exit the gastropod host. They have a small and spiky rod of a tail and a stylet-shape structure in the oral sucker. The cercaria is very active and moves around in the riverbed and on the rocks, with motion resembling that of a caterpillar, searching for the second intermediate host, the crayfish. Many freshwater crayfish species can act as the second intermediate host, most commonly *Cambarus* and *Orconectes* genera. It is assumed that the cercaria may also reach the crayfish when they use infection-carrying snails as food. Metacercaria, the stage infective for the definitive host, grow in the crayfish tissues. The definitive host receives the infection by eating an infected crustacean. The infection can also happen through a paratenic host. The digestive juices of the host break down the cyst of metacercaria. The liberated larvae penetrate the intestinal wall into the peritoneum and the abdominal cavity, from where they continue migration through the diaphragm and the pleura toward the lungs. The juvenile stages meet in the lungs forming fluke cysts.

The parasite appears to avoid solitary life: the larva may arrest its development, and the maturation and the formation of the cyst continue only when the parasite has met a companion of same species. The prepatent period is 5–7 weeks. Live flukes have been found in lungs up to 4 years after infection. An illustrated life cycle of *P. kellicotti* is presented in Fig. 3.17.

Distribution

Paragonimus species are encountered in the Americas, Asia, and Africa.

Importance to Canine Health

The infection can be totally without signs. The most common manifestations of the infection include cough, exercise intolerance, and dyspnea. If a parasite cyst ruptures, pneumothorax may complicate the condition. Cases of sudden death without any preceding signs and attributed to the disease have been described in the literature.

Diagnosis

The diagnosis is based on finding large, operculated eggs, typical of the species, in sputum, broncho-alveolar lavage (BAL) or fecal samples. Methods based on sedimentation work best for fecal analysis. A much less uncertain diagnosis than that obtained with sedimentation is achieved using centrifugation and flotation. Sugar or magnesium sulfate solutions can be used as the flotation solution. The egg may be distinguished from those of similar trematodes and Pseudophyllidae worms (such as Diphyllobothrium) by recognizing the thickening of the junction of operculum. The worm cysts can be visible in radiography. They are commonly located in the dorso-caudal lobes and appear as multisegmented cystic structures or patchy consolidations.

Treatment and Prevention

Praziquantel or fenbendazole are commonly used to treat the *Paragonimus* infection. Both substances are used for longer than the label dosage. Treatment success has been described with a dose of praziquantel 3 times daily for 3 days and with a daily fenbendazole dose continuing for 10 days.

Morphology of *Paragonimus kellicotti*

The length of adult *P. kellicotti* is 7–12 mm. The width of the worm is 4–6 mm. *Paragonimus* is dorso-ventrally flat, but quite thick, about 3.5–5 mm. The surface of the worm is covered with scaly protrusions. The worm has a clearly visible oral and ventral sucker, both of the same size. The oral

Continued

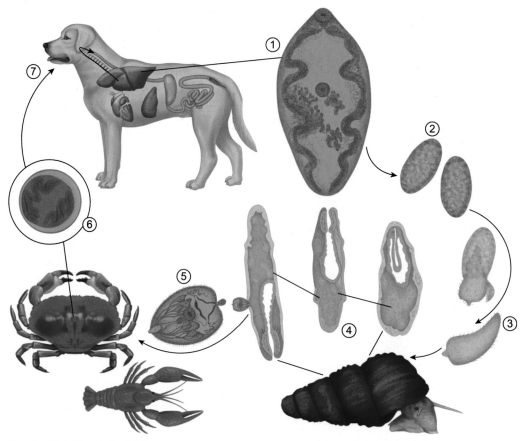

FIG. 3.17 Life cycle of *P. kellicotti*: (1) adult *Paragonimus* flukes live encapsulated in lung tissue; (2) the eggs are transferred with sputum to the pharynx and then swallowed into the alimentary tract and passed in feces into the external environment; (3) *Paragonimus* eggs must reach freshwaters. The miracidium larva hatching from the egg must find the first intermediate host, an aquatic gastropod; (4) the following life cycle stages that involve asexual reproduction of the parasite take place in the gastropod. The miracidium first develops into a sporocyst, in which redia and then masses of cercariae are formed; (5) the cercariae exit the gastropod intermediate host. The have a small, spiky, rod-like tail and a stylet-shaped structure in the oral cavity. The cercaria is very active and it moves in the riverbed and on the rocks in a manner reminiscent of a caterpillar, searching for the second intermediate host, the crayfish; (6) metacercaria, the stage infectious for the definitive host, develops in the crayfish tissues; and (7) the definitive host is infected by eating a parasite-carrying crayfish or the crab. The infection may also happen via a paratenic host. The prepatent period is 5–7 weeks.

Morphology of *Paragonimus kellicotti*—cont'd

sucker is located ventrally close to the front end of the worm and the ventral sucker (acetabulum) slightly above the midline of the worm. The pharynx is well developed and the main branches of the intestine extend close to the end of the worm. The testes are lobular, symmetrical to each other, and located at the caudal end of the worm, at the border of the third and fourth quarters. The genital pore is close to the ventral sucker, posterior from it. The lobular ovary is located anterior to the testis, slightly to the left of the central axle. The uterus forms a tight, rosette-shaped curving structure left from the ventral suction orifice. There is a duct connection between the uterus and the genital atrium, the space joining the female and male genitals. There are numerous vitellar follicles, and they appear to fill a major part of the lateral and dorsal part of the worm, from the level of the pharynx all the way to the rear. The general morphology and internal organs of *P. kellicotti* are presented in Fig. 3.16.

METORCHIS SPP.

- A liver fluke of fish-eating carnivores, also dogs and humans.
- Two intermediate hosts: a snail and a cyprinid fish.
- Length of the adult 2–3 mm; eggs have opercula.
- Most cases are subclinical, but bile obstruction may cause signs, even death.
- Diagnosis is based on the detection of eggs in the fecal sample.

Identification

Metorchis spp. (Fig. 3.18) belongs to the liver fluke family Opistorchidae. The length of the adult worm is about 2–3 mm. Worms have both a ventral and an oral sucker, a very short or absent esophagus, two testes (anterior smaller than

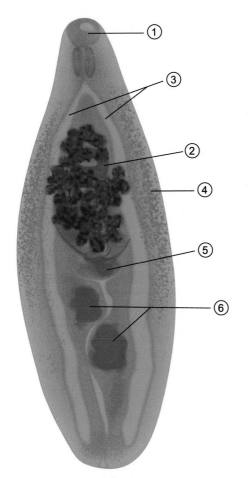

FIG. 3.18 General morphology and internal organs of *Metorchis* sp. (1) oral sucker, (2) ventral sucker, (3) intestine (caecum branches), (4) vitellaria (5) ovary (6) testes.

the posterior), and an ovary anteriorly to the testes. Egg length varies between 27 and 34 μm and egg width between 16 and 22 μm, and the eggs have opercula.

Life Cycle

Several *Metorchis* species have been reported to infect dogs and cause clinical signs to them. The life cycle is indirect with two intermediate hosts: a snail and a cyprinid fish, which metacercariae are infective to definitive hosts, fish-eating carnivorous animals, including dogs and humans. The prepatent period is 2–4 weeks.

Distribution

Different *Metorchis* species are distributed in different geographical locations. For example, *Metorchis conjunctus* is prevalent in North America, whereas *Metorchis orientalis* appears in the Far East. *Metorchis bilis*, nowadays genetically identified as a single species together with *Metorchis albidus* and *Metorchis crassiusculus*, is found in Europe.

Importance to Canine Health

Most cases are subclinical and presumably underdiagnosed. The possible signs are caused by bile obstruction due to worms and the following liver damage and hepatic dysfunction. Cholelithiasis, ascending cholangitis, pancreatitis, and cholangiocarcinoma due to irritation and immune reaction are possible consequences. Liver abscesses have been reported, and even death.

Diagnosis

Metorchis eggs are secreted in feces, and can be found with flotation techniques, but the method is rather insensitive and the eggs cannot be specified morphologically. PCR methods and sequencing may be used, if it is necessary to identify the eggs to species level. Clinical cases may be indirectly suspected if there is a fish-eating history of the canine patient with elevated liver enzyme values that give an indication of liver dysfunction. For research purposes, ELISA tests have been successfully used in dogs. From fish samples, metacercariae can be isolated with artificial digestion method.

Treatment and Prevention

Metorchis infection is treated with praziquantel (25–30 mg/kg). The length of the course varies. Even a single dose might be enough, but in human cases of liver abscesses, for example, the treatment has been continued for several weeks. A canine abscess case report describes a 6-day treatment p.o. with 30 mg/kg BID. The feces were examined for eggs, and the clinical recovery and the laboratory results were used as indicators. Because the abscess situation is often complicated with bacterial infection, prolonged course of antibiotics for 4–6 weeks is used in humans, and may also be advisable in dogs in addition to the drainage of the cysts.

The infection occurs only after eating raw or undercooked cyprinid fish, so excluding these from the dog's diet prevents infections. In addition, deep-freezing destroys the metacercariae from the fish. Kennel epidemics have been reported after feeding dogs for years with low commercial value fish.

HETEROBILHARZIA AMERICANA

- A blood fluke of mesenteric and portal veins in mammal definitive hosts.
- Indirect life cycle involving freshwater snails as intermediate hosts.

- Has distinct male and female individual organisms, but the female lives in the abdominal groove of the male.
- Infection occurs through skin penetration by the cercariae.
- The clinical signs are skin reactions or inflammatory changes caused by the eggs released in veins, and signs related to them.
- Diagnosis is based on the detection of eggs in the fecal sample.

Identification

Infections of *H. americana* trematodes are diagnosed especially in raccoons and coypus (nutrias), but also in other mammals such as dogs. The *Heterobilharzia* are digenetic trematodes, which live in the hepatic portal veins and the veins of the omentum. In contrast to many other trematodes, the parasite is dioecious (male and female reproductive organs are in separate individuals). The worms are 9–17 mm long. The male is bigger, but the female is usually longer than the male. The genders are in close contact, since the female lives at the abdominal side of the male, in the groove, called the gynecophoral canal. In the gynecophoral canal of one male, several females can live simultaneously. Blood flukes living in the blood vessels include parasites of Schistosoma family (Fig. 3.19), which are important human pathogens. The eggs of *Heterobilharzia* are thin-walled and about $87 \times 70\,\mu m$ in size. They lack the operculum lid, common in other trematodes. A fully

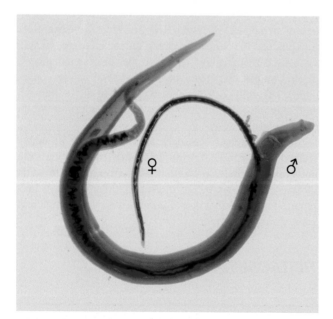

FIG. 3.19 A typical Schistosomatidae blood fluke. The worms live in blood vessels. The male is the larger sex. The egg-filled female is longer than the male. The female worm lives in a groove called the gynecophoral canal at the abdominal side of the male.

developed miracidium larva can be seen in the eggs that exit the host in feces.

Life Cycle

The worms live in veins of the omentum and the hepatic portal veins. The eggs laid by the female penetrate from the blood vessels to the gut wall. The immune response of the organism pushes the eggs in the intestinal lumen, from where they exit to the environment in feces. If the eggs end up in waterways, miracidium, the actively mobile larva, is freed from the egg. The larvae infect the freshwater snail (*Lymnaea cubensis*, *Pseudocuccinea columella*), acting as an intermediate host. The asexual reproduction of the parasite takes place in the hepato-pancreas of the snail, resulting in sporocysts and further daughter sporocysts. The gastropod stage lasts about 25 days. Masses of cercaria, the stage infective to the definitive host, develop inside the daughter sporocysts. The cercariae are capable of active movement. They exit the gastropod and search for an animal suitable as a definitive host. Cercaria can swim both forward and backward, and their swimming motion is directed toward the surface and light. Shadows and currents obstruction the light reveal that there may be a host species in the vicinity, and stimulate the cercaria to swim toward the potential host. The cercariae recognize skin by detecting temperature, surface lipids, and fatty acids. They attach to the skin, drop their tails, and search for a place suitable for penetration. A suitable spot is usually in a skin fold or a pore. Movement and grasping are facilitated by the small, thorny protrusions of the larval surface. From its glandular structures, the cercaria oozes protolytic enzymes on the skin, penetrating the skin in a few hours. The larvae travel in the blood into the liver, where further development takes place. From the liver, the larvae continue into the portal and omental veins. The laying of eggs starts about 12 weeks after infection. The illustrated life cycle of *H. americana* is presented in Fig. 3.20.

Distribution

H. americana trematodes are endemic in the southern and southwestern parts of the United States, especially in Texas and Louisiana. Several other trematodes of Schistosomatidae family may infect dogs and are found especially in Asia and Africa.

Importance to Canine Health

The pathogenicity of *Heterobilharzia* is associated with the tissue damage and inflammation caused migration phase and the inflammatory changes caused by the eggs. The eggs may disperse into different parts of the organism, and they are often targeted by a granulomatous inflammatory

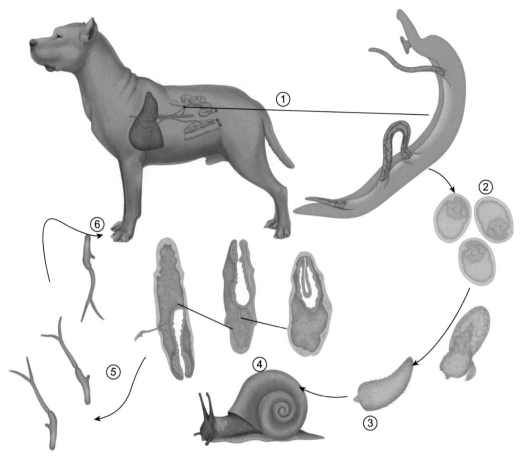

FIG. 3.20 Life cycle of *Heterobilharzia americana*: (1) adult worms live in veins of the omentum and the hepatic portal veins; (2) the eggs laid by the female penetrate from the blood vessels into the intestinal lumen, from where they exit to the environment in faeces; (3) if the eggs end up in waterways, miracidium, the actively mobile larva, hatches from the egg. The miracidium infects the freshwater snail, acting as an intermediate host; (4) the asexual reproduction of the parasite takes place in the hepato-pancreas of the snail, resulting in sporocysts and further to daughter sporocysts; (5) masses of cercaria, the stage infective to the definitive host, develop inside the daughter sporocysts. The cercariae are capable of active movement. They exit the gastropod and search for an animal suitable as a definitive host. After recognizing the skin of their potential host, they attach to the skin, drop their tails, and search for a place suitable for penetration; and (6) the larvae travel in the blood into the liver, where further development takes place. From the liver, the larvae continue into the portal and omental veins. The prepatent period is about 12 weeks.

response. As the result of the inflammation, the worm egg regularly dies, but scar tissue and calcification grow at the affected tissues, leading into dysfunction of the organ. The changes are most often seen in the gut wall and the liver. The clinical signs of the invasion are commonly somnolence, weight loss, vomiting and/or diarrhea or diminished appetite. In the analysis of blood, lymphopenia and hypercalcemia are most typical findings. Sensitization to skin-penetrating cercariae may lead to skin reactions similar to those caused by swimmer's itch. They have been described especially in humans.

Diagnosis

Heterobilharzia eggs may be detected by analyzing a fecal sample with sedimentation method or direct microscopy. Physiological saline should be used for sedimentation, since the eggs hatch rapidly when in contact with water. Flotation methods are not suitable for *Heterobilharzia* diagnosis. The diagnosis is often based on the pathological analysis of a tissue biopsy or autopsy findings. In histopathology, eggs, and the granulomatous inflammatory reaction provoked by them, scar tissue and calcifications are seen.

Treatment and Prevention

Treating the infection is often difficult, since the signs usually result from chronic inflammatory changes and tissue damage. The most common treatment is the combination of praziquantel (10 mg/kg 3 times daily for 3 days) and fenbendazole (24 mg/kg daily for 7 days).

Many Trematodes Infect Dogs

Trematodes are not usually very specific of their definitive hosts. Many, apart from the ones listed here, may infect dogs. For instance, *Pseudamphistomum truncatum* may be passed in fish to dogs. Other canine infecting trematodes, as listed in the literature, include *Opisthorchis* species (Fig. 3.21) (e.g., *O. tenuicollis*, *O. felineus*, and *O. viverrini*, *Metagonimus yokogawai*, *Cryptocotyle lingua*), *Echinochasmus* spp. (Fig. 3.22) (e.g., *E. schwartzi*, *E. perfoliatus*, *E. japonicus*, *E. liliputanus*), *Plachiorchis* species (Fig. 3.23), and *Sellacotyle mustelae* (Fig. 3.24). Their life cycle includes a gastropod as the first and a freshwater fish as the second intermediate host.

Many blood flukes representing several species are common endoparasites of waterfowl. The cercariae of these parasites may cause a water-borne transient skin reaction in the skin of mammals, especially humans. This condition is referred as swimmer's itch or cercarial dermatitis. Adult worms are schistosome trematodes that reside in the circulatory system of waterfowl. The eggs produced by the females are voided within the feces of the bird. In water, a free-living larval stage, the miracidium, emerges. It has to find the first intermediate host, a freshwater snail. In the snail, the parasite undergoes several cycles of asexual reproduction, another free-living stage, the cercaria (Fig. 3.25), as an end-result. Cercariae leave the snail and use their tail-like forked appendage to swim. They try to locate their definitive host, a bird. The cercaria penetrates through the skin of the bird, drops its tail, and enters the circulatory system of the host and continues its development. If a cercaria accidentally comes into contact with the skin of a swimmer—the swimmer could also be a dog—it penetrates the skin, but cannot migrate further and dies rapidly. In humans, these attempts to invade the skin often result in a skin reaction. The reaction is initially associated with mildly itchy spots on the skin, each spot representing a site where a cercaria tried to penetrate the skin. Repeated exposure to the cercariae will worsen the immunologic reaction, often presented as an intensively itchy papular dermatitis. It is unclear if the swimmer's itch type of skin reaction occurs in dogs, but it is likely.

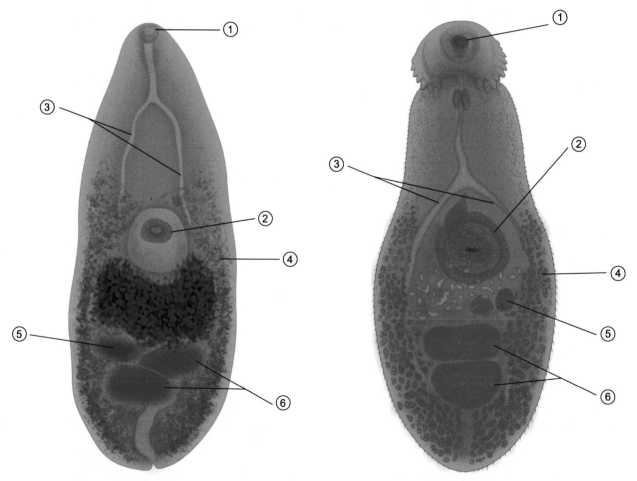

FIG. 3.21 General morphology and internal organs of *Cryptocotyle lingua*. (1) oral sucker, (2) ventral sucker, (3) intestine (caecum branches), (4) vitellaria (5) ovary (6) testes.

FIG. 3.22 General morphology and internal organs of *Echinochasmus* sp. (1) oral sucker, (2) ventral sucker, (3) intestine (caecum branches), (4) vitellaria (5) ovary (6) testes.

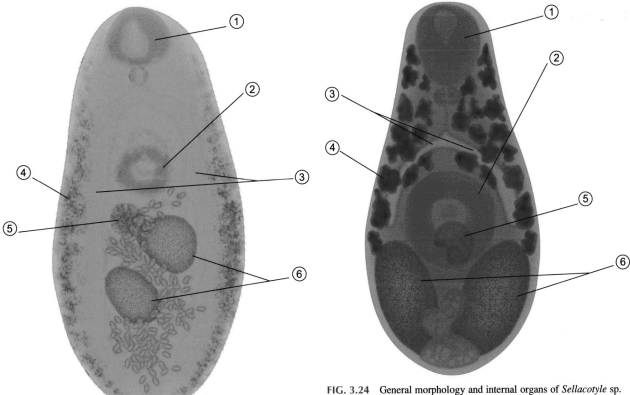

FIG. 3.23 General morphology and internal organs of *Plachiorchis* sp. (1) oral sucker, (2) ventral sucker, (3) intestine (caecum branches), (4) vitellaria (5) ovary (6) testes.

FIG. 3.24 General morphology and internal organs of *Sellacotyle* sp. (1) oral sucker, (2) ventral sucker, (3) intestine (caecum branches), (4) vitellaria (5) ovary (6) testes.

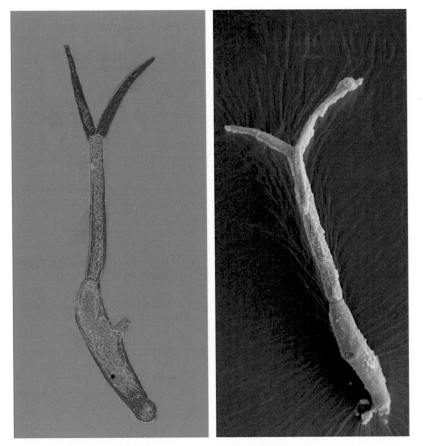

FIG. 3.25 The cause of swimmer's itch as observed under microscope and SEM. The causative agent is a cercaria of schistosome trematode of waterfowl. With the aid of its forked tail, the cercaria can swim and locate a host. Proteolytic enzymes enable the cercaria to penetrate the skin of the host. Upon penetration, the cercaria docks its tail. If a cercaria accidentally comes into contact with the skin of a mammal, it cannot infect it, but may cause a skin reaction. This is referred to as swimmer's itch or cercarial dermatitis.

FURTHER READING

Aiello SE, Moses MA, editors: *The Merck veterinary manual*, Rahway, NJ, 2016, Merck & Co.

American Association of Veterinary Parasitologists: http://www.aavp.org/wiki/trematodes-2/trematodes-small-intestine (Accessed January 2018).

American Association of Veterinary Parasitologists: Heterophyes heterophyes. http://www.aavp.org/wiki/trematodes-2/trematodes-small-intestine/echinostomatidae/echinochasmus-perfoliatus (Accessed January 2018).

American Association of Veterinary Parasitologists: Mesostephanus milvi. http://www.aavp.org/wiki/trematodes-2/trematodes-small-intestine/cyathocotylidae/mesostephanus-milvi (Accessed January 2018).

Arrellano L: *Paragonimus kellikotti*, Animal Diversity Web, University of Michigan http://animaldiversity.org/accounts/Paragonimus_kellicotti (Accessed January 2018).

Barr S, Bowman D: *Blackwell's five-minute veterinary consult clinical companion: canine and feline infectious diseases and parasitology*, ed 2, Oxford, 2012, Wiley-Blackwell.

Blair D, Xu ZB, Agatsuma T: Paragonimiasis and the genus Paragonimus, *Adv Parasitol* 42:113–222, 1999.

CABI: *8th international training course on identification of Helminth parasites of economic importance*, UK, 1996, International Institute of Parasitology.

Chai J, Darwin Murrell K, Lymbery A: Fish-borne parasitic zoonoses: status and issues, *Int J Parasitol* 35:1233–1254, 2005.

Conboy G: Helminth parasites of the canine and feline respiratory tract, *Vet Clin North Am Small Anim Pract* 39:1109–1126, 2009.

Doanh P, Yukifumi Nawa Y: *Clonorchis sinensis* and *Opisthorchis* spp. in Vietnam: current status and prospects, *Trans R Soc Trop Med Hyg* 110:13–20, 2016.

Dunn AM: *Veterinary helminthology*, ed 2, London, 1978, Heinemann.

El-Gayar AM: Studies on some trematode parasites of stray dogs in Egypt with a key to the identification of intestinal trematodes of dogs, *Vet Parasitol* 144:360–365, 2007.

Fang F, Li J, Huang T, Guillot J, Huang W: Zoonotic helminths parasites in the digestive tract of feral dogs and cats in Guangxi, China, *BMC Vet Res* 11:211, 2015. https://doi.org/10.1186/s12917-015-0521-7.

Flowers JR, Hammerberg B, Wood SL, et al: *Heterobilharzia americana* infection in a dog, *J Am Vet Med Assoc* 220:193–196, 2002.

Freeman R, Stuart P, Cullen J, et al: Fatal human infection with mesocercariae of trematode *Alaria americana*, *Am J Trop Med Hyg* 25:803–807, 1976.

Fürst T, Keiser J, Utzinger J: Global burden of human food-borne trematodiasis—a systematic review and meta-analysis, *Lancet Infect Dis* 12:210–221, 2012.

Guildal J, Clausen B: Endoparasites from one hundred Danish red foxes (Vulpes vulpes), *Norw J Zool* 21:329–330, 1973.

Gunn A, Pitt S: *Parasitology—an integrated approach*, ed 1, Oxford, 2012, Wiley-Blackwell.

Headley S, Scorpio D, Vidotto O, Dumler S: *Neorickettsia helminthoeca* and salmon poisoning disease: a review, *Vet J* 187:165–173, 2011.

Horák P, Kolarová L, Adema C: Biology of schistosome genus trichobilharzia, *Adv Parasitol* 52:155–233, 2002.

Hung N, Madsen H, Fried B: Invited review: global status of fish-borne zoonotic trematodiasis in humans, *Acta Parasitol* 58:231–258, 2013.

Jacobs D, Fox M, Gibbons L, Hermosilla C: *Principles of veterinary parasitology*, Chichester, 2016, Wiley Blackwell.

Johnson E: Canine schistosomiasis in North America: an underdiagnosed disease with expanding distribution, *Comp Cont Ed Vet* 32: E1–E4, 2010.

Kumar V: *Trematode infections and diseases of man and animals*, Dordrecht, 1999, Springer.

Lemetayer J, Snead E, Starrak G, Wagner B: Multiple liver abscesses in a dog secondary to the liver fluke *Metorchis conjunctus* treated by percutaneous transhepatic drainage and alcoholization, *Can Vet J* 57:605–609, 2016.

Lin R, Tang J, Zhou D, et al: Prevalence of *Clonorchis sinensis* infection in dogs and cats in subtropical southern China, *Parasit Vectors* 4:180, 2011.

Mehlhorn H: *Encyclopedic reference of parasitology*, ed 2, Berlin/Heidelberg, 2001, Springer.

Millemann RE, Knapp SE: Biology of *Nanophyetus salmincola* and "salmon poisoning" disease, *Adv Parasitol* 8:1–41, 1970.

Nesvadba J: Dicrocoeliosis in cats and dogs, *Acta Vet Brno* 75:289–293, 2006.

Olsen O: *Animal parasites—their life cycles and ecology*, Baltimore, MD, 1974, University Park Press, pp 237–240.

Paulsen P, Forejtek P, Hutarova Z, Vodnansky M: *Alaria alata* mesocercariae in wild boar (Sus scrofa, Linnaeus, 1758) in south regions of the Czech Republic, *Vet Parasitol* 197:384–387, 2013.

Persson L, Christensson D: Endoparasiter hos rödräv i Sverige, *Zool Rev* 33:17–24, 1971 (in Swedish).

Roberts L, Janovy J, editors: *Gerald D. Schmidt & Larry S. Roberts' foundations of parasitology*, ed 8, New York, 2009, McGraw-Hill, pp 291–292.

Rodriguez JY, Camp JW, Lenz SD, Kazacos KR, Snowden KF: Identification of *Heterobilharzia americana* infection in a dog residing in Indiana with no history of travel, *J Am Vet Med Assoc* 248:827–830, 2016.

Saari S, Westerling B, Nikander S: Madot tappoivat suden Hämeessä: kuolemaan johtanut *Alaria* sp. -imumatoinfektio sudella, *Suom eläinlääkäril* 104:716–721, 1998 (in Finnish).

Schmidt G, Roberts L: *Foundations of parasitology*, St Louis, MO, 1989, Times Mirror/Mosby College Publishing, pp. 260–264.

Schuster R, Heidrich J, Pauly A, Nöckler K: Liver flukes in dogs and treatment with praziquantel, *Vet Parasitol* 150:362–365, 2007.

Shoop W, Corkum K: Migration of *Alaria marcianae* (Trematoda) in domestic cats, *J Parasitol* 69:912–917, 1983.

Sitko J, Bizos J, Sherrard-Smith E, Stanton D, Komorová P, Heneberg P: Integrative taxonomy of European parasitic flatworms of the genus Metorchis Looss, 1899 (Trematoda: Opisthorchiidae), *Parasitol Int* 65:258–267, 2016.

Soulsby EJL: *Helminths, arthropods and protozoa of domesticated animals*, ed 7, London, 1982, Balliére Tindall.

Taylor M, Coop R, Wall R: *Veterinary parasitology*, ed 4, Oxford, 2016, Wiley Blackwell.

Willingham A, Ockens N, Kapel C, Monrad J: A helminthological survey of wild red foxes (Vulpes vulpes) from the metropolitan area of Copenhagen, *J Helminthol* 70:259–263, 1996.

Yamaguti S: *Synopsis of digenetic trematodes of vertebrates*, (vol. 1), Tokyo, 1971, Keigaku Publishing Company, p 1074.

Ye C, Yang Z, Zheng H: Fatal multi-organ *Clonorchis sinensis* infection in dog: a case report, *Vet Parasitol* 195:173–176, 2013.

Zajac A, Conboy G: *Veterinary clinical parasitology*, ed 8, West Sussex, 2012, John Wiley & Sons.

Chapter 4

Cestoda (Tapeworms)

Parasitic worms of the dog are classified as flatworms (Platyhelminthes), roundworms (Nematoda), thorny-headed worms (Acantocephala) and ringed worms (Annelida). Flatworms are further separated into tapeworms (Cestoda) and flukes (Trematoda). Tapeworms (Cestoda) are flat, tape-like worms with parenchymatous bodies. Adult tapeworms typically have a body structure consisting of a scolex, a neck, and a strobila made of a few to a large number of proglottids, which are often called "segments" (Fig. 4.1). The head, or scolex, contains structures, which enable the worm to attach to the gut wall of its definitive host. Such structures may include sucking grooves, suckers, and hooks. The major part of the tapeworm consists of the segmented part called the strobila and may be up to several meters long, depending on the species. Segments contain both male and female reproductive organs. Thus, they are hermaphrodites and capable of self-fertilization, as well as cross-fertilization. Each proglottid is equipped with muscle fibers, a nervous system, and an osmoregulatory system. Tapeworms do not have a digestive tract. Instead, they absorb their nutrients from the gut contents of the host directly through their outside surface or tegument.

New segments are constantly formed in the neck of the worm and along the length of the tapeworm proglottids mature and increase in size. Hence, the most distal segments are occupied by a uterus filled with embryonated eggs. These gravid proglottids detach from the tail end of the worm and are passed in the feces. They disintegrate and the eggs are released.

The scolex and its morphology are distinctive parts of an adult tapeworm and can be utilized in the identification of tapeworms. However, in a clinical setting the scolex is usually unavailable, as it is inside the host. Therefore, the diagnosis is usually based on finding segments or eggs in feces of the host.

As a rule of thumb, the tapeworm cannot be directly transmitted from one dog to another. The parasite has to develop and the transmission must happen via one or several intermediate hosts.

Cestodes important in veterinary medicine belong to the order Cyclophyllidea or Pseudophyllidea, which have differences in life cycles and morphology. Diagnostically, the major difference is how the eggs pass from the parent. Cyclophyllidea tapeworms, which comprise most canine tapeworms, lack a uterus opening for egg release. The eggs are distributed within the segments that separate them from the distal part of the worm.

Thus, eggs of the Cyclophyllidea cestodes are not found free in large numbers in the feces. Consequently, they are not detected with sufficient sensitivity, for instance, with the flotation methods used in fecal analysis. If the segments of the species are macroscopic, they can be seen by the naked eye on the surface of stools or around the anus of a dog.

Pseudophyllidea cestodes have a route leading out of the uterus for secreting the eggs directly into the fecal mass inside the intestine. Empty segments are released in chains. Thus, the Cyclophyllidea eggs are usually easily found in routine fecal analysis.

Tapeworms Lack an Alimentary Tract

Tapeworms have no intestine, mouth, or anus. A tapeworm utilizes so-called contact digestion to absorb nutrients. It purloins the nutrients from its host through its outer membrane, or tegument, utilizing both self-produced as well as the host's digestive enzymes. The surface of the worm is covered with small villi, which increase absorbing surface area substantially. Tapeworms are known to secrete into their habitat in the host's gut molecules, which, in addition to other functions, induce the contraction of intestinal wall musculature. Thanks to this, the alimentary tract cannot mechanically eliminate the worm and the contact between the gut contents and the tegument of the worm is prolonged, enabling the worm to optimize the nutrient uptake.

The tegument is resistant to both acids and alkalis, and is replaced continuously with a fast turnover time. As a part of the food uptake, tapeworms might absorb certain host enzymes and use them to break down nutrients. In addition, tapeworms are capable of increasing the acidity of the gut contents and secreting trypsin inhibitors. These features help the worm to survive in conditions where it is at risk of being digested by the host.

Canine Parasites and Parasitic Diseases. https://doi.org/10.1016/B978-0-12-814112-0.00004-0

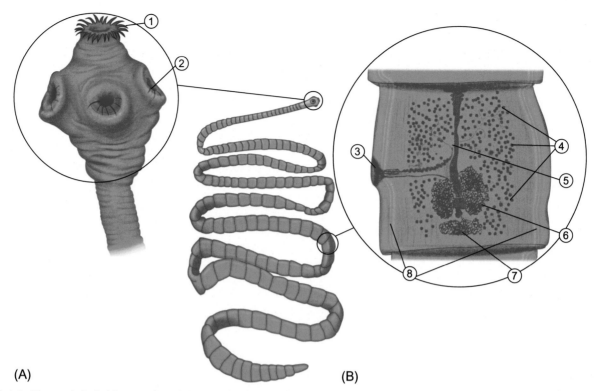

FIG. 4.1 The morphological features of a typical cestode. (A) The scolex is a head contains structures that enable the worm to attach to the gut wall of its definitive host. Such structures may include hooks (1) and suckers (2). (B) Each segment or proglottide contains both male and female reproductive organs, muscle fibers, a nervous system, and an osmoregulatory system, including: genital opening (3), testes (4), uterus (5), ovaries (6), vitelline glands (7), and osmoregulatory canal (8).

TAENIA SPECIES, Taeniid Tapeworms

- A genus consisting of several tapeworm species residing in the small intestine of the definitive host, a dog.
- Indirect life cycle: dog gets infected by ingestion of the metacestode larval stage of the tapeworm in the tissues of intermediate hosts.
- Morphologically characterized by a ribbon-like body composed of a large strobila with numerous segments.
- The intermediate hosts vary depending on *Taenia* species and are often rodents, lagomorphs, or ruminants.
- Canine infections are rarely associated with clinical signs.
- Diagnosis is based on the detection of taeniid eggs or proglottids in the fecal sample.

Identification

The size and morphology of adult taeniid cestodea vary for each species, but the worms can be very large, up to meters in length. Taenias belong to the tapeworm order Cyclophyllidea, which have the characteristic of producing egg-containing proglottids to the environment in the feces of the definitive host. The morphology of the scolex and the proglottids is specific for each *Taenia* species. The eggs of all *Taenia* tapeworms are typically round or somewhat oval, and about 30 μm in diameter. The species cannot be identified from the morphology of the eggs. Inside the egg, three pairs of hooks of an oncosphere larva can be seen.

Life Cycle

The dog and other canids are often the definitive hosts of *Taenia* tapeworms. Adult worms live in the small intestine of the definitive host and multiply sexually. The proglottid has a genital pore, but typically for Cyclophyllidea cestodes, there is no uterine pore for secreting eggs. The adult proglottids detach from the posterior end of the worm, and they and the eggs inside end up in the external environment, where the intermediate host, usually a herbivorous animal, ingests the proglottids of eggs with forage into its alimentary tract. The oncosphere larva is released from the egg in the small intestine, and it travels in the lymph and blood circulation into the target organ. The larval metacestode stage develops in the intermediate host. In some species it is microscopic, and in some a very large larval cyst. The dog is infected by eating the infective meat or offal of the intermediate host, containing metacestodes.

Distribution

The geographical distribution of *Taenia* species depends of the abundance of host and intermediate species in each area. Intermediate hosts are most often rodents and lagomorphs, but some *Taenia* species utilize larger domestic animals, such as ruminants, pigs, or horses, as intermediate hosts. The following *Taenia* species have been found in dogs: *T. crassiceps*, *T. endothoracicus*, *T. hydatigena*, *T. krabbei*, *T. madoquae*, *T. martis*, *T. multiceps*, *T. ovis*, *T. parenchymatosa*, *T. pisiformis*, *T. polyachanta*, *T. retracta*, *T. serialis*, *T. talicei*, and *T. taxidiensis*. The following have zoonotic potential: *T. crassiceps*, *T. multiceps*, and *T. serialis*.

Importance to Canine Health

Taenia infections are typically subclinical in the dog, i.e., in the definitive hosts. If any signs manifest, they are associated with the alimentary tract: diarrhea, abdominal pain, and sometimes vomiting. A severe infection can lead to an intestinal obstruction. Proglottids that actively move around the anal region may cause irritation and pruritus. Scratching and rubbing the affected areas may lead to local inflammation.

Diagnosis

Taeniid proglottids can be seen in canine feces, on the skin around the anus, or in the fur. Since proglottids are capable of autonomous motion and can be seen by the naked eye, they may attract the attention of the dog's owner. An expert parasitologist may identify the species on the basis of the proglottid morphology. *Taenia* eggs are found in the flotation analysis of feces, but the method is not very sensitive in the diagnosis of Cyclophyllidea tapeworms, because most eggs are inside the proglottid and not loose in the fecal mass. The egg morphology is not diagnostic, and if it is necessary to identify the species, the diagnosis can be made in an analytical laboratory with PCR and sequencing methods. However, it is common to treat the canine tapeworm infection without a species-specific diagnosis.

Treatment and Prevention

Canine taeniosis is controlled with drugs effective against cestodes. Apart from cestode drugs praziquantel and epsiprantel, several benzimidazoles, niclosamide, and nitroscanate are effective. Treating dogs is necessary to prevent infections in the intermediate hosts, which may include humans, because the tapeworms may survive and produce eggs for over a year, and the pathology and symptoms of intermediate hosts are usually more severe than those of the definitive host. When production animals act as intermediate hosts, the infections also causes economical losses from organ condemnation, decreased carcass weight and milk yield. An important measure is to prevent the dogs from eating uncooked infective meat and offal of the intermediate hosts. If *Taenia* cysts are found in the organs of intermediate hosts in meat inspection, the organs are rejected. As an intermediate host is required for the completion of the life cycle, *Taenia* is not contagious directly between dogs.

TAENIA HYDATIGENA

T. hydatigena is a large tapeworm, up to 5 m long. Its distribution is worldwide. Of common domestic animals, ruminants, pigs, and horses may act as intermediate hosts, as well as a number of wild ruminants that ingest the eggs along with forage. The metacestode stage, *Cysticercus tenuicollis*, is easily found in meat inspection. It is cyst-like, thin-walled, and filled with liquid; it is usually found in the thoracic or abdominal cavity (Figs. 4.2 and 4.3). The dog receives the infection by eating offal that contains these large, fluctuating cysts. The prepatent period lasts about 7 weeks. An adult *Taenia* resides in the small intestine of the dog. The adult scolex has two rings of rostellar hooks and gravid proglottids are longer than their width (Fig. 4.4), $10–14 \times 4–7$ mm. Each proglottid has only one genital pore, located laterally. Other specific morphological features used for the morphological differentiation of *Taenia* species are, for instance:

(1) The size and shape of the rostellum hooks (Fig. 4.5): In *T. hydatigena* there are 26–44 hooks and their length is 170–220 μm in the ring or larger hooks and 110–160 μm in the ring of smaller hooks;

(2) The number and location of testes: In *T. hydatigena* there are 600–700 testes in one layer, none of them is located posterior to the vitellary glands, and they are fused in the anterior part of the proglottid; and

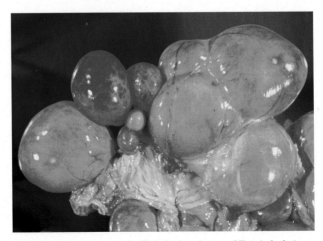

FIG. 4.2 *Cysticercus tenuicollis* is the larval stage of *Taenia hydatigena* in the intermediate host, infective for the dog. Its cystic structures, consisting of numerous liquid-filled cysts, are found especially on the fascia of abdominal organs of ruminants. The infection is usually mild and subclinical in the intermediate host. A small, light lump, containing the invaginated scolex of the future tapeworm, can be seen in some cysts.

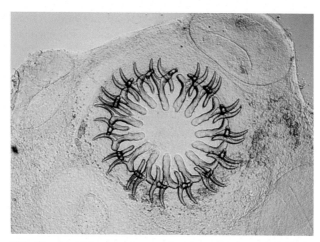

FIG. 4.3 One of the parasitic cysts of the figure in the top of the page cut open. Each cyst has the invaginated scolex of the future adult tapeworm. The figure shows part of the sucker of the scolex and the hooks of the rostellum.

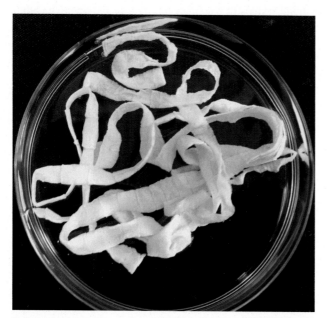

FIG. 4.4 The strobila of *T. hydatigena* showing proglottids that are longer than their width.

(3) The lateral branches of uterus: *T. hydatigena* has about 10 of them. The eggs are typical for *Taenia*, round or oval and about 30 μm in diameter (Fig. 4.6).

Infections are usually asymptomatic but there are clinical signs, if large amounts of tapeworms obstruct the intestine. The life cycle of *T. hydatigena* is shown in Fig. 4.7.

TAENIA PISIFORMIS

The length of *T. pisiformis* varies between 50 and 100 cm. There are 34–48 large rostellum hooks, the largest being over 220 μm (Fig. 4.8). The number of testes is 600–950, occurring in 2–4 layers; they are located laterally but merging in the anterior and posterior end of the proglottid. The intermediate hosts of *T. pisiformis* are most commonly lagomorphs and more rarely rodents. The larvae migrate in the intermediate host via the liver to the abdominal cavity, forming metacestode cysts, or cysticerci. They are infective for dogs and other canids and about as big as a pea. The prepatent period is about 8 weeks.

Taenia ovis

The length of adult *T. ovis* varies between 45 and 110 cm. There are 24–36 rostellar hooks. The length of the larger hooks varies between 156 and 202 μm, and that of the hooks in the ring of smaller hooks between 89 and 157 μm. The size of a gravid proglottid is 15–20 × 5–10 mm. A mature proglottid can be distinguished from those of other *Taenia* species from the number of lateral branches that separate from the uterine main body (there are many: 20–25 lateral branches) and from a pronounced, laterally located genital pore. There are 350–570 testes present in one layer and they extend to the level of ovaries in the posterior part of the proglottid. Testes locate laterally but merge in the anterior part of the proglottid. The most common intermediate host of *T. ovis* is the sheep. The metacestode stages, cysticerci, infectious for dogs, are about 6 mm long when in the infective stage. They are located in striated muscle of the heart and skeletal muscles. The prepatent period in dogs is 6–9 weeks.

TAENIA MULTICEPS

The length of *T. multiceps* ranges from 40 to 100 cm. The rostellum has 22–32 hooks. The length of the larger hooks varies between 150 and 177 μm and the length of the hooks in the ring of smaller hooks between 90 and 136 μm. There are fewer testes than in taeniid tapeworms generally (280–300 in two layers). There are few testes anterior from the ovaries, and they merge in the anterior part of the proglottid. The size of the gravid proglottid is 5–10 × 3–5 mm. *T. multiceps* is best known for its metacestode stage. The most common intermediate host is sheep, and less frequently goats or cattle. The larva of the parasite migrates to the ovine spinal cord or brain, where a metacestode cyst, or coenurus, typical for the species, develops in 6–8 months following the infection. A coenurus is a single parasitic cyst, filled with opaque and viscose liquid. Its germinal epithelium possesses a great number of invaginations formed by scolex structures of future adult tapeworms. This is an end-result of asexual reproduction that takes place in the intermediate host where one larval oncosphere has multiplied into a cyst with a great number of potential future tapeworms. The coenurus may grow up to the size of a hen's egg and cause neurological signs e.g., weakness, problems with eyesight and seizures, in the intermediate host, making it easy prey for predators. After being eaten by a dog, the maturation takes 4–5 weeks. *T. multiceps* is

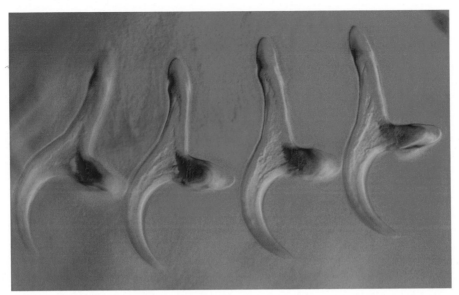

FIG. 4.5 Hooks from the rostellum of the *T. hydatigena* scolex. The amount, size, measurements, and proportions (handle, blade, and guard) of the rostellar hooks can be used in identification.

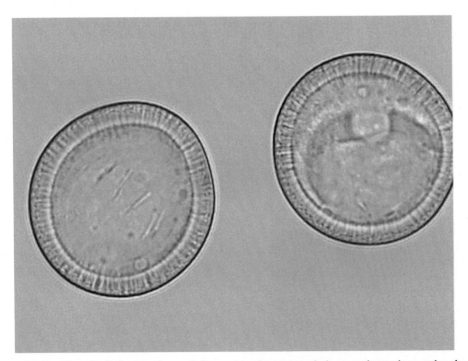

FIG. 4.6 *Taenia* eggs. The lamellar and radially striated outer shell or embryophore surrounds the oncosphere or hexacanth embryo. Three hook pairs shaped like the letter f are typical for the oncosphere. It is important to note that these eggs are found free only after disintegration of the gravid tapeworm segment.

a zoonotic parasite and it infrequently may cause central nervous system symptoms in humans too.

TAENIA SERIALIS

The length of *T. serialis* is 20–72 cm. There are 26–34 rostellum hooks. The length of the larger hooks ranges between 145 and 175 μm and the length of the hooks in the ring of smaller hooks between 90 and 136 μm. There are 350–500 testes in 2–3 layers and they join in the anterior part of the proglottid. The size of the gravid proglottid is 6–10 × 3–5 mm. The most common intermediate hosts are hares and rabbits. Metacestoid stages of *T. serialis* have rarely been found also in goats, horses, and humans. The metacestoid stage is coenurus and this develops mostly in the connective tissue between the intermediate host's muscles.

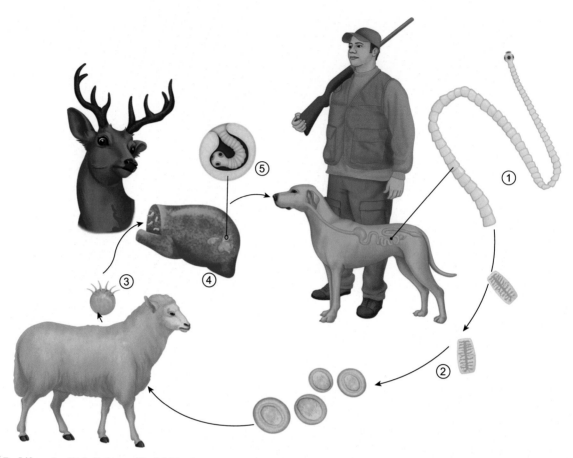

FIG. 4.7 Life cycle of *T. hydatigena*: (1) adult *Taenia* tapeworms live attached to the canine small intestine. Mature, egg-containing proglottids are shed from the caudal part of the worm and exit the dog in its feces; (2) the proglottids disintegrate in the environment and the eggs are released. The intermediate host ingests eggs with the forage; (3) the oncosphere larva is freed from the egg in the intermediate host and penetrates its organs; (4) fluctuating *C. tenuicollis* metacestodes are formed typically in the omentum or liver. They are infective for the definitive host; and (5) the dog gets the infection by eating, e.g., metacestode-containing abattoir waste. The prepatent period is about 7 weeks.

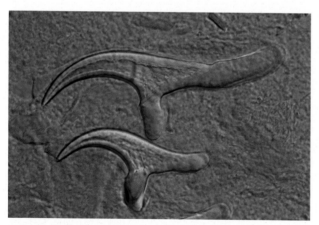

FIG. 4.8   The hooks of the scolex of *Taenia pisiformis*.

TAENIA CRASSICEPS

T. crassiceps has 28–34 rostellum hooks. The length of the larger hooks varies between 172 and 299 μm and the length of the hooks in the ring of smaller hooks is 121–155 μm.

The hook base, shaped like a handle, is much shorter than its arching claw-like blade. There are two layers of testes (200 − 220) laterally, joining at the anterior and posterior part of the proglottid. Moles, mice, squirrels, and other rodents usually act as intermediate hosts. The metacestode stage of the parasite, *Cysticercus*, grows in the subcutaneous tissue of the intermediate host. The *Cysticercus* of *T. crassiceps* differs from all others in being capable to reproduce asexually by budding in the intermediate host, forming daughter cysticerci. Another unique feature of the species is that the dog can act as an intermediate host too. If the dog gets proglottids or eggs from the environment or from its own parasite invasion into the alimentary tract, typical oval and fluctuating *Cysticercus* cysts may grow into its subcutaneous tissue. The length of the cysts is usually 5–9 mm and the width 3–4 mm. Thanks to budding, they can be numerous. Cases have been reported of massive occurrences of cysticerci and daughter cycticerci in dogs' thoracic and abdominal areas, leading to the death of these dogs. Cysticerci of *T. crassiceps* can in rare cases also be found in humans.

ECHINOCOCCUS GRANULOSUS-Complex (*E. GRANULOSUS* G1-G3, *E. EQUINUS* G4, *E. ORTLEPPI* G5, and *E. CANADENSIS* G6-G10)

- A genus consisting of tiny tapeworm species residing in the small intestine of the definitive host.
- Indirect life cycle, dog ingests the metacestode larval stage—hydatid cyst—of the tapeworm in the tissues of intermediate hosts and gets infected.
- Usually less than 5 mm in length; body composed of a short strobila with few segments.
- The intermediate hosts vary within the *E. granulosus* complex and are often ruminants or horse.
- *E. granulosus* possesses low clinical significance to canine medicine but is very significant to public health.
- Diagnosis is based on the detection of taeniid eggs (morphologically indistinguishable from the eggs of *Taenia* spp.). Diagnostic tests based on coproantigen or PCR are required for specific diagnosis.

Identification

An adult *Echinococcus* tapeworm (Fig. 4.9) is only about 0.5 cm long and it consists of scolex with two rings of hooks (Fig. 4.10) and three or four proglottids, the last of which is the largest. The proglottids have one genital pore and the posterior proglottid as typical, with round and smooth-surfaced taeniid eggs inside. The most central layer of the egg shell, the so-called embryophore, is radially striated. The six hooks of the oncosphere can be discerned inside the egg. The diameter of eggs is about 30 μm. Metacestodes, the larval forms found in the organs of the intermediate host, usually in the lungs and liver, grow into about 5–10 cm large (sometimes larger), fluid-filled hydatid cysts (Fig. 4.11). The outer wall of the cyst is layered and contains smaller daughter cysts and protoscolexes, the early forms of the worms' heads (Fig. 4.12).

Life Cycle

Depending on the *Echinococcus* species, dogs and wild canids are definitive hosts and ruminants, horses, pigs, and cervids act as intermediate hosts of the parasite. Humans can be infected as well, but as dead-end intermediate hosts. The dog is infected by eating offal of an intermediate host, containing metacestode stages of the tapeworm. Once it gets into the definitive host, the parasite attaches itself into the small intestine, usually in the anterior part. Its cervical scolex sheds proglottids that mature while progressing to caudal direction. The prepatent period is about 40 days, after which the posterior gravid proglottid

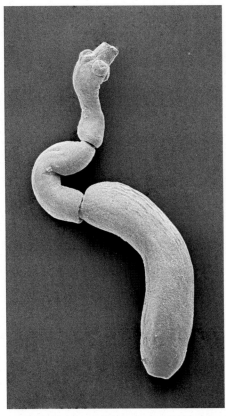

FIG. 4.9 *Echinococcus granulosus* in scanning electron microscopy. At less than 5 mm long, it is one of the smallest tapeworms. The length of the gravid posterior proglottid accounts for over 50% of the total length of the strobila.

of the worm dislodges and is replaced at about 1-week intervals. An *Echinococcus* lives about 7 months. The oncosphere larva inside the egg may stay infective in the environment for up to 2 years. Herbivorous animals act as intermediate hosts and they become infected by ingesting eggs in their feed. The hatched oncospheres migrates in blood or lymph to the liver or the lungs, where, during the following months, they form larval cysts that are infective for the definitive host. The larval stage undergoes asexual reproduction, resulting in the increase of the larval stages and the volume of the cyst. 3 months after the infection, the cyst is about 5 mm in diameter, and after half a year, about 20 mm. For instance, a cyst attached to the abdominal wall may contain up to 16 L of liquid. This is made possible by the volume of the abdominal cavity, allowing almost limitless expansion compared to other tissues. The fecundity of an adult *Echinococcus* is rather poor compared to those of many other worms. The tapeworm population carries out a major part of its reproduction in the intermediate host, in which a parasitic cyst formed by one oncosphere gradually develops into a hydatid cyst, which acts as an effective asexual production facility. Eating an infected intermediate host ensures that the small intestine of the definitive host be

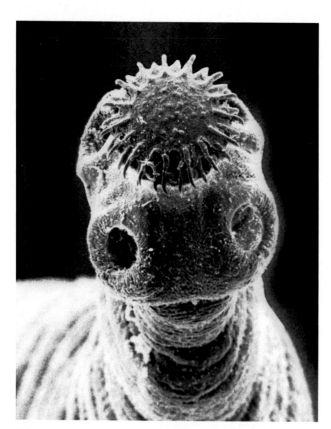

FIG. 4.10 The scolex of *E. granulosus* in scanning electron microscopy. Two of the four suckers of the parasite and the hooks forming the crown-like structure of the rostellum are clearly visible.

will be colonized by an *Echinococcus* population of thousands of tapeworms. A hydatid cyst with its infective protoscolexes inside the intermediate host becomes infective for the dog in about 5–6 months. The life cycle of *E. granulosus* is shown in Fig. 4.13.

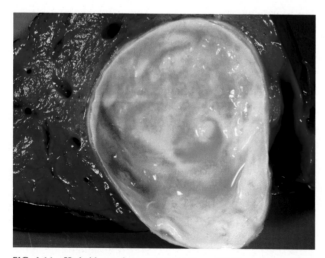

FIG. 4.11 Hydatid cyst, the metacestode stage of *Echinococcus* and thus, a source of infection for the dog, found in the liver of an equine intermediate host. Small and light nodules, visible in the internal wall of the cyst, are so-called daughter cysts.

Distribution

The tapeworms of *E. granulosus* complex are distributed widely in the world. The local genotypes depend on the availability of host species.

Importance to Canine Health

Dogs, the definitive hosts of *Echinococcus* tapeworm, do not show clinical signs of infection. The intermediate hosts, whose infection is diagnosed at autopsy or during the meat inspection, also do not usually show signs. In contrast, the symptoms can be severe in humans.

Morphology of the Cestodes in the *Echinococcus granulosus* Complex

Echinococci belong to the smallest tapeworms. The length of *E. granulosus* is 2–5 mm. The worm attaches to the intestinal wall with its rostellum equipped with two rings of hooks. The hooks of the first ring are larger (45–49 µm) than those of the second ring (17–31 µm). In total, there are 30–60 hooks. The worm has usually three proglottids, less frequently four. The gravid, most posterior proglottid accounts for over 50% of the total length of the strobila. In each mature proglottid, there are 25–50 testes, fewer than in tapeworms generally. The testes are located anteriorly, and in regard to the female genitals, laterally. The genital pore is unilateral, locating in the mid-part of the proglottid or posterior to it. The ovary has two branches and is located in the posterior part of the proglottid. The vitellary gland is compactly located in a clearly defined area, posterior of the ovary. The uterus consists of a medially located main trunk, from which branches protrude out laterally. These do not branch further into smaller parts. The metacestoid stage of the parasite is the hydatid cyst. This is typically a liquid-filled, single-compartment parasite cyst, which grows about 1–5 cm a year, depending on the species of the intermediate host and the location of the cyst within the intermediate host. The cyst may be infertile. In this case, no larval stages of the tapeworm are inside it. In a classical case, the cyst wall has three layers. The innermost layer is consists of germinal epithelium, enabling the asexual reproduction of the parasite. Daughter cysts shed loose from the germinal epithelium and are free in the cyst contents. These protoscolexes are also developed directly front the germinal epithelium of the cyst. In the definitive host, the protoscolex forms the scolex and hooks of the tapeworm.

Diagnosis

Since the proglottids are small and infrequently found in canine feces, they are difficult to detect. The echinococci are also rarely found in autopsy due to their small size. Since echinococci belong to Cyclophyllidea cestodes, which have no specific opening for secreting eggs from the proglottids, eggs are not readily found in coprological

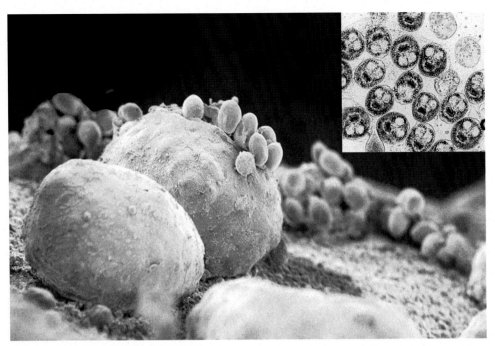

FIG. 4.12 A scanning electron image of the wall of the hydatid cyst. Daughter cysts and protoscolexes being squeezed out of them can be seen. Each protoscolex holds potential to develop into an *Echinococcus* tapeworm, if the hydatid cyst reaches the intestinal tract of a definitive host. The *square* figure shows the protoscolexes of the *Echinococcus* in light microscopy. Hooks are clearly visible inside each protoscolex.

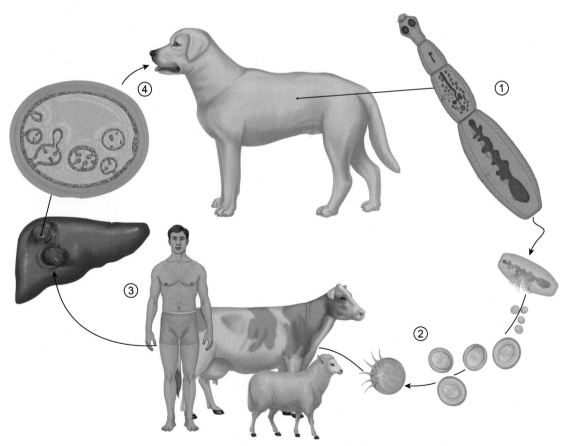

FIG. 4.13 Life cycle of *E. granulosus*: (1) adult echinococci live in the small intestine of the dog. The posterior proglottid degenerates, is shed loose, and is transferred to the environment at about 1-week intervals; (2) herbivores acting as intermediate hosts ingest *Echinococcus* eggs in their feed. The oncosphere hatches in their intestinal tract; (3) the larva migrates in blood or lymph to the liver or the lungs, in which it develops in 5–6 months into a hydatid cyst, infectious to the dog; and (4) the dog is infected by eating the offal of the intermediate host, containing hydatid cysts, and the metacestoid of the parasite forms. The prepatent period is about 40 days.

examination—for instance, with the flotation methods. If eggs are found in fecal analysis, their species cannot be morphologically specified from those of other taeniid eggs. ELISA assays have been developed to detect antigen in feces. A coprological PCR assay is available for detecting the DNA of the *Echinococcus*.

Treatment and Prevention

The anticestode substances praziquantel and epsiprantel are effective against canine *Echinococcus* infections as a single dose. If the infection is confirmed, the stools of the dog should be collected and discarded in household waste for 2 days after treatment. This prevents eggs getting into the environment. It is wise to emphasize good hand hygiene among the dog's handlers. The life cycle of the parasite can be disrupted by stopping the dog from eating abattoir waste and the organs of game. Frequent treatments against tapeworms in endemic areas also prevent eggs from being secreted into the environment and further to intermediate hosts. Controlling the population of stray dogs has been reported to reduce the number of infections in humans.

E. granulosus Is a Zoonotic Parasite

E. granulosus causes cystic echinococcosis. The human is infected directly from the feces of the definitive host of the parasite or from drinking water or food contaminated with canine feces. The hydatid cyst develops usually for years or even decades in the human body without causing symptoms. The infection becomes clinical, when the growing cyst starts to cause pressure lesions in the surrounding tissues. Depending on the location of the cyst, the person may have respiratory symptoms or an enlarged liver, and consequently an extended abdominal cavity. The growing hepatic cyst is associated with vague pains of the upper abdomen, nausea, and vomiting. Gradually, with passing years, the cyst may calcify. The liquid inside is a powerful antigen. If it leaks to surrounding tissues, an allergic reaction, even anaphylactic shock, often ensues.

ECHINOCOCCUS MULTILOCULARIS, Fox Tapeworm

- A tiny tapeworm species residing in the small intestine of canines.
- Indirect life cycle, infection by ingestion of the metacestode larval stage—alveolar hydatid cyst—in the tissues of intermediate hosts.
- Only a few millimeters in length; body composed of a short strobila with few segments.

- Several rodent species can serve as intermediate hosts.
- Low clinical significance in canine medicine but very significant to public health as it may afflict humans with serious, potentially deadly, alveolar hydatid disease.
- Diagnosis is based on the detection of taeniid eggs (morphologically indistinguishable from the eggs of *Taenia* spp.). Diagnostic tests based on coproantigen or PCR are required for specific diagnosis.

Identification

An adult *E. multilocularis* is a slender tapeworm only a few millimeters long. It consists of a scolex with four suckers and two rings of hooks, and three to five proglottids, of which the most posterior one is the largest Fig. 4.14). The proglottid has one genital pore and the last proglottid holds a few hundred typical, round taeniid-type eggs (Fig. 4.15). Of the three layers of the eggshell, the middle one is the thickest; this is radially striated and called the embryophore. The six hooks of the oncosphere larva can be seen inside the egg in pairs. The diameter of the egg is about 30 µm.

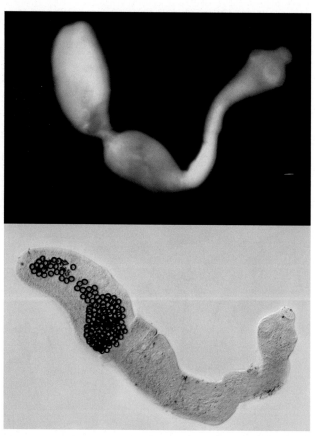

FIG. 4.14 *Echinococcus multilocularis* under stereomicroscope. Its length varies between 1.2 and 3.7 mm. This small and slender tapeworm is very difficult to detect with the naked eye, e.g., at autopsy. The dark and round material present in the posterior proglottid are eggs.

FIG. 4.15 Eggs of *E. multilocularis*. They are of the *Taenia*-type and cannot be distinguished morphologically from, e.g., the eggs of *Taenia* species. A thick outer membrane, called the embryophore, can be clearly seen. This protects the round oncosphere larva. There are three pairs of f-shaped hook structures in the oncosphere.

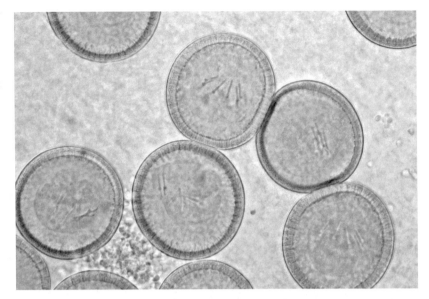

Life Cycle

Dogs and wild canids act as definitive hosts and moles, among others, act as natural intermediate hosts. The life cycle is usually sylvatic, taking place in wild fauna. Humans can also be infected and act as dead-end intermediate hosts. A dog is infected by eating offal of an infected intermediate host, infected with parasitic metacestode stages. Once in the definitive host, the alveolar hydatid cyst releases larvae, which attach the cranial part of the small intestine. Their scolex starts budding proglottids, which mature while traveling caudally. The prepatent period is about 40 days, after which the last, gravid proglottid releases and regenerates at about 1-week intervals. The oncosphere larva, living in the shelter provided by the egg, is robust and can survive in the environment for up to 2 years. The herbivorous animals, intermediate hosts, ingest the eggs with their feed. The hatched oncosphere migrates in blood or lymph into the liver, or more seldom into the lungs, where a polycystic structure grows in between surrounding tissues during the following months (Fig. 4.16). This phase of asexual reproduction is an important for parasitic survival, since the fecundity capacity of an adult tapeworm is quite limited and the life span short, only 3–4 months. In infrequent cases, larval stages may end up elsewhere in the organism with circulation as metastases. The dog can also rarely act as an intermediate host with cysts in its tissues. Its life cycle is shown in Fig. 4.17.

Distribution

E. multilocularis is endemic in the northern hemisphere. The distribution is variable and depends, for instance, on

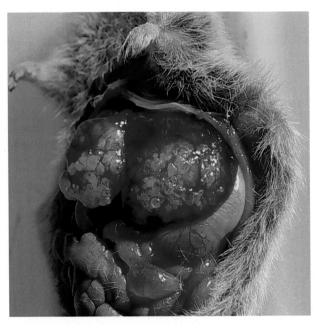

FIG. 4.16 The so-called alveolar hydatid cyst is the metacestode stage of *E. multilocularis* and is infective for the dog. The parasite reproduces asexually in the intermediate host, forming structure consisting of tightly packed parasitic cysts, which penetrate the surrounding tissues in a manner resembling that of a malignant tumor. The intermediate host becomes severely ill due to liver damage, and becomes easy prey for the definitive host, such as a dog or fox. Similar lesions may develop into human viscera. The figure depicts a grey red-backed vole with a dissected abdomen. The parasitic cysts have destroyed the liver, seen in the middle, almost entirely. *(Reproduced with permission from Heikki Henttonen.)*

the abundance of suitable definitive and intermediate host species. The prevalence is highest in foxes. In many countries of Central and Western Europe, about 50% of them carry the infection.

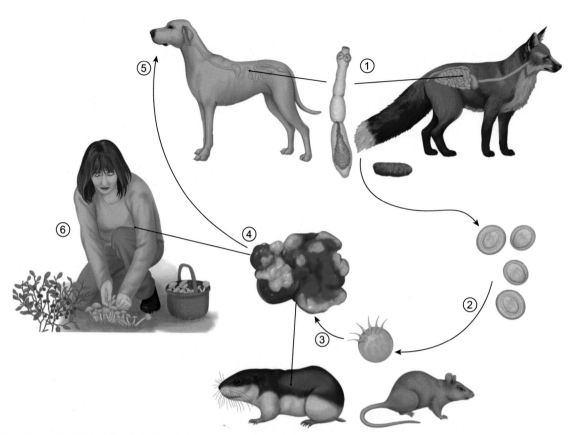

FIG. 4.17 Life cycle of *E. multilocularis*: (1) adult echinococci are attached to the canine small intestine. They are very short tapeworms consisting of a few proglottids. The posterior, gravid proglottid is released and regenerates at about 1-week intervals; (2) the robust oncosphere is protected inside the egg and can stay infective in the environment for long periods. The herbivores, acting as intermediate hosts, ingest the *Echinococcus* eggs into their alimentary tract in their feed; (3) moles and other animals, including humans, are intermediate hosts and may be infected from eggs; (4) the hatched oncosphere migrates in blood or lymph into the liver and more rarely into the lungs, where over the following months they form polycystic structures of hydatid cysts that penetrate into surrounding tissues; and (5) the dog is infected by eating visceral organs of the intermediate host, infected by larval metacestodes. The prepatent period is about 40 days.

Morphology of *Echinococcus multilocularis*

The echinococci belong to the smallest tapeworms. The length of *E. multilocularis* is 1.2–3.7 mm. This small and slender tapeworm is very difficult to see with the naked eye, e.g., at autopsy. The worm attaches into the gut wall with its rostellum, which has two rings of hooks. The hook size varies between 20 and 35 μm. The tapeworm has three to five proglottids. The gravid, most posterior proglottid is the largest, but in contrast to *E. granulosus*, its length is less than 50% of the total length of the worm. There are 16–35 testes, fewer than in tapeworms in general. The testes are mainly located posteriorly and laterally in regard to the female genitals. The cirrus sac is oval or pear-shaped. The genital pore is located in each proglottid unilaterally, in the middle part or anterior from it. The ovary has two branches and is located in the posterior part of the proglottid. The vitellary glands are situated as a compact and well-defined structure, posterior from the ovary. The bag-like uterus is in the anterior part of the proglottid and has no side branches. The metacestode stage of the parasite is an alveolar hydatid cyst, which usually develops in the liver and rarely in the other organs. In the hydatid cyst of *E. granulosus*, the germinal epithelium that generates new larvae is in the internal wall of the cyst. *E. multilocularis* has germinal epithelium at the internal and external wall, while the most productive location for cyst formation is in the external wall. As a result of this asexual reproduction, a parasitic polycystic mass is formed. This space-occupying mass pushes into surrounding tissues without forming a capsule around it. Cysts are usually small, about 1–10 mm, at most 30 mm. They are filled with jelly-like transparent liquid. The formation of the cysts stimulates the growth of fibrous tissue in the area.

Importance to Canine Health

Echinococcus infection in the alimentary tract of a dog is asymptomatic. Neither does the intermediate hosts show signs while the cysts are gradually growing. At certain point, the infection will result in hepatic failure in the intermediate host, making it easy prey for predators. The infection is often detected at autopsy, not before. The symptoms in humans can be serious.

Diagnosis

The small size of the proglottids makes their detection in feces difficult. Since echinococci are Cyclophyllidea tapeworms that have no pores for secreting eggs, too few eggs reach the fecal mass to be found reliably, e.g., with flotation assays. Also, cannot be morphologically distinguished from those of other taeniid tapeworm eggs. In the autopsy of canid definitive hosts, sedimentation techniques or scrapings from of the gut can be used to look for echinococci. ELISA assays have been developed to detect fecal *Echinococcus* antigens and coprological PCR methods for detecting DNA of *Echinococcus* origin.

Treatment and Prevention

The anticestode substances praziquantel and epsiprantel are effective against canine *Echinococcus* infections at a single dose. If the infection is confirmed, the stools of the dog should be collected and discarded in household waste for 2 days after treatment. This prevents the eggs getting into the environment. It is wise to emphasize good hand hygiene among the dog's handlers. If food items collected from the nature, such as forest berries of mushrooms, may have been contaminated with the feces of the definitive host, they must be washed or heated thoroughly before consumption. The excellent cold tolerance of the eggs makes them very resilient parasites adapted the harsh climate conditions of the northern hemisphere. They remain infective in a home freezer and prolonged storage in −70°C is needed to suppress them. High temperatures (over 70°C) and drying kill them. The life cycle of the parasite can be disrupted by preventing the dogs from eating prey or abattoir waste. Frequent treatments against tapeworms in endemic areas also prevent eggs from being secreted into the environment and further to intermediate hosts, especially humans. However, since the parasite has a large sylvatic reservoir, full *Echinococcus* control is impossible in endemic areas. Certain *Echinococcus*-free countries demand documented tapeworm medication from the imported dogs.

E. multilocularis Is a Zoonotic Parasite

Alveolar echinococcosis (AE) disease is caused by the larval stage of *E. multilocularis*. A human receives an infection either from ingesting eggs from the fecal material from the definitive host or from drinking water or food contaminated by canine feces. For instance, berries and mushrooms contaminated by tapeworm-carrying fox or raccoon dog feces are frequently discussed in context of the epidemiological risks of *E. multilocularis*. The infection is not passed from an intermediate host to humans. The majority of infected humans never get parasitic cysts in their body, and the growth of alveolar hydatid cysts in humans is usually very slow. When a polycystic mass is detected, it is commonly years after infection, the pathology and the symptoms associated may already be serious, depending on the location and spread of the cyst. Primary symptoms are usually upper abdominal discomfort, pain, nausea, and vomiting.

When the alveolar hydatid cyst grows bigger, hepatic insufficiency may result in ascites, weight loss, and jaundice. Due to the expansive nature of cysts, the surgical removal of *E. multilocularis* cysts is more difficult than removing the more compartmentalized cysts of *E. granulosus*-group. Indeed, the growth of *E. multilocularis* cyst resembles the growth of a malignant tumor and even comes with a risk of metastasizing. An alveolar hydatid cyst is almost always sterile in humans; that is, echinococcal protoscolex larvae are not found inside the cysts. Alveolar hydatidosis is considered as one of the most lethal parasitic helminthiases in humans. The disease is quite well controlled with modern therapies, but as recently as in the 1970s, life expectation after the diagnosis was about 3 years. However, alveolar hydatidosis remains a life-threatening parasitic disease, and 70%–100% of untreated cases are still fatal.

DIPYLIDIUM CANINUM, Flea Tapeworm

- A tapeworm species often referred as a flea tapeworm residing in the small intestine and infect dogs by ingestion of the metacestode larval stage—cysticercoid—of the tapeworm in the tissues of insect intermediate hosts.
- Up to 50 cm in length; body composed of a large strobila with numerous segments that are longer than wide.
- Cat flea (*Ctenocephalides felis*) is the main intermediate host, but also biting lice (*Trichodectes canis*) can serve as intermediate hosts.
- *D. caninum* is rarely associated with clinical signs in dogs.
- Diagnosis is based on the detection of double-pored proglottids and identifying typical egg packets filled with taeniid eggs with microscope.

Identification

D. caninum is a pinkish or yellowish tapeworm. It lives in the small intestine of a dog (or cat). The adult cestode is up to 50 cm long. Suckers are clearly visible in the scolex of the worm, together with a rostellum with four rows of hooks (Fig. 4.18). The strobila consists of 60–175 proglottids that are wider than their length. The posterior end sheds proglottids with visible genital pores on both sides (Figs. 4.19 and 4.20). Hence, it is sometimes referred as the double-pored dog tapeworm. The proglottides are filled with typical egg pouches 100–200 μm large. They contain 1–30 round eggs of taeniid type. With light microscopy, the embryo and its hooks can be seen inside a single egg (Fig. 4.21).

> **Morphology of *Dipylidium caninum***
>
> *D. caninum* belongs to midsized Cyclophyllidea cestodes. The worm is able to retract its holdfast organ, the rostellum, to the safety of the scolex. Rostellum has three or four rows of thorn-shaped hooks. Apart from the rostellum, attachment is facilitated by four pairs of suckers. There are several proglottids (Fig. 4.20), and these are arranged in a chain referred as craspedote so that each slightly extends over the subsequent one. Especially the segments at the tail end of the worm are longer that their width. The genitals are paired. The genital pores are situated laterally at both edges of each proglottid just below the midline. The cirrus sac is pear-shaped. There are many testes. Ovaries are paired. The vitelline glands are located posterior to the ovaries and the vagina is at the ventral or posterior side of the cirrus sac. In the gravid proglottids, the uterus forms pouches and capsules with 1–30 taeniid eggs (Fig. 4.21) inside each of them.

Life Cycle

The tapeworm is attached to the intestinal wall with the scolex hooks and suckers. Gravid and egg-filled mature proglottids are being released from the posterior part of the worm and moved out in fecal mass. The proglottids are also capable to some extent of autonomic moving, and they can be seen writhing at the proximity of the anus. The life cycle of the *Dipylidium* tapeworm requires an intermediate host. The most important intermediate host of the worm is the cat flea (*C. felis*), which is infective to dogs too. Adult fleas and proglottides of *Dipylidium* rarely meet, but the flea larvae like to ingest the egg packages protruding from desiccated cestode proglottids. It is likely that also the canine chewing louse (*T. canis*) can act as an intermediate host. In other flea species (for instance dog flea, *Ctenocephalides canis*), the development of the larval stage stops and never reaches the stage needed for infection a dog. Outside the host, the proglottid of the tapeworm dries quickly, but remains infectious to the intermediate host. The eggs remain infective at 30°C for about 2.5 months and at 15°C for 3.5 months. In refrigeration, in physiological saline the larval stage stays infective for about a week. In the intermediate host, the larval stage is released from the egg and it penetrates the intestinal tract of

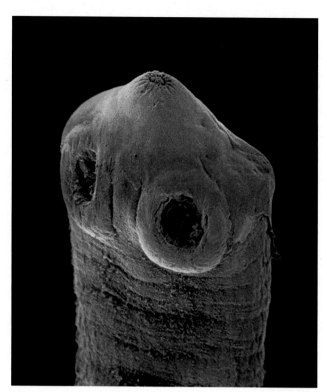

FIG. 4.18 Head of scolex of the *D. caninum* in scanning electron microscopy. The hooked rostrum or rostellum is almost totally retracted. Two of the tapeworm's four suckers are visible.

the flea larva with the aid of the hooks and the enzymes it secretes. The larval stage infective for the dog is called cysticercoid and develops in the body cavity of the intermediate host. The development of the cysticercoid takes 9–15 days in a warm environment (about 30°C), and longer in colder conditions. If the environment is cool, the intermediate host must be in contact with the warm-blooded mammalian skin for about a week. The dog is infected when it eats an infected flea or louse with the cysticercoids. The development into an adult tapeworm takes about 3 weeks in the dog. Its life cycle is shown in Fig. 4.22.

> **Dipylidiosis Is a Zoonosis**
>
> The flea tapeworm is capable of developing in adulthood also in the human gut. The infection requires that a human ingests an infected flea (intermediate host) or a cysticercoid from the flea. Dipylidiosis is most common in little children who are in close contact with a dog. If the dog has recently crushed a flea with its teeth, cysticercoids may be present in the dog's saliva. Since the worms reach adulthood in the human, alive and writhing cestode proglottids may be found in the soiled nappy or perianal area. The human infection is usually accidental and typical human dipylidiosis is caused by a single worm. The infection is usually subclinical. Abdominal pain, diarrhea, general irritability, and itching of the anal region have been described in the literature.

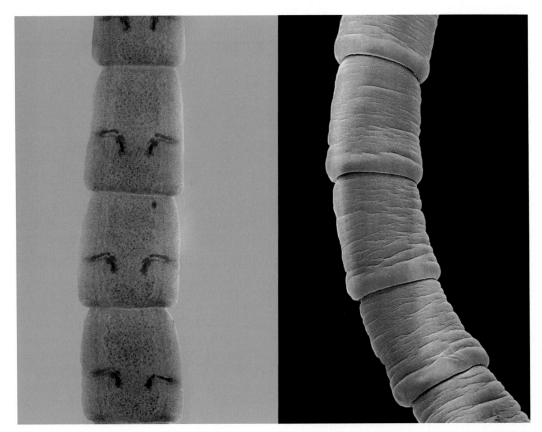

FIG. 4.19   Stained proglottids of *Dipylidium caninum* in light microscopy and scanning electron microscopy. Genital pores are located laterally at the edges of each proglottid, slightly below the central line. The structures stained darker are the ovaries and pore structures of the genitals. Scanning electron microscopy shows that the proglottids are located so that each anterior proglottid slightly extends over the subsequent posterior one.

Distribution

Since fleas are found everywhere in the world, *D. caninum* is ubiquitous. It is also one of the most important and prevalent feline cestodes. It is also found in humans, albeit rarely.

Importance to Canine Health

Single cestodes very rarely cause clinical signs in canines. The most common signs are itching caused by proglottids moving in the anal area and other irritation. The discomfort leads into rubbing of the caudal area and subsequent trauma. Massive *Dipylidium* infections are very rare. They may be associated with gastro-intestinal signs such as diarrhea or constipation.

Diagnosis

Diagnosis is based on the recognition of species-specific proglottids and egg packets. The *Dipylidium* proglottids are elongated and oval, resembling cucumber seeds. A proglottid is placed on the objective glass with a drop of water, covered with a cover slip, and viewed in a microscope. The proglottid releases into the water between the glass surfaces egg packages typical to the species. A fecal sample examined parasitologically by flotation method gives almost always a negative result for *D. caninum*.

Treatment and Prevention

Most anticestode drugs are efficacious against worms found in the gut of the primary host. These substances include praziquantel, epsiprantel, and nitroscanate. The intermediate host plays an important role in *D. caninum* infection. The dog will be quickly reinfected unless the anticestode treatment is complemented with an efficient flea control.

MESOCESTOIDES SPP.

- A tapeworm residing in the small intestine and infect dogs by ingestion of the metacestode larval stage—tetrathyridium—of the tapeworm in the tissues of intermediate hosts.
- Up to 70 cm in length; body composed of a large strobila with numerous segments. The scolex is lacking a rostellum.
- The indirect life cycle involves coprophagic arthropods as a first intermediate hosts and several animal species, e.g., reptiles, amphibians, birds, and mammals can serve as second intermediate hosts.

- Intestinal *Mesocestoides* infection is typically sub-clinical. In rare circumstances, the tetrathyridium stages may invade into the peritoneal cavity of the dog and cause peritonitis.
- Diagnosis is based on the detection of mobile proglottids crawling in the feces. When the proglottid is placed between the object and cover glasses and squeezed lightly, the parauterine organ can be identified by microscope.

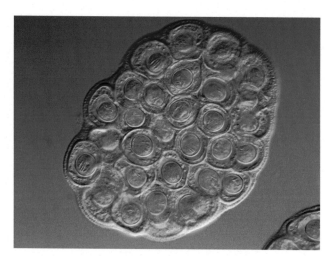

FIG. 4.21 The egg package full of taeniid eggs, typical for *D. caninum.*

Its proglottids are elongated and a few millimeters wide (Fig. 4.24). The size of the strobila depends on the worm burden. If there are many individual worms, they are usually smaller and the strobila is more narrow and shorter. Mature proglottids are released from the posterior part of the strobila into the fecal mass. When outside the dog, the proglottids may move independently. Proglottids are often numerous in the feces of an infected dog and they may be present around its anus. On fresh feces, proglottids are often seen in upright position moving their elongated anterior part and soon crawling away from the fecal mass. A proglottid is recognized as belonging to *Mesocestoides* with the microscope on the basis of ventromedially located genital pore and clearly visible ball-like parauterine organ locating centrally in the segment. Inside the egg, a hooked oncosphere can be seen. In the life cycle, the oncosphere is followed by cysticercoids, infective to the second intermediate host, which are found in the first intermediate host, usually a coprophagic arthropod. Tetrathyridium larvae, found in the second intermediate host, are white, irregularly shaped, and a few millimeters long (Fig. 4.25) Suckers and calcareous particles can be seen. There are also larvae that lack suckers.

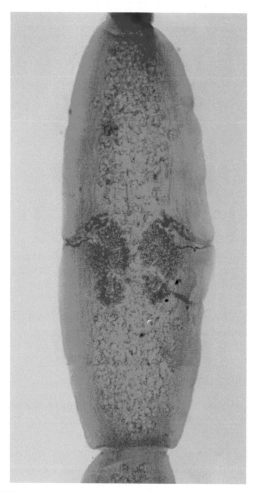

FIG. 4.20 A mature proglottid of *D. caninum* in light microscopy. The proglottid is stained for better visibility of the organs. The genital pores at the both sides of the proglottid and the tubule structures leading into them are clearly seen in the photo. Ovaries are seen as structures that are stained *darker red*. There are numerous testes. They are light, transparent bulbous structures, filling two quarters at the center and extending through the whole proglottid.

Identification

Mesocestoides belongs to Cyclophyllidea cestodes that carry their eggs to the environment within the proglottids. The scolex is of medium size and it has four suckers but no hooks (Fig. 4.23). A full-sized worm is 25–70 cm long.

Life Cycle

The life cycle of *Mesocestoides* is not fully known, but it is recognized that at least two intermediate hosts are needed. Dogs, cats, wild carnivores, and humans can act as definitive hosts. The worm attaches to the small intestine with its scolex and the proglottids mature rapidly. The prepatent period is 2 weeks at its shortest. Mature, egg-carrying proglottids detach from the posterior part of the worm. Inside eggs, the first-stage larva, the oncosphere, develops. This is infective for the first intermediate host. It is believed that several coprophagic arthropods, such as *Oribatidae* mites or beetles, are suitable first intermediate hosts. A cysticercoid develops in the first intermediate host. Since the oncosphere is not

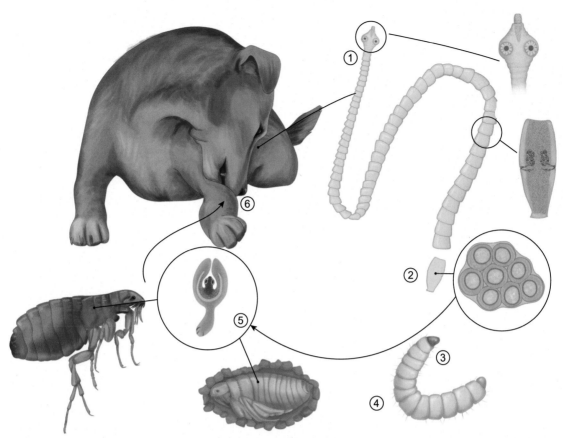

FIG. 4.22 Life cycle of *D. caninum*: (1) the adult tapeworm, attached to the canine intestinal wall with the scolex hooks and suckers, sheds mature proglottids from the posterior part of the worm, and they move out in the fecal mass; (2) the proglottides are to some extent capable of independent movement. The proglottids contain egg packages trapped inside uterine folds, each usually holding 1–30 eggs; (3) an intermediate host, the cat flea, is needed for the life cycle of the flea flatworm. The flea larva feed on the proglottids of the tapeworm and the egg packages within; (4) the larval stage, the flatworm, is released from the eggshell in the intermediate host and it penetrates the flea larva intestinal tract using its hooks and secreted enzymes; (5) the larval stage infectious for the dog, cysticercoid, grows in the body cavity of the intermediate host; and (6) the dog is infected when it eats the flea with its cysticercoid. The development into an adult flatworm takes about 3 weeks in a dog.

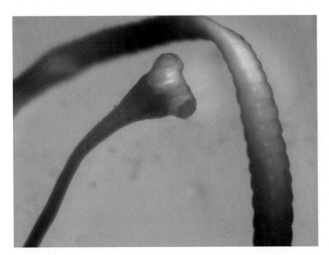

FIG. 4.23 Scolex of a *Mesocestoides* worm and proglottids of the strobila.

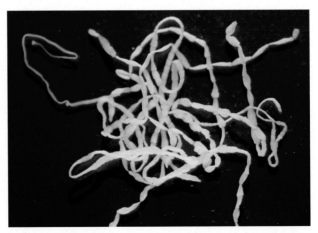

FIG. 4.24 *Mesocestoides* tapeworms, mainly the strobila parts. In the upper left corner, the anterior end with a scolex can be seen.

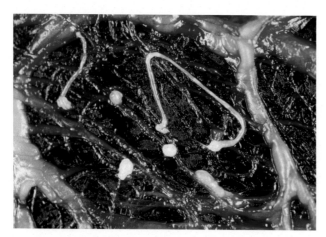

FIG. 4.25 Tetrathyridium larval stages, typical for *Mesocestoides*, on the omentum of a raccoon dog. In tetrathyridium stage the larva is in a small and tight bundle, which is visible as a light-colored ball. The photo is not fully authentic, since the bundle of two larvae has been unraveled to display the worm-like structure of the larva.

directly infective for vertebrate hosts, dogs cannot receive a *Mesocestoides* infection directly from the feces of another dog. When the cysticercoid reaches the alimentary tract of the second intermediate host, the development of the cysticercoid into a third larval stage, a tetrathyridium, proceeds. It multiplies asexually by cellular division. A reptile, amphibian, bird, or mammal, e.g., a rodent, can act as a second intermediate host. The history of an infected dog often tells that it likes to prey and eat small animals in the nature. In addition to its role as the definitive host, the dog may also act as a second intermediate host. The condition is manifested by the occurrence of large numbers of tetrathyridium larvae in the abdominal cavity, instead of the intestine. It is not known whether this sort of infection is the result of the dog eating the first intermediate host or an untypical result from eating the second intermediate host. Most reported human infections have been caused by eating insufficiently heated frog's legs. Dogs, however, do not pose a direct infection risk to humans. The life cycle of *Mesocestoides* is shown in Fig. 4.26.

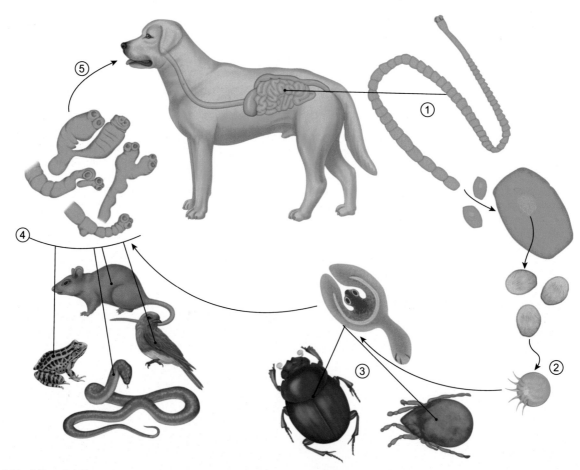

FIG. 4.26 Life cycle of *Mesocestoides* spp.: (1) *Mesocestoides* attaches to the small intestine of the definitive host and proglottids containing mature eggs are shed from the posterior part of the worm; (2) the eggs are secreted to the environment inside the proglottid and the first-stage larva, oncosphere, develops in them. The oncosphere infects the first intermediate host; (3) it is assumed that several coprophagic arthropods, e.g., Oribatidae mites or beetles, can act as first intermediate hosts. A cysticercoid metacestode develops in the first intermediate host; (4) when the cysticercoid reaches the intestine of the second intermediate host, the third larval stage, tetrathyridium, develops. It multiplies asexually by division. A reptile, amphibian, bird, or mammal, e.g., a small rodent, can act as a second intermediate host; and (5) a dog becomes infected by eating the second intermediate host and the worm-like tetrathyridium stage it contains. The prepatent period is 2 weeks at its shortest.

Distribution

Mesocestoides species are found in Asia, Africa, Europe, and the United States, especially the western states. The parasite has been reported to become more common in many parts of Europe during the last decades, mostly in foxes. The infection is relatively common and recurring in dogs that are allowed to eat small wild animals.

Importance to Canine Health

An intestinal *Mesocestoides* infection is typically sub-clinical. The dog is brought to the veterinarian, usually due to the owner's aversion to the presence of the moving and crawling tapeworm proglottids in feces. The colonization of the small intestine by the adult worms may occasionally cause diarrhea and illthrift. The entry of tetrathyridium stages into the dog's abdominal cavity does not usually cause clinical signs. They are accidentally found, e.g., during autopsy or abdominal surgery. Clinical signs of tetrathyridiosis in dogs may include the signs associated with peritonitis. In very rare cases, tetrathyridium larvae start to multiply uncontrollably in canine abdomen, leading to canine peritoneal larval cestodiasis (CPLC), a serious disease with a guarded prognosis. A dog with CPLC often ends up euthanized despite treatment attempts. The initial observations are often abdominal edema—in male dogs especially scrotal edema—as a result of fluid accumulation. The CPLC is often associated with the underlying immunocompromising condition, i.e., a consequence of the body's lowered defenses against infections.

Diagnosis

A dog owner can see the plentiful mobile proglottids crawling in the feces (Fig. 4.29). The history of the dog often points toward *Mesocestoides* infection, especially in areas where main differential diagnosis, a tapeworm

Morphology of *Mesocestoides*

The scolex is oval and slightly angular. It has four suckers. The rostellum with its hooks is absent. The immature proglottids of the anterior end are wider that their length. The genital opening is ventromedially located. Each proglottid has male and female genitals. Testicular structures are numerous, dozens for each proglottid, and they are laterally located along the total length of the proglottid. The vitellary glands are tightly backed in two foci. The ovary is also in two lobes. The vitellaria and the ovary are located adjacent to each other in the proximity of the posterior edge of the proglottid. The developing eggs are packed in the thick-walled parauterine organ with no opening for egg secretion (Figs. 4.27 and 4.28). This is why *Mesocestoides* eggs are not found in the fecal examination of eggs. The gravid proglottid is longer than its width. The taeniid-type eggs within the parauterine organ are slightly oval and about $27 \times 35\,\mu m$ large. The oncosphere larva within the egg has three pairs of f-shaped hooks that can be seen in light microscopy.

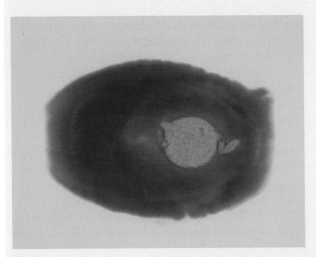

FIG. 4.27 The *Mesocestoides* diagnosis is confirmed by detecting proglottids in canine feces by microscopy. A round structure with a tail-like extension can be seen within the proglottid. This is the parauterine organ that acts as an egg repository for the tapeworm.

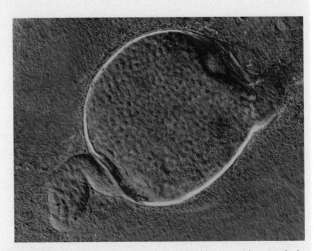

FIG. 4.28 The parauterine organ, typical for *Mesocestoides* cestode, in a close-up photo.

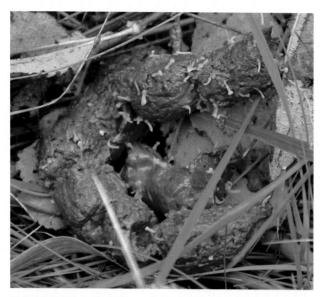

FIG. 4.29 In a typical *Mesocestoides* infection, the canine fecal mass contains many proglottids. In fresh feces, the proglottids are mobile and pointing with their elongated anterior part toward upright. *(Reproduced with permission from Erik Lindholm.)*

infection caused by *D. caninum*, is not common. The diagnosis is confirmed when the proglottid is placed between the object and cover glasses and squeezed lightly. In microscopy, a round structure with a tail-like appendix can be seen. This is the parauterine organ, which serves as a storage of eggs (Figs. 4.27 and 4.28). The proglottid sample need not be stained or otherwise processed for diagnosis. The result of fecal flotation analysis is usually negative, unless proglottids have broken down, releasing eggs in the fecal mass. The abdominal *Mesocestoides* infection is diagnosed by tapping abdominal effusion fluid or taking a biopsy of visceral organs, in which tetrathyridiums of about 1 mm length or calcifications typical for cestodes can be detected. Sometimes larval stages can be seen in cytological samples. Fecal analysis for eggs is not diagnostic for *Mesocestoides* infection.

Treatment and Prevention

When proglottids have been detected, one dose of a drug effective against cestodes, such as praziquantel or epsiprantel, is sufficient. When assessing the efficacy of treatment, the short prepatent period of the parasite needs to be taken into account: it takes only 2 weeks for proglottids to reappear in feces, if the dog is reinfected soon after the treatment. Pets in rural environments are more at risk due to hunting or scavenging on small vertebrates infected with tetrathyridia. The infection may be prevented by preventing the dog from doing that. Dog-to-dog infections do not take place. In cases of abdominal *Mesocestoides* infection, the primary treatment of fenbendazole

for up to 8 weeks has been reported to control the larval stages. In addition to medical treatment, the parasite mass and abdominal transudate has to be often removed surgically. The prognosis of symptomatic abdominal infection is guarded.

HYMENOLEPIS SPECIES

- A genus consisting of small tapeworm species residing in the small intestine of the definitive host.
- Intestinal parasites of the rats and other rodents, which are capable to infect humans and presumably canines too. The literature about dog cases is scarce.
- Usually indirect life cycle, dog ingests the metacestode larval stage—cysticercoid—in the tissues of arthropod intermediate host. *Hymenolepis nana* is an exception among the cestodes, as it can develop directly in the same host.
- *Hymenolepis* spp. possesses low clinical significance to canine medicine, but is significant to public health.

Identification

There are three medically relevant *Hymenolepis* (syn. Rodentolepis) species that are capable of infecting humans (and presumably canines too, although the literature about dog cases is scarce): *H. diminuta* (the rat tapeworm), *H. nana* (the dwarf tapeworm), and *H. microstoma* (the mouse bile duct tapeworm). *Hymenolepis* species belong to Cyclophyllidea cestodes which secrete their eggs into the external environment within the proglottids.

The length of adult *H. diminuta* is about 20–60 cm, *H. nana* about 2–4 cm, and *H. microstoma* about 3–8 cm. In the scolex they all have four suckers and a retractable rostellum. In *H. nana* the rostellum has 20–30 hooks, whereas *H. diminuta* lacks hooks. The segments are significantly wider than long. Genital pores are located unilaterally, and each mature segment contains both male and female reproductive organs, single ovary and especially three clearly defined testes are considered typical for *Hymenolepis* (Fig. 4.30).

The typical *Hymenolepis*-looking eggs of *H. diminuta* and *H. microstoma* are spherical about 60–80 μm in diameter, and they have a thick striated outer membrane and thinner inner membrane of embryophore in the middle (Fig. 4.31). The six paired hooks of the oncosphere larva can be seen inside. The eggs of *H. nana* are slightly smaller, about 40–60 μm in diameter.

Life Cycle

The natural definitive hosts for *Hymenolepis* are rodents (mostly mice and rats), but occasionally they infect also

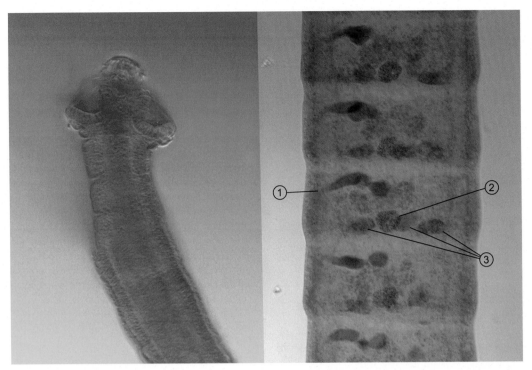

FIG. 4.30 A scolex and a part of the strobila of *Hymenolepis nana* as seen in a stained specimen. In the scolex, four suckers and a retractable armed rostellum are present. The segments of strobili are significantly wider than long. Genital pores are located unilaterally (1), and each mature segment contains both male and female reproductive organs, single ovary (2) and especially three clearly defined testes (3) are considered typical for *Hymenolepis*. *(Specimen from the collection of the Department of General Biology and Parasitology, Medical University of Warsaw, Poland.)*

FIG. 4.31 The eggs of *H. nana* is spherical about 40–60 μm in diameter, and they have a thick striated outer membrane and thinner inner membrane of embryophore in the middle. The six paired hooks of the oncosphere larva can be seen inside.

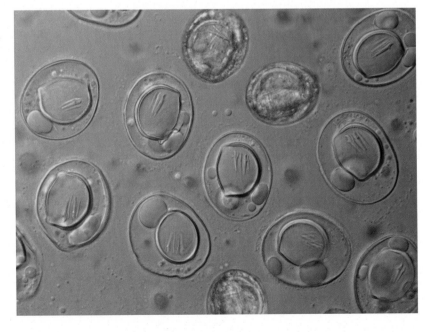

dogs and humans. The intermediate hosts are grain beetles (genus Tribolium and Tenebrio), fleas, or other insects. The cysticercoid metacestode stage develops in these hosts after they ingest *Hymenolepis* eggs. A dog becomes infected through eating the infected insects, either directly or in contaminated water or food. *H. nana* is an exception among the cestodes as it has an option of a direct life cycle. The direct life cycle may take place either feco-orally from secreted eggs without any intermediate or as an autoinfection, where eggs hatch within the intestine and initiate a new generation without ever exiting the host. During the direct life cycle, the oncospheres from the ingested eggs or the eggs voided by intestinal tapeworms are released. The oncospheres (hexacanth larvae) penetrate the intestinal villus and develop into cysticercoid larvae. In favorable conditions, the cysticercoids return to the intestinal lumen, evaginate their scolices, and attach to the intestinal mucosa. A morphologically identical variant of *H. nana*, namely *H. nana* var. *fraterna*, infects rodents and uses arthropods as intermediate hosts.

In the small intestine, or in the case of *H. microstoma*, in the bile ducts, of the definitive host the worm matures in about 2–4 weeks and starts producing eggs to the environment. They are immediately infective and can only survive for about 2 weeks outside the host.

Distribution

Hymenolepis species are found worldwide, but more commonly in warm climate areas. *H. nana* is common in humans (especially children) due to its direct feco-oral life cycle where the sanitation and rodent-control are poor. In such areas, dogs may be at higher risk too.

Importance to Canine Health

Typically of cestodes, *Hymenolepis* does not usually cause clinical signs to the definitive host. In cases where they appear, diarrhea, abdominal pain, or weight loss might be exhibited.

Diagnosis

The eggs can be found with flotation methods from the fecal sample of the dog. Sample collection over several days is recommended.

Treatment and Prevention

As a medical treatment in diagnosed cases, cestoda specific drugs (praziquantel, epsiprantel) can be used. Reinfections are unfortunately common in highly endemic areas, at least in humans. Accidental canine *H. diminuta* infections from eating insects might be difficult to prevent, but as a general method for prevention of *Hymenolepis*-infections, an effective rodent-control should be practiced.

H. nana and *H. diminuta* Are Zoonotic Parasites

Both *H. nana* and *H. diminuta* are zoonotic and able to develop patent infections in the human intestine. Human infections are often associated with the poor hygiene. Hence, although both tapeworm species are ubiquitous, hymenolepiosis (hymenolepiasis) is more common in children in

---

developing countries. The source of infection can be contaminated food, e.g., cereals or flour. The infective contamination can be small beetles present in flour containing cysticercoids of the tapeworms. These intermediate hosts have gained the infection, e.g., by ingesting rat feces. *H. nana* infections are more common than *H. diminuta* infections in humans. This is because *H. nana* it is capable of completing its life cycle without an intermediate host and the disease can be spread directly from person to person by eggs in feces or within one person as a result of internal autoinfection. In adults, *Hymenolepis* infection is usually innocuous and more of a nuisance than a health problem. However, in small children, heavy *H. nana* infection can be associated with pathological changes and clinical signs. Adult tapeworms residing in the intestinal lumen are usually harmless. However, when the infection takes place without an intermediate host, there is an additional developmental phase, from larva to cysticercoid, required in the host. The larvae burrow into the wall of the intestine and, if they are present in large quantities, can inflict severe damage. Heavy infections with *H. nana* can cause abdominal pain, nausea, vomiting, diarrhea, weight loss, and anal pruritus.

DIPHYLLOBOTHRIUM LATUM, Fish Tapeworm or Broad Tapeworm

- A tapeworm residing in the small intestine of the definitive hosts.
- Indirect life cycle, infect dogs by ingestion of the metacestode larval stage—plerocercoid—of the tapeworm in the tissues of fish.
- One of the longest worms infecting dogs, up to several meters in length; body composed of a large strobila with numerous segments. The scolex is lacking a rostellum and suckers; grooved structures of the scolex serve as a holdfast organ instead.
- The life cycle involves an aquatic copepod as a first intermediate host and several freshwater fish species as a second intermediate host.
- Intestinal *Diphyllobothrium* infection is typically subclinical although in humans the infection has been associated with B12 vitamin deficiency and pernicious anemia.
- Diagnosis is based on the detection of typical operculated eggs in fecal analysis. The empty proglottid chains passed in feces intermittently may attract the attention of the dog owner.

Identification

D. latum, the fish tapeworm or broad tapeworm, belongs to Pseudophyllidea tapeworms. It is large; an adult may be up to 20 m long. In a dog, it is usually shorter. The scolex has sucking grooves (bothria) for attachment to the intestine, but there are no suckers or hooks. The proglottids are light and wider than their length, about 2 cm (Figs. 4.32 and 4.33). A darker bulge that contains the branched uterus and the eggs within it can be seen in the middle of the chain of proglottids. Apart from the genital pore, the proglottid has another opening, thorough which the eggs continue to be secreted into the fecal mass, where they can be seen in microscopy. Once the proglottids have been emptied of eggs, they are shed and removed in stools, often in chains (Fig. 4.34). The eggs resemble trematode eggs: they are large, about 70 × 50 μm and oval and they have a lid, or operculum, in the other end (Fig. 4.35). The eggs of another

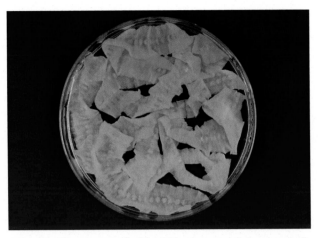

FIG. 4.34 The empty proglottids of fish tapeworm exit the gut typically in chains. The proglottids are light and wider than their length, about 2 cm, and a darker bulge consisting of the branched uterus can be seen in their center.

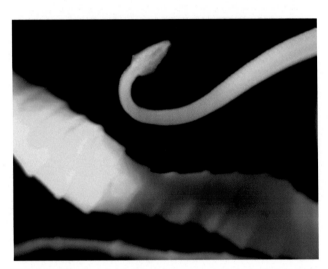

FIG. 4.32 Scolex or head of the fish tapeworm and the proglottids, wider than their length.

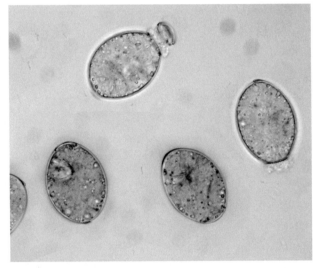

FIG. 4.35 The eggs of the fish tapeworm resemble those of trematodes. They are oval and large, about 70 × 50 μm. They have a lid, known as an operculum, in the other end.

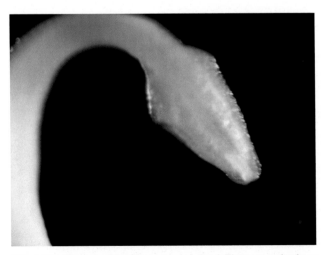

FIG. 4.33 Close-up of the fish tapeworm's head. There are no hooks or suckers. The worm attaches to the gut wall with two grooved structures (bothriae) of the scolex.

Pseudophyllidea tapeworm, *Spirometra*, have a sharper end and are somewhat smaller.

Life Cycle

Many fish-eating mammals, such as dogs, cats, wild carnivores, and humans, can act as definitive hosts of the fish tapeworm. A human is the preferred host, since the eggs produced in the human intestine are more robust than those produced in the other hosts. The life cycle requires two intermediate hosts. When the eggs reach a water environment, they hatch to release the ciliated larval form, coracidium. This must rapidly reach the first intermediate host, the copepod crustacean, since it cannot survive for long. In the copepod, the following life cycle stage is developed, the procercoid larva. When a fresh-water fish, the second intermediate host of the parasite, eats the crustacean, plerocercoid larvae are formed in its muscles. The plerocercoid is infective for the definitive host, when it eats raw fish. The scolex attaches to the small intestine and the continuous production of the proglottids starts in the neck region of the scolex. While the proglottids mature, they move further away from the scolex with the lengthening proglottid chain. Eggs are found in the feces of the definitive host about 4 weeks after infection. The life cycle of *D. latum* is shown in Fig. 4.36.

Distribution

D. latum is endemic in the northern hemisphere, Scandinavia, Russia, Japan, and North America. Many human infections are diagnosed annually, although they are rarer than before.

Importance to Canine Health

Fish tapeworm infection usually occurs without clinical signs in dogs. Although the worm does not damage the intestine, it absorbs nutrients intended for the host through its tegument. This may cause signs. Due to its large size, the worm has a large surface area, which makes a significant loss of nutrients possible for the host. The host loses weight and may suffer vomiting and diarrhea. Pernicious anemia, caused by vitamin B12 deficiency, has been described in humans in association with fish tapeworm infection. Some sources claim it can also cause anemia in dogs.

Diagnosis

D. latum infection can be diagnosed by analyzing stool samples of the definitive host, because Pseudophyllidea tapeworms secrete their eggs loose to the intestine content. Typical eggs are found with, e.g., flotation and sedimentation methods. The empty proglottid chains detached in

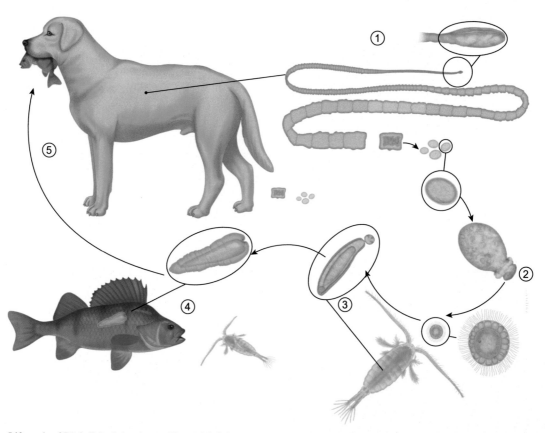

FIG. 4.36 Life cycle of *Diphyllobothrium latum*: (1) an adult fish tapeworm lives in the small intestine of the definitive host. The scolex of the worm is equipped with grooves (bothria) for attachment in the gut wall. The eggs are liberated into the fecal mass through the uterine opening. The empty proglottid chains are released and exit in feces; (2) the eggs are carried in feces into waterways, where coracidium larvae are hatched; (3) the larvae reach the body of the first intermediate host, a copepod crustacean. The next stage, procercoid larvae, develops in the copepod; (4) when the copepod is eaten by the second intermediate host, a fish, plerocercoid larvae, infectious for the definitive host, develop in the muscles of the fish; and (5) a dog is infected by eating raw or undercooked fish. The scolex attaches in the small intestine and starts to produce the strobila with its proglottids. The prepatent period is about 4 weeks.

feces may attract the attention of dog owners (Fig. 4.33). It is important to reach a definite diagnosis because the infection of fish tapeworms requires an exceptionally large dose of dewormer.

Treatment and Prevention

D. latum infection may be treated with praziquantel, but this requires the use of an eightfold dose compared to ordinary cestode control. It is preferable to give the drug orally, although injectable praziquantel is available too. This ensures a sufficient and timely concentration of the substance in the worm's location: the intestinal lumen. The worm absorbs the drug the same way it absorbs nutrients, through its tegument. For prevention, it is essential to cook or thoroughly freeze (−10°C for at least 24–48h in every spot of the fish) freshwater fish given to the dog. The distribution of the parasite has been limited by adequate waste treatment: untreated sewage is no longer allowed to reach waterways.

Morphology of *Diphyllobothrium latum*

The fish tapeworm is a hermaphrodite, typical of cestodes. Each proglottid is equipped with both female and male genitals. The proglottids of fish tapeworm are wider than their length and arranged as a craspedote-type chain: the posterior part of a proglottid partly covers the anterior part of an adjacent proglottid. A fully mature proglottid has laterally numerous small testes structures that appear round, and vitellum (yolk), necessary for egg maturation, in vitellary glands. The genital pore is situated above halfway point of the proglottid. Pores provide a connection from both the female as well as from male genitals to a single hemispherical genital atrium. The opening to the vagina is located posteriorly to the cirrus sac, the end point of the male genitals with a cirrus. The ovary is in the posterior part of the proglottid and forms a butterfly-shaped figure. The uterus is shaped as a rosette and its opening for egg secretion is situated posterior from the genital pore.

Broad Tapeworm in Humans

As in dogs, the main source of *D. latum* infection is an ingestion of the plerocercoid of *D. latum* by consuming raw fish or roe. Dogs cannot be a direct source of infection for their owners, and vice versa. The fish tapeworm *D. latum* is considered native to Fenno-Scandinavia, western Russia, and the Baltics, but it can be found globally. In endemic countries, the infection is becoming rare due to preventive measures, mainly by people avoiding eating raw fish. *D. latum* infection is usually asymptomatic, but heavy infection may result in weight loss, dizziness, abdominal pain, diarrhea, and loss of appetite. The broad tapeworm is famous for its

feature to derive vitamin B12 from its host's intestinal content. This may lead to severe vitamin B12 deficiency and even to a megaloblastic anemia. This type of anemia is indistinguishable from pernicious anemia and may present as pallor, gasping for breath during exertion, and neurologic symptoms such as coordination disturbances.

SPIROMETRA SPECIES

- A tapeworm residing in the small intestine of the definitive hosts.
- Indirect life cycle, infects dogs by ingestion of the metacestode larval stage—plerocercoid (sparganum)—of the tapeworm in the intermediate host.
- The worm's body is up to 1.5m in length and is composed of a large strobila with numerous segments. The scolex lacks a rostellum and suckers; grooved structures of the scolex serve as a holdfast organ.
- The life cycle involves an aquatic copepod as a first intermediate host and several vertebrates, e.g., frogs and snakes serve as a second intermediate host. Life cycle may involve paratenic hosts. Many vertebrate species may serve as paratenic host.
- Clinical signs in the definitive host are usually not apparent.
- Diagnosis is based on the detection of typical operculated eggs in feces, e.g., with flotation and sedimentation methods.

Identification

The Spirometras are Pseudophyllidea tapeworms as is *Diphyllobothrium*, which the *Spirometra* closely resembles. The adult worm can grow to the length of 1.5m. The mature proglottids have a genital pore and a uterine opening for secreting eggs. The uterus is spiral, in keeping with the parasite's name. The eggs of *Spirometra* species are oval-shaped with a distinct operculum at one pole that is slightly cone shaped. The length of plerocercoid larvae (sparganums), found in the second host species, including the dog, vary from a few millimeters up to 10cm. They are light colored and resemble crimpled tapes.

Life Cycle

Dogs, cats, and wild carnivores act as definitive hosts for the *Spirometra*. The life cycle requires two intermediate hosts. The first one is a tiny copepod crustacean living in waters, and the second one is an amphibian, fish, reptile, bird, or mammal. They can also act as paratenic hosts of this parasite. When a dog is infected by eating the plerocercoid phase inside the second host, the larva attaches into the gut wall and start to produce proglottids from the scolex. The proglottids mature in the same manner as in other tapeworms and are conceived while moving toward the tail of the worm. The eggs that develop inside the proglottids are secreted into fecal mass, through the uterus opening. The prepatent period is 15–18 days. The empty proglottids are released from the tail of the worm. In the environment, the larval stage grows inside the egg in a few weeks, depending on the temperature (e.g., 29°C, 8–14 days). Once the eggs reach the waterways, a ciliated larva, the coracidium, hatches from them. This is eaten by a copepod. A procercoid stage develops in the crustacean intermediate host within 2–3 weeks. It is infective for the second-stage intermediate hosts. If the dog gets the infection from the first hosts, copepods, by drinking water or from the paratenic hosts, and acts as the second intermediate host instead of definitive host, plerocercoid larvae spread into its subcutis, muscle fascia, and thoracic and abdominal cavity, forming cystic growths.

Sparganosis

The old name for *Spirometra* larva found in the second intermediate host is sparganum. This gives the name to sparganosis, the infection caused by a plerocercoid larva. Humans may get sparganosis too. In man, the plerocercoids may stay viable for up to 20 years. Humans may get the infection in endemic areas by drinking water contaminated with feces and consequently ingesting infected copepod crustaceans. Infections from other intermediate hosts are possible as well. In these cases, a human acts as a paratenic host for the parasite. People are educated about the need to cook potential *Spirometra* sources properly before eating or using them for medicinal purposes. The larvae have been found in different body parts, for instance in the thoracic and abdominal cavity and the visceral organs, subcutaneous tissue, eye, urinary tract, scrotum, and central nervous system. In a case report, sparganosis was suspected in a man because his eye had been treated in China with a poultice made of raw frog meat. An abnormality (larva) found in the brain scan changed location during the 4-year follow-up, until it was surgically removed.

Distribution

Spirometras, infective for dogs, are endemic especially in northern and southern America and Asia; however, they are also found in other continents. The most common species in dogs are *Spirometra mansoni* and *S. mansonoides*.

Importance to Canine Health

Typical of tapeworms, the canine *Spirometra* infection is subclinical and does not damage the intestine of the definitive host, although the worm can survive and produce eggs for years. However, if the dog enters the life cycle of *Spirometra* at the wrong stage and acts as a second intermediate host, the signs depend on which tissues the plerocercoid larvae colonizes. For instance, they can cause an inflammation of the thoracic or abdominal cavity. A large number of plerocercoids in the musculoskeletal organs may manifest as pain and lameness.

Diagnosis

The *Spirometra* eggs are secreted from the uterine opening of the proglottid into the fecal mass, in which they can be detected, e.g., with flotation or sedimentation techniques. Detecting the species of plerocercoids on the basis of their morphology is difficult and requires expertise. The easiest and most specific method of determining the species is to use PCR methods.

Treatment and Prevention

Treating the tapeworm infection of the intestine of the definitive host can be done with an increased dose of praziquantel. If the exposure is constant, the treatment can repeated at the intervals of the prepatent period (3 weeks). In contrast, the infection caused by plerocercoids is more difficult to manage with anthelmintics. Praziquantel, fenbendazole, and nitazoxanide have been tried with poor results. Plerocercoids can be surgically removed. To prevent plerocercoid infection, dogs in endemic areas should be given only clean drinking water and prevented from drinking from waterways. The infection as a definitive host can be prevented if dogs are not allowed to hunt potential intermediate or paratenic hosts of *Spirometra*, or to eat their meat uncooked. Canine or feline feces should not let contaminate waterways. Untreated surface water should not be used as drinking water. However, preventing fecal contamination of natural waters is almost impossible due to drainage waters.

Morphology of *Spirometra*

Spirometras belong in medium or large Pseudophyllidea cestodes. The scolex is elongated and resembles a digit or spoon. There are no suckers in the head. The groove-like bothria structures that are located on both edges of the scolex, aid in attaching to the gut wall. The mature proglottids are usually wider than their length. There are many testes. The openings of the cirrus and the vagina are separate and close to each other. The ovary has two compartments. The uterus is curled into a spiral in the middle part of the proglottid. The last proglottids of the tail of the parasites often split in the middle before coming loose. This part of the worm resembles an open zipper. Indeed, *Spirometra* is often called a zipper worm.

FURTHER READING

Aiello SE, Moses MA, editors: *The Merck veterinary manual.* Rahway, NJ, 2016, Merck & Co.

Al-Sabi M, Chriél M, Jensen T, Enemark H: Endoparasites of the raccoon dog (*Nyctereutes procyonoides*) and the red fox (*Vulpes vulpes*) in Denmark 2009–2012—a comparative study, *Int J Parasitol Parasites Wildl* 2:144–151, 2013.

Arora H: Hymenolepiasis. *Medscape, drugs & diseases, pediatrics: general medicine.* https://emedicine.medscape.com. (Accessed September 2018).

Barr S, Bowman D: *Blackwell's five-minute veterinary consult clinical companion: canine and feline infectious diseases and parasitology,* ed 2, Oxford, 2012, Wiley-Blackwell.

Bennett H, Mok H, Gkrania-Klotsas E, et al: The genome of the sparganosis tapeworm *Spirometra erinaceieuropaei* isolated from the biopsy of a migrating brain lesion, *Genome Biol* 15:510, 2014.

Boreham R, Boreham B: *Dipylidium caninum*: life cycle, epizootiology and control, *Comp Cont Ed Pract Vet* 12:667–676, 1990.

CABI, International Institute of Parasitology: *8th international training course on identification of helminth parasites of economic importance,* UK.

Cho S-H, Kim T-S, Kong Y, Na B-K, Sohn W-M: Tetrathyridia of *Mesocestoides lineatus* in Chinese snakes and their adults recovered from experimental animals, *Korean J Parasitol* 51:531–536, 2013.

Companion Animal Parasite Council: Intestinal parasites—*Diphyllobothrium* spp. https://www.capcvet.org/guidelines/diphyllobothrium-spp/. (Accessed January 2018).

Cunningham L, Olson P: Description of *Hymenolepis microstoma* (Nottingham strain): a classical tapeworm model for research in the genomic era, *Parasit Vectors* 3:123, 2010.

Dunn AM: *Veterinary helminthology,* ed 2, London, 1978, Heinemann.

Dvorak J, Jones A, Kuhlman H: Studies on the biology of *Hymenolepis microstoma* (Dujardin 1845), *J Parasitol* 47:833–838, 1961.

Eckert J, Deplazes P: Biological, epidemiological, and clinical aspects of echinococcosis, a zoonosis of increasing concern, *Clin Microbiol Rev* 17:107–135, 2004.

Eckert J, Conraths F, Tackmann K: Echinococcosis: an emerging or re-emerging zoonosis? *Int J Parasitol* 30:1283–1294, 2000.

European Scientific Counsel Companion Animal Parasites: *ESCCAP guidelines; Worm control in dogs and cats,* ed 3, July 2017. (Accessed January 2018).

Franssen F, Nijsse R, Mulder J, et al: Increase in number of helminth species from Dutch red foxes over a 35-year period, *Parasit Vectors* 7:166, 2014.

Georgi J, Georgi M: *Canine clinical parasitology,* Philadelphia, 1992, Lea & Febiger.

Guardone L, Macchioni F, Torracca B, Gabrielli S, Magi M: *Hymenolepis diminuta* (rat tapeworm) infection in a dog in Liguria, Northwest Italy, *Parassitologia* 52:244, 2010.

Gunn A, Pitt S: *Parasitology—an integrated approach,* ed 1, Oxford, 2012, Wiley-Blackwell.

Haukisalmi V: Checklist of tapeworms (Platyhelminthes, Cestoda) of vertebrates in Finland, *ZooKeys* 533:1–61, 2015.

Jacobs D, Fox M, Gibbons L, Hermosilla C: *Principles of veterinary parasitology,* Chichester, 2016, Wiley Blackwell.

Kashiide T, Matsumoto J, Yamaya Y, et al: Case report: first confirmed case of canine peritoneal larval cestodiasis caused by Mesocestoides vogae (syn. M. corti) in Japan, *Vet Parasitol* 201:154–157, 2014.

Kruse D, Herhilan S. Fargo D: *Diphyllobothrium latum*, Animal Diversity Web, University of Michigan. animaldiversity.org/accounts/Diphyllobothrium_latum/. (Accessed January 2018).

Lass A, Szostakowska B, Myjak P, Korzeniewski K: The first detection of *Echinococcus multilocularis* DNA in environmental fruit, vegetable, and mushroom samples using nested PCR, *Parasitol Res* 114:4023–4029, 2015.

Lavikainen A: *A taxonomic revision of the Taeniidae Ludwig, 1886 based on molecular phylogenies,* Nummela, 2014, Oasis Media Finland Oy.

Lee S, We J, Sohn W, Hong S, Chai J: Experimental life history of Spirometra erinacei, *Kisaengchunghak Chapchi* 28:161–173, 1990.

Loos-Frank B: An up-date of Verster's (1969) 'taxonomic revision of the genus *Taenia Linnaeus*' (Cestoda) in table format, *Syst Parasitol* 45:155–183, 2000.

Mehlhorn H: *Encyclopedic reference of parasitology,* ed 2, Berlin/Heidelberg, 2001, Springer.

Olsen O: *Animal parasites—their life cycles and ecology,* Baltimore, 1974, University Park Press, pp. 237–240.

Patten PK, Rich LJ, Zaks K, Blauvelt M: Cestode infection in 2 dogs: cytologic findings in liver and a mesenteric lymph node, *Vet Clin Pathol* 42:103–108, 2013.

Pugh R: Dipylidium caninum *in intermediate hosts: with special reference to the hosts' susceptibility to infections,* Brisbane, 1985, University of Queensland.

Pugh R: Effects on the development of *Dipylidium caninum* and on the host reaction to this parasite in the adult flea (*Ctenocephalides felis* felis), *Parasitol Res* 73:171–177, 1987.

Roberts L, Janovy J, editors: *Gerald D. Schmidt & Larry S. Roberts' foundations of parasitology,* ed 8, New York, 2009, McGraw-Hill, pp 291–292.

Saari S: *Koiranhesimato (*Dipylidium caninum*)—tuontikoirien tuliainen* (vol. 99), 1993, Suomen Elainlääkäril, pp. 749–753 (in Finnish).

Soulsby EJL: *Helminths, arthropods and protozoa of domesticated animals,* ed 7, London, 1982, Balliére Tindall.

Tamura Y, Ohta H, Kashiide T, et al: Case report: protein-losing enteropathy caused by Mesocestoides vogae (syn. M. corti) in a dog, *Vet Parasitol* 205:412–415, 2014.

Taylor M, Coop R, Wall R: *Veterinary parasitology,* ed 4, Oxford, 2016, Wiley Blackwell.

Thompson R: Review: neglected zoonotic helminths: *Hymenolepis nana, Echinococcus canadensis* and *Ancylostoma ceylanicum, Clin Microbiol Infect* 21:426–432, 2015.

Zajac A, Conboy G: *Veterinary clinical parasitology,* ed 8, West Sussex, 2012, John Wiley & Sons.

Chapter 5

Nematoda (Roundworms)

Nematodes infecting dogs can be microscopic, such as *Trichinella* and *Strongyloides stercoralis*, or substantial, such as the almost snake-like giant kidney worm, *Dioctophyma renale*. Nematodes are dioecious (separate sexes) and generally demonstrate sexual dimorphism. Female roundworms are usually bigger than the male. Nematodes are typically longish and cylinder shaped, with tapering ends. Nematodes have a distinct fluid-filled body cavity or pseudocoelom with high internal pressure. The cross-section is round. Nematodes have an elastic but firm outer membrane, or cuticle, which permits some nutrients to be absorbed through it. The cuticle contains openings for secretion. Underneath the cuticle there is a layer called hypodermis with four ridges or cords projecting toward the body cavity. Two lateral cords serve as a stem for an excretory canal, while the nerves run along the dorsal and ventral cords. A prominent nerve ring surrounding the esophagus is another vital part of the nervous system.

Somatic muscles are attached to the hypodermis and are in four sections separated by hypodermal cords. Two types of muscle arrangement occur in nematodes: platymyarian and coelomyarian. Muscle arrangement plays a role in diagnostics, especially in histopathology, when transversal sections of nematodes are studied.

Nematodes have a complete digestive system with an anterior mouth and a posterior anus. The mouth may be equipped with specialized structures, such as lips, sensory organs, and chitinous teeth or plates for feeding or attaching to the host. These structures are used in morphological identification of nematodes. The pharynx is situated at the anterior end of the nematode. The esophagus is very muscular. Strong esophageal muscles and a valve between the esophagus and intestine are morphological adaptations and developed to function against the high pressure levels in the pseudocoelom. The shape of the esophagus plays an important role in identification of nematodes. The intestine of nematode is a simple tube. Digestion occurs rapidly and feces are expelled from the anus.

The reproductive organs of the nematodes occupy a large portion of the body cavity in sexes. Males usually have a single set of reproductive organs. A tubular testis is connected to a seminal vesicle, which is connected to a vas deferens leading to a cloaca, where the anus is also located. In addition to their gonads, many nematode males have in their caudal end a bell or funnel-shaped widening of the cuticle, copulatory bursa, with which the male attaches to the female during copulation. The bursa is supported by finger-like structures, called bursal rays. In addition, many males have a separate pair of spicules or a single spicule, organs for copulation, and a gubernaculum, a structure that guides the exertion of the spicules. Since there is much interspecies variation between the structures of copulation bursas and spicules, these morphological differences are often used for the detection of the species.

Females often have several sets of reproductive organs. Tubular ovaries are connected to an oviduct that is connected to a uterus. Eggs are expelled from the uterus through a vulva located separately from the anus. There is a lot of interspecies variation in the location of the vulva. A basic morphology of a typical nematode is illustrated in Fig. 5.1.

Some nematodes produce eggs into a dog's feces, some larvae, and some produce microfilarial larvae into the circulation or the surrounding tissues as a result of reproduction. Most produce eggs. The egg, larval, and microfilarial morphologies are of diagnostic value.

Nematodes usually have a direct life cycle, but lungworms, for instance, have a life cycle requiring an intermediate host.

TOXOCARA CANIS, Dog Roundworm

- Spaghetti-like, large worms up to 18 cm long.
- Very common intestinal ascarid roundworm of canines, zoonotic.
- Infection through the placenta or milk to puppies, or from eating infectious eggs or a paratenic host.
- Clinical signs are most severe in puppies and may include ill thrift, respiratory or digestive tract signs; in adult dogs the infection is usually innocuous.
- Diagnosis is based on the detection of typical eggs in a fecal sample.
- Common reason for anthelmintic treatment of dogs.

Canine Parasites and Parasitic Diseases. https://doi.org/10.1016/B978-0-12-814112-0.00005-2

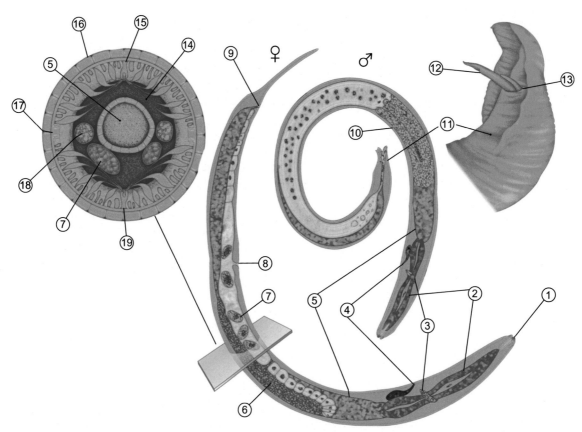

FIG. 5.1 A basic morphology of a typical female and male nematode. A cross section and the caudal part of the male are presented as details: (1) oral opening and lip structures; (2) esophagus; (3) nerve ring; (4) excretory pore; (5) intestine; (6) ovary; (7) uterus; (8) genital pore; (9) anus; (10) testis; (11) copulatory bursa; (12) spicules; (13) cloacal opening; (14) pseudocoeloma; (15) dorsal epidermal and nerve cord; (16) cuticle; (17) lateral epidermal and nerve cord; (18) oviduct; and (19) ventral epidermal and nerve cord.

Identification

Adult *T. canis* roundworms are spaghetti-like, large worms with a round cross-section. The females may be up to 18 cm and the males up to about 10 cm long (Fig. 5.2). The eggs are microscopical, typical for ascarids (Fig. 5.3). They are round with a thick, rough shell. Their size is about $75 \times 90\,\mu m$. Migrating larvae are about $300\,\mu m$ long.

Life Cycle

Ascarids have a complex life cycle. The routes of the life cycle are affected by several factors, such as the age and immunological status of the host and the infection route. Canids act as definitive hosts for the parasite. The sexual reproduction of the adult worms takes place in the canid small intestine. The eggs are not infectious immediately. Instead, even in suitable conditions it takes at least 2 weeks before the egg has reached the infective stage with the larval form L3 inside it. Sticky and thick-shelled eggs remain infectious for extended periods even in demanding conditions. Infectious eggs find their way from the

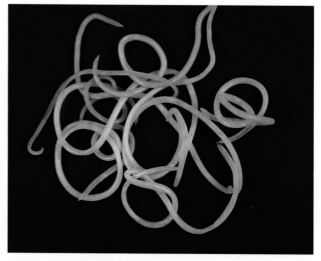

FIG. 5.2 Dog roundworms. Males can be distinguished from the females on the basis of the umbrella hook in the tail.

environment into the alimentary tract of the next canid. There the eggshells are digested in a few hours and the larvae are released. The larvae molt twice and mature to adults. The adult worms copulate and begin reproduction. In an infection,

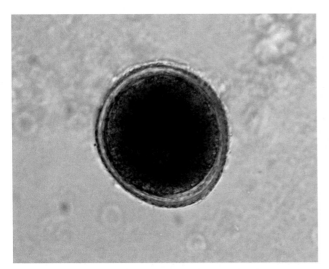

FIG. 5.3 A typical *Toxocara* egg: round or subglobular and surrounded by a thick and rough shell. Bile of the host stains the egg with a yellowish-brown color.

not all larval stages mature immediately and reproduce. Instead, a major part of them migrate from the intestine through the liver and pulmonary circulation to different parts of the body. Small puppies, typically under 16 weeks of age, display the so-called hepato-tracheal migration, in which the larvae migrate to liver and further via the heart, lungs, and respiratory tract to the pharynx, from where the puppy swallows the larvae into the alimentary tract. The first larvae reach the intestine after migration lasting 1–2 weeks. The larvae mature in the intestine and start to produce eggs. In older dogs, the larvae do not usually penetrate the respiratory tract, but instead spread to all parts of the dog to settle in the hypobiotic dormant stage. This is called somatic migration. However, research has also shown that infections in adult dogs, caused by few infective eggs, lead not necessarily to a somatic migration, but instead to the development of adult, reproductive worms.

It is crucial for *Toxocara* epidemiology that the parasite may migrate from the bitch to the puppy transplacentally before birth and via suckling as galactogenic infection soon after whelping. The hypobiotic larval stages activate in the dam at the last third of the gestation and move through the placenta to the puppy's lungs to wait for the birth and access via pharynx to the intestine. The larvae emerging from hypobiosis in the dam also migrate to the mammary gland and further to the sucking puppies via the transmammary route. The transmammary transmission does not usually include larval migration in the puppy, but instead the complete larval development takes place in the intestine. Infective eggs may end up from the environment also to the bodies of paratenic host animals, e.g., small rodents. No parasite development happens in the paratenic host. Instead, the infection survives up to 10 years in the form

of hypobiotic L3 larvae and may further transfer to a dog that eats the rodent or other suitable paratenic host. In addition to rodents, many other species can act as paratenic hosts, such as pigs, birds and humans. The survival of the parasite larvae in the paratenic host varies widely depending on the species. The *Toxocara* larvae seem to favor nerve tissue in the paratenic host. The paratenic host may transfer the *Toxocara* infection further to its offspring. An infection obtained from a paratenic host does not usually include a migratory phase. The prepatent period associated with *Toxocara* infection varies from 2 to 4 weeks depending on the infection route. If the puppy was infected at the fetal stage transplacentally, worm eggs appear in the feces at the earliest when the puppy is 16–21 days old. When infective eggs are ingested, the migration and maturation last about 4 weeks. The prepatent period associated with an infection obtained by eating a paratenic host is the shortest, often about 2 weeks. An illustrated life cycle of *T. canis* is presented in Fig. 5.4.

Morphology of *Toxocara canis*

Dog roundworms resemble spaghetti. The length of the male is 4–10 cm. The female is larger: 5–17 cm (Fig. 5.2) The dog roundworm has a complete alimentary tract that starts from the mouth surrounded by three lips (Figs. 5.5 and 5.6) and ends up in the cloaca, which is joined by the male spicules (length 0.75–1.3 mm). The lips are lined with a row of small, tooth-like protrusions (Fig. 5.6). In the front end at both sides, there are small, wing-like structures: the cervical alae (Fig. 5.5). There is a bulb at the junction of the esophagus and the intestine (Fig. 5.7). The tip of the male tail is bent into a hook resembling the handle of an umbrella, and there is a finger-like protrusion at the end of the tail (Fig. 5.8). The female has a straight tail. To the naked eye, *T. canis* resembles its close relative *Toxascaris leonina*. The most easily detected differences are the bulb between the esophagus and intestine and the shape of the finger-like male tail tip and the eggs.

Distribution

T. canis is the most common canine intestinal worm in the world. The prevalence varies between the regions and depend, for instance, on the culture of dog management. In areas with lots of stray dogs and lacking anthelmintic usage, the prevalence is high. The climate also influences the prevalence. Although the eggs survive in winter under the snow, their development to the infective stage stagnates or is arrested. The development continues with rising temperatures. Apart from the temperature, the infectivity is dependent on humidity. Drought is adverse for *Toxocara* eggs.

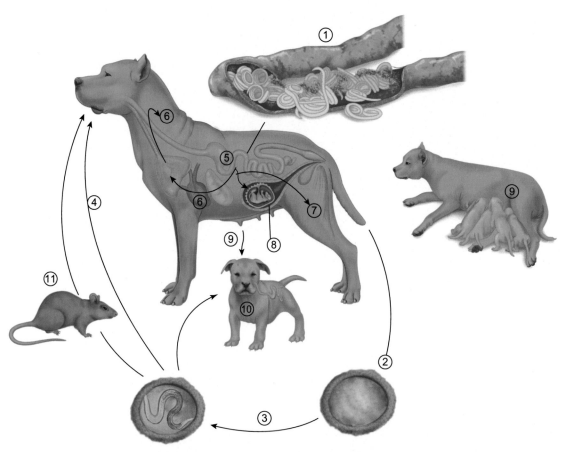

FIG. 5.4 Life cycle of *Toxocara canis*: (1 and 2) adult roundworms live in a dog's small intestine and female worms produce eggs that are voided to the environment in feces; (3) during the next weeks, infective larval forms develop inside the egg; (4) infective eggs find their way into the alimentary tract of a canid; (5) the eggshell breaks down in the stomach and the larva is released; (6) hepato-tracheal migration takes place in young puppies: larvae travel via the liver, heart, and respiratory organs to the pharynx, where the puppy swallows them into the alimentary tract, where they mature; (7) the larvae do not usually penetrate the respiratory organs in dogs over 16 weeks of age. Instead, they disperse to different parts of the body and settle in various places as hypobiotic dormant forms; (8) *Toxocara* infection may pass from the pregnant bitch to fetuses already before birth transplacentally, once the hypobiotic larvae have activated close to the end of the gestation; (9) the infection may also take place when the larvae that have activated postpartum migrate to the mammary gland and the bitch's milk; (10) the transplacentally acquired larval forms wait for the birth in the lungs of the puppy and after the birth are coughed up and swallowed to the gut to mature. The bitch may be reinfected when cleaning the puppies; and (11) infective eggs may reach the paratenic host's body also from the environment. The infection stays dormant in them and may be further passed to the definitive host, when it eats the tissues of the paratenic host.

Importance to Canine Health

Puppies experience the worst clinical signs. During the pulmonary stage, respiratory signs may manifest: irritation of respiratory tract, cough, rales, and even pneumonia. When the infection passes on to the alimentary tract, the signs change: vomiting, diarrhea, distended abdomen—despite weight loss—and pain start to affect the puppy. If the infection is severe, the adult worms may even penetrate the intestine, causing peritonitis and death (Fig. 5.9). In adult dogs, the infection is typically subclinical. There are no respiratory signs, but diarrhea, weight loss, and general malaise have occasionally been associated with *Toxocara* infection also in adult dogs.

Diagnosis

A quick diagnosis may be made if a worm with characteristic morphology is spotted in the dog's stools or vomits. Usually the diagnosis is reached with a method based on microscopy of eggs that have been extracted from feces (Fig. 5.3). However, according to a study, up to one-third of ascarid eggs found in fecal samples of dogs are in fact those of the feline roundworm, *Toxocara cati*. The feline roundworm does not infect dogs, but dogs like to eat cat's stools, and the eggs travel through the intestine to be detected in fecal analysis. Their feline origin cannot be reliably distinguished in microscopy, because the morphology is similar. In uncertain cases, the diagnosis

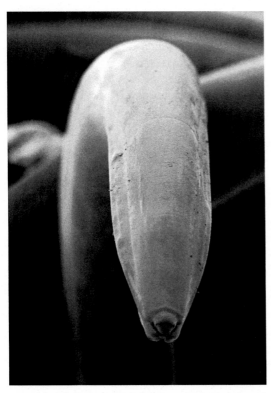

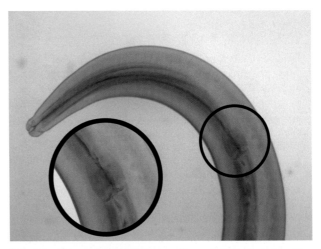

FIG. 5.7   The anterior end of a dog roundworm in light microscopy. *Toxocara canis* differs from its close relative *Toxascaris leonina* by having a bulge at the end of the esophagus.

FIG. 5.5   The anterior end of *Toxocara canis* in scanning electron microscopy. The lip structures surrounding the mouth and the cervical alae at the sides of the front end are clearly visible.

may be supported by polymerase chain reaction (PCR) techniques. The migrating larval forms of *Toxocara* can sometimes be found in histological samples or in bronchoalveolar lavage (BAL) samples or they can be seen in endoscopy (Fig. 5.10), when alimentary tract signs are studied. Besides finding worms in the intestine in autopsy, the tracts and inflammatory reaction caused by migrating larvae may be seen in many organs, e.g., in the liver and kidneys, as light necrotic spots.

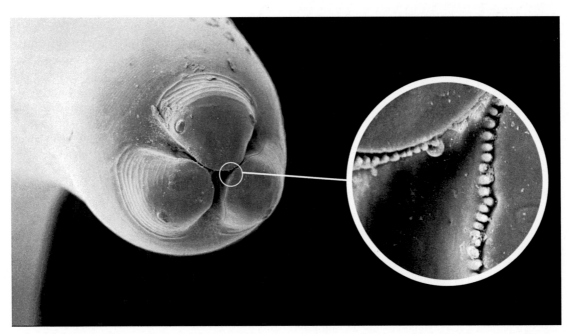

FIG. 5.6   The anterior end of a dog roundworm in scanning electron microscopy. The mouth is surrounded by three lips—one dorsal and two ventro-lateral—with sensory papillae. The round figure displays a detail of the ridge of tooth-like structures surrounding the margin of lips.

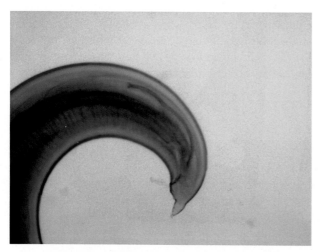

FIG. 5.8 The finger-like protrusion in the tip of the dog roundworms tail in light microscopy.

Treatment and Prevention

The intestinal *Toxocara* roundworms are easily managed with many different anthelmintics such as benzimidazoles, pyrantel, nitroscanate, and macrocyclic lactones. Resistance remains rare, although single cases of pyrantel resistance have been reported in countries with widespread use of this substance. Getting rid of hypobiotic larvae is a challenge. Fenbendazole, a member of the benzimidazole group, has been rather effective in preventing immigration into puppies, when given to the bitch daily from pregnancy day 40 on up to day 14 postpartum. However, an intensive dosing of this sort is rarely used except in kennels with a recognized roundworm problem. In practice, the puppy infection is managed by dosing the puppies from the age of 2 weeks in 2-week intervals until the puppy is passed on to new owners, and thereafter in the new home monthly until the age of 6 months. Analyzing worm eggs in the feces of the puppy is not much use, because the puppy may manifest severe signs already during the prepatent period of the parasite, when there is no egg secretion. Adult dogs have traditionally been given anthelmintics regularly, e.g., twice a year. Nowadays it is thought that one-size-fits-all instructions are not feasible, and a risk-based individually tailored parasite control should be practiced instead. The infection pressure and the zoonotic character of the parasite should be considered in the management of dog roundworms. A dog in a kennel needs more frequent dosing than a single dog living in home. The risk of human toxocariasis should certainly be taken into account, when the dog lives in a household with small children. The need for anthelmintics of an adult dog can be determined with the analysis of worm eggs in the feces. The frequency of fecal tests should be determined in cooperation with a veterinarian and considering the infection pressure. The fact that puppies secrete the majority of *Toxocara* eggs supports their frequent deworming. Environmental infections can be controlled by removing dog stools immediately to household waste before they have become infective. This is especially important in population centers and in the areas with a high density of dogs. Good waste handling prevents canine and human infections and is inherent in proper dog husbandry in maintaining general wellbeing. Cleaning the yard frequently, preferably weekly, of canine stools prevents the infections of family members. Hands should be washed meticulously after handling dogs and soil. Children should be prevented from eating gravel of dirt. Stools must be removed regularly in kennels. After the premises are washed, they should be allowed to dry, since moisture is advantageous for *Toxocara* eggs. Removing stools from pens diminishes the infection pressure. The yard soil should be replaced occasionally, since *Toxocara* eggs can survive in the soil for years.

TOXASCARIS LEONINA

- Large, spaghetti-like ascarid roundworm of carnivores, up to 10 cm long.
- Often found as a coinfection together with *Toxocara*.
- Infection from infectious eggs or paratenic hosts, not through placenta or milk.
- Infections are mostly asymptomatic.
- Diagnosis is based on the detection of typical eggs in a fecal sample.

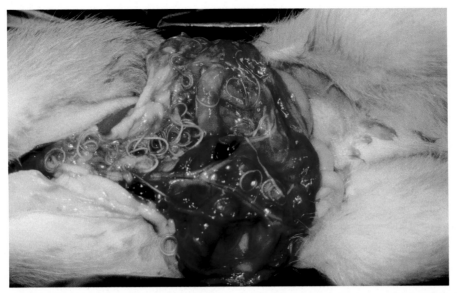

FIG. 5.9   The dissected abdomen of a puppy that died of a severe *Toxocara* infection. The roundworms had caused an intestinal obstruction, which had led to rupture of the gut and severe peritonitis. *(Photo by Marina Hultholm, reproduced with permission.)*

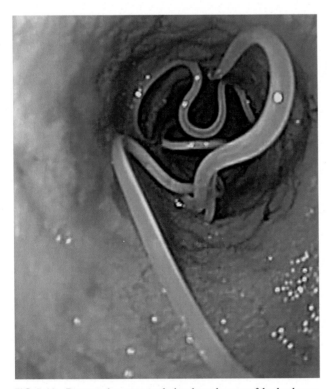

FIG. 5.10   Dog roundworms seen during the endoscopy of the duodenum. *(Photo by Thomas Spillmann, reproduced with permission.)*

Identification

Adult *Toxascaris* roundworms are large, spaghetti-like, cream-colored or pinkish worms with round cross-cut. They resemble *T. canis*, the other canine roundworm. Females can be 10 cm and males 7 cm long. Lancet-like wings, cervical alae, are located at the sides of the head. The mouth is

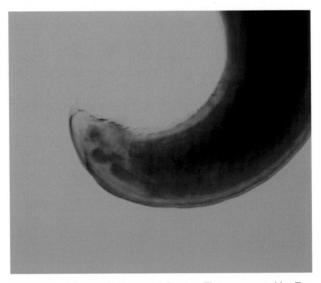

FIG. 5.11   Tail of male *Toxascaris leonina*. The worm resembles *Toxocara canis*, but the tail tip of the male has no finger-like appendage.

surrounded by three lips. The *Toxascaris* male lacks the finger-like caudal appendage (Fig. 5.11) of *Toxocara* as well as the posterior bulb of the esophagus. The eggs are typical thick-walled roundworm eggs, but have a smoother surface and are more transparent and oval than those of *Toxocara*. The size of eggs is about 85 × 75 μm (Fig. 5.12).

Life Cycle

The dog is infected by eating an infective egg or a paratenic host, e.g., a small rodent, with larval forms in its organs. The infection does not happen transplacentally or via milk. Unlike *Toxocara*, *T. leonina* does not migrate in the body

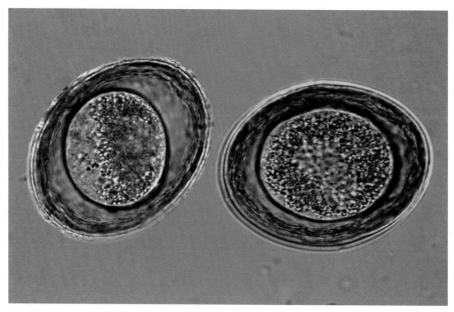

FIG. 5.12 The oval egg of *Toxascaris leonina* has a smooth exterior. Typical dimensions are 75 × 85 μm. *(Photo by Antti Oksanen, FINPAR, reproduced with permission.)*

of the definitive host. Instead it develops on the mucosa of the small intestine. Adult worms can be detected in the intestine about 6 weeks after infection. The prepatent period is about 9 weeks. The eggs produced by the female pass into the environment in feces. In suitable conditions, they develop into the infective stage rapidly, in about a week. Thereafter they can infect the following definite or paratenic host animal.

Distribution

Toxoascaris is endemic all over the word, but especially it parasitizes dogs, foxes, cats, and many wild canids and felids in cool climates. It is less common than *Toxocara* roundworm. The two species may also cause a mixed infection.

Importance to Canine Health

Puppies less than 2 months of age are not usually infected due to the manner of infection and the prepatent period. Clinical signs, if any, are limited to those of the alimentary tract, mostly diarrhea. The signs are caused by the mechanical damage of adult worms in the lining of the intestine, the immune response associated with the infection or possible secondary infections. In rare cases, the infection can be fatal, especially in puppies. However, *Toxascaris* is substantially less pathogenic than *Toxocara*.

Diagnosis

The diagnosis is done by analyzing a fecal sample with the flotation method and with the microscopical detection of

eggs produced by the female. *Toxascaris* eggs are more oval and have a smoother cell than *Toxocara* eggs. Otherwise they resemble each other. PCR methods have been developed for *Toxascaris* diagnosis, but usually the diagnosis is based on the morphological features of the egg.

Treatment and Prevention

Several anthelmintics are efficacious against *Toxascaris* (see *T. canis*). Benzimidazoles, pyrantel, and piperazine are most commonly used. Infections are prevented by removing dog stools from the environment and preventing the dog from eating paratenic hosts. Isolated and rare cases have shown that *Toxascaris* can infect humans. The infection risk is not considered great.

Morphology of *Toxascaris leonina*

The length of an adult *T. leonina* male is 2–7 cm in length and 1.5–2 mm thick. Females are larger, with a length of 2–10 cm and a thickness of 1.8–2.0 mm. Morphologically the worm closely resembles *T. canis*. Both species have cervical alae at the sides of the head. Those of *Toxascaris* are more pronounced and they give the worm a spear-like figure. Both species have three lips surrounding the mouth: a dorsal and two latero-ventral lips. When the worms are made transparent, for instance, with lactophenol, differences in the form of the esophagus can be detected: *T. canis* has a distinct bulb at the end of the esophagus. This is missing in *Toxascaris*. The tail ends cylindrically and the tip of the tail is missing the finger-like appendage typical for *Toxocara* (Fig. 5.11). The spicules of *T. leonina* are 0.7–1.5 mm long and almost identical to each other. The genital pore of the male is located closer to the anterior end or the worm, at the junction of the first and the second third. The genital pore of the *Toxocara* is more anterior, at the junction of first and second quarter. Another important morphological difference involves the eggs of the two species: *Toxocara* eggs are round or almost round and rough-textured on the surface. The egg of *T. leonina* is more oval and smooth-celled (Fig. 5.12). The dimensions are 75–85 × 60–75 μm.

BAYLISASCARIS PROCYONIS, Raccoon Roundworm

- Large, spaghetti-like ascarid roundworm of raccoons; can infect dogs; zoonotic.
- Infection caused by infectious eggs acquired from contaminated ground or by eating a paratenic host.
- Since dogs can act as a definite as well as a paratenic host, clinical signs and the damage done depends on the organs affected. Larvae may migrate to the canine brain.
- In raccoon habitats, the soil may be heavily contaminated with eggs.
- Patent infection can be treated with many anthelmintics, but migrating larvae survive the medication.

Identification

Baylisascaris is an ascarid roundworm of raccoons. It infects also dogs and can mature into an egg-producing adult in them. Adult *Baylisascaris* females can be 20–22 cm and males 9–11 cm long. Eggs are typical for roundworms: they have a thick surface and they are at one-cell stage in fresh stools. The egg is slightly smaller than that of *Toxocara*, about 80–85 × 65–70 μm in diameter. The larval stages migrating in the tissues are large, 60 μm in diameter and in histological cross section they have distinctive lateral alae on both sides of the larva. Several other animals, such as the badger, skunk, and bear, have their own *Baylisascaris* species, but since raccoons live close to human habitation in many countries, their *Baylisascaris* pose a specific risk to humans and dogs.

Life Cycle

The life cycle in the definitive host, the raccoon, is typical for a roundworm: the adults live in the small intestine and the females produce a substantial number of eggs that are extracted in fecal mass into the environment. Up to 250,000 eggs or more in a gram of raccoon feces have been counted. Depending on the prevalent climatic conditions,

the eggs become infective in a few weeks, after which the definitive host or the many mammals suitable for the role of the paratenic host can get the infection. The infection may be transferred to dogs also through eating the tissues of a paratenic host. In some dogs the infection proceeds into a patent stage, in which eggs are secreted in feces. People may be infected from the eggs, which can survive a long time in the soil. Migrating larvae may cause symptoms similar to those of *Toxocara* larvae. Children are typically in greatest risk, because their behavior exposes them to the worm eggs and their immunity is still immature. In contrast to *Toxocara*, the *Baylisascaris* larva continues growing while migrating in humans and causes more tissue damage due to its increasing size.

Distribution

B. procyonis is found in regions endemic for the raccoon in North America, Central Europe, and Japan. In some areas, almost all raccoons carry the infection. About 100 species of paratenic hosts, including rodents, have been recognized. The parasite is expected to infect dogs in increasing numbers. This is a concern since dogs and humans are in close contact and the parasite can cause serious symptoms in humans.

Importance to Canine Health

Since a dog can act in the role of the definitive host as well as the paratenic host, the clinical signs depend on which role is current. In the role of a definitive host, the dog may display signs of emesis and diarrhea, due to the adult worms living in the intestine, although definitive hosts usually do not show signs. In heavy infections, large *Baylisascaris* may also cause an intestinal obstruction. In the role of the paratenic host, the dog can primarily display neurological signs due to the tendency of larvae to seek after nerve tissue. Isolated larvae that stray into the central nervous system can cause severe inflammatory lesions and a serious disease, such as eosinophilic meningoencephalitis. Paralysis, ataxia, blindness, and somnolence have been reported in dogs.

Diagnosis

A patent infection in dogs can be diagnosed by seeking *Baylisascaris* larvae in a fecal sample, for instance, with the flotation method. The larval stages in tissue can be recognized morphologically. A PCR method suitable for analyzing tissue, feces, and soil is commercially available. The human infection is diagnosed from tissue biopsy or the presence of antibodies in serum. The latter also helps to distinguish the infection from *Toxocara* infection.

Treatment and Prevention

In areas endemic for raccoon, the soil may at places be severely contaminated with *Baylisascaris* eggs, because the raccoons tend to defecate in certain spots. The stools should be removed near housing before the eggs reach their infective stage, and dogs and children should not be given access to places of fecal contamination. The paratenic host may also serve as an infection source in endemic areas, and dogs should not be allowed to eat them. While intestinal *Baylisascaris* are easily removed with many anthelmintics effective against nematodes, similarly to *Toxocara*, larval stages migrating elsewhere in the organism are difficult or impossible to kill with anthelmintics. The dogs that are considered to be under heavy infection pressure are treated every month with a substance effective against nematodes.

STRONGYLOIDES STERCORALIS

- Nematode infecting humans, some strains also pathogenic to dogs.
- One of the smallest canine nematodes, up to 2.5 mm long.
- Canine infection is caused by parthenogenetic females and their offspring; sexual reproduction takes place in the environment as a part of the nonparasitic phase.
- Larvae cause infection to puppies orally, transcutaneously, or through milk. Auto-infection is possible.
- Infection is often asymptomatic.
- Diagnosis is based on detection of larvae in a fecal sample.
- The efficacy of the treatment should be monitored with fecal analysis; hygiene instructions must be given due to zoonotic potential.

Identification

The *Strongyloides* species infectious to the dog is *S. stercoralis*. It is among the smallest nematode worms of dogs. Females, eggs, and larvae are found in canine intestine (Figs. 5.13 and 5.14). Males are not present as all the adults are parthenogenetic females. The females are transparent and tiny nematodes, about 2–2.5 mm long (Fig. 5.15). The larva is 200–250 µm long. A genital primordium can be distinctly seen with light microscopy (Fig. 5.16). The eggs are oval and their size is 50–60 × 30–35 µm. Inside them, an embryonated larva can be seen.

> **Morphology of *Strongyloides stercoralis***
>
> The parthenogenetic females are transparent and reach a length of 2–2.5 mm (Fig. 5.15). Six lip-like structures surround the hexagonal mouth. They have a long, cylindrical esophagus that extends from the anterior part to the junction of the first and second third of the worm. The tail end is thin and sharp. The uterus has two compartments and contains a

> **Morphology of *Strongyloides stercoralis*—cont'd**
>
> small number of developing eggs. The genital pore and the anus are located in the posterior third. The genital pore is close to the junction of the middle and posterior third, the anus close to the tip of the tail. The larva is 200–250 µm long. It has a rhabditiformic esophagus, which is a type of esophagus with a narrow, long segment between posterior bulb and slight mid-length swelling, and tubular buccal cavity, which is significantly shorter than the width of the larval body. A genital primordium can be distinctly seen with light microscopy (Fig. 5.16). The eggs are oval and their size is 50–60 × 30–35 µm. Inside them, an embryonated larva can be seen.

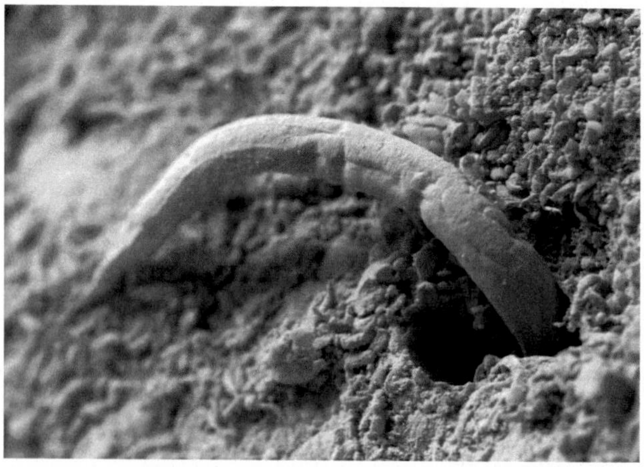

FIG. 5.13 A SEM micrograph showing female *S. stercoralis* embedded in the mucosa of the small intestine.

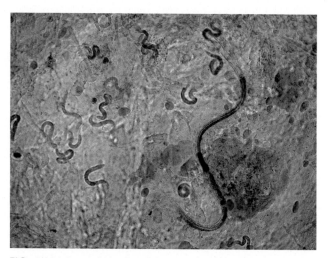

FIG. 5.14 A scraping taken from the intestinal mucosa of a puppy infected with *S. stercoralis*. Adult small female nematodes, eggs, and larvae are present. *(Reproduced with permission from Dillard K, Saari S, Anttila M: Case report—Strongyloides stercoralis infection in a Finnish kennel, Acta Veterinaria Scandinavica, 49:37, 2007, https://doi.org/10.1186/1751-0147-49-37.)*

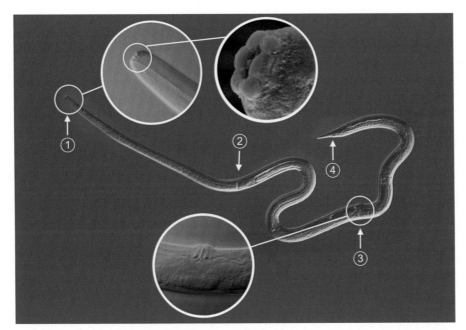

FIG. 5.15 *Strongyloides stercoralis* female in light and scanning electron microscopy. An adult parasitic female possesses long cylindrical esophagus that occupies the anterior third of the body. The genital opening (vulva, depicted in a detail) and anus are located in the posterior third of the body and the tail is narrowly tapered. The anterior end of a parasitic female *S. stercoralis* is depicted as observed under SEM. Hexagonal oral opening surrounded by six well-defined lips is clearly visible. (1) Anterior part with oral opening, (2) posterior end of the esophagus, (3) genital pore, and (4) anus as observed under SEM. *(Reproduced with permission from Dillard K, Saari S, Anttila M: Case report—Strongyloides stercoralis infection in a Finnish kennel, Acta Veterinaria Scandinavica 49:37, 2007, https://doi.org/10.1186/1751-0147-49-37.)*

Life Cycle

Nematodes of the *Strongyloides* genus have many characteristics that separate them from other nematodes. Their life cycle has typically two forms: a parasite stage, in which females reproducing via parthenogenesis maintain the population, and the cycle of sexual reproduction taking place in the environment, without a host animal. In addition, the *Strongyloides* are capable of autoinfection. This means that the offspring of the worms in the intestine can infect the same definitive host without the cycle stages taking place in the environment. All adult stages parasitizing the dog are thus females reproducing via parthenogenesis. They live in the folds of the mucosa and lay embryonated eggs, which hatch into L1-stage larvae (rhabditiformic larvae). The larvae exit the intestine in feces into the environment, where they develop either into L3 larvae (filariformic larvae) or they continue their development into adult *Strongyloides* living in the environment. An infective L3 larva infects the dog either orally or transcutaneously. The larva migrates in the dog into its predilection site small intestine, where it develops via the L4 stage into an adult female. The infection can be carried from the bitch to its puppies in

FIG. 5.16 First stage larva of *S. stercoralis*. It is 200–250 μm long. Genital primordium (*arrow*) is prominent.

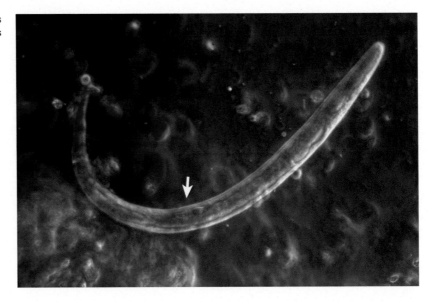

milk. There is no transplacental transmission. The parasitic life cycle of the *Strongyloides* is called a homogonic life cycle. If the environmental conditions are favorable for the worm, it changes into a nematode living independently in the environment and reproduces via a heterogonic life cycle. This means that the L1 larvae develop in the environment via molting into adult females and males, which reproduce. The eggs laid by the female develop into infective L3 larvae.

The rhabditiformic L1 larvae living in the canine intestine can very rapidly develop into infective L3 larvae, which can penetrate through the colonic mucosa or the anal skin. After the migration phase, the larvae end up maturing in the small intestine. This so-called autoinfection happens especially in the early stage of the infection, in small puppies and in immunocompromised dogs. *S. stercoralis* also infects people, although it appears that the strains adjusted to life in dogs are seldom pathogenic for humans. An illustrated life cycle of *Strongyloides stercoralis* is presented in Fig. 5.17.

Distribution

S. stercoralis is traditionally associated with tropical and subtropical conditions. However, many distribution studies and case reports indicate that the parasite can also live and reproduce in cool regions.

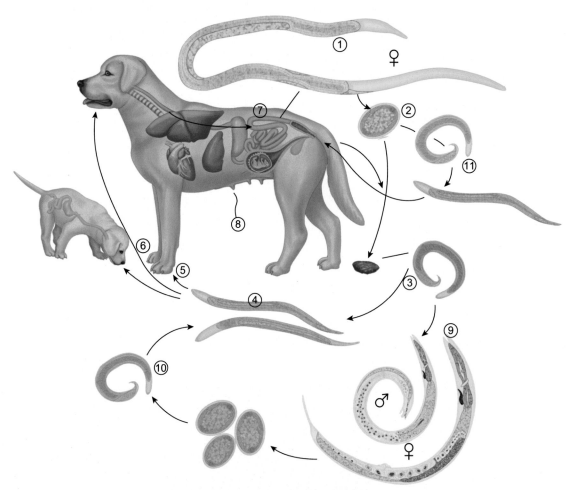

FIG. 5.17 Life cycle of *Strongyloides stercoralis*: (1) all adult parasites are parthenogenetic females that reside in the crypts of small intestine; (2) their embryonated eggs hatch in the crypts or the intestinal lumen; (3) the L1 rhabditiform larvae are voided in feces and give a rise either to L3 infective filariform larvae (L3i) or develop into free living adult nematodes depending on environmental conditions; (4) the L3i develops no further if it does not gain access to a new host. The L3i enters the dog percutaneously (5) or perorally (6); (7) the larvae migrate to the small intestine and molt first to L4 and then to the parthenogenic adult female; (8) the puppies can be infected via milk if the bitch has migrating L3 larvae. Transplacental infection does not occur. This parasitic life cycle of *S. stercoralis* is referred as the homogonic life cycle. If the environmental conditions are optimal, an alternative route of the life cycle (heterogonic life cycle) can take place; (9) noninfective rhabditiform larvae develop to free-living adult male and female worms that copulate and produce eggs; (10) noninfectious rhabditiform larvae hatching from the eggs will develop to L3i; and (11) during passage through the host intestinal tract, rhabditiform larvae may rapidly undergo molts into L3i. These larvae can penetrate through the wall of large intestine or perianal skin of the host, resulting in migration ending in the small intestine. The process is called autoinfection and it is favored especially in neonatal or immunocompromised hosts.

Importance to Canine Health

Canine *Strongyloides* infection is usually subclinical. Young dogs may often display diarrhea and mucous, loose stools, which may be blood-tinged. In a small puppy, severe infection may lead to weight loss and arrested growth. The puppy's appetite and activity remain normal especially in the early stages of the infection. In severe autoinfection and in immunocompromised dogs, there may be lots of migrating larva, which may stray into aberrant tissues. The result is often dyspnea, fever, and diarrhea. In these cases, the infection may be fatal.

Diagnosis

The L1 stages of *Strongyloides* larvae are often found in the direct microscopy of an unprocessed fecal sample. The use of the Baermann method to find the larvae improves the diagnostic possibilities significantly. In contrast, finding *Strongyloides* eggs in samples handled with the flotation method is rare and unlikely. Examining the contents of the duodenum produces larvae more likely than examining feces. Adult females, eggs, and larvae can be found by scraping the mucosa of the intestine (Fig. 5.14) and sometimes in biopsies taken from the intestine (Fig. 5.18). Adult worms are exceptionally small, but seeing eggs inside the worms helps to avoid confusing an adult *Strongyloides* with the larva of other types of nematodes. The samples from the suspected cases should be handled with caution, as the sample may contain infective L3 larvae with a possible zoonotic capability through the transcutaneous route.

Treatment and Prevention

According to the literature, *S. stercoralis* infections in dogs have been treated at least with levamisole, ivermectin, albendazole, and fenbendazole. Because there is no registered drug for canine *S. stercoralis* infection, the efficacy of any selected treatment should be confirmed first with 2–3 weekly Baermann examinations, followed with monthly controls for 6 months. All infected fecal material should be removed from the environment as household waste to diminish the infection risk of other dogs and humans. Using gloves or other protection when handling the feces and washing hands frequently, when in contact with a *Strongyloides*-infected dog, is recommended.

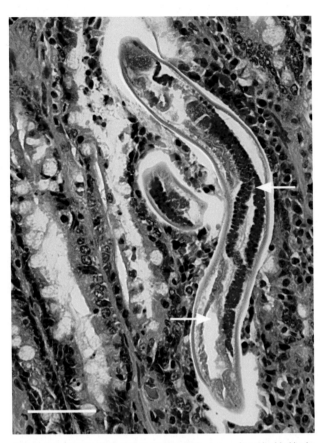

FIG. 5.18   Longitudinal section of a female *S. stercoralis* embedded in the mucosa of the intestine. The tissue sample has been stained with hematoxylin-eosin. The *upper arrow* points to the bifurcated uterus, typical for the species and the *lower arrow* points to the intestine. Bar = 50 μm. *(Reproduced with permission from Dillard K, Saari S, Anttila M: Case report—Strongyloides stercoralis infection in a Finnish kennel, Acta Veterinaria Scandinavica 49:37, 2007, https://doi.org/10.1186/1751-0147-49-37.)*

S. stercoralis Is a Zoonotic Parasite

S. stercoralis is an important human intestinal parasite in the tropics. It does appear that the species includes strains that have adapted to living in dogs as well as those preferring humans. Consequently, it is rare that the human gets an infection from a dog. Human *Strongyloides* infection shares many similar features with canine one. The subclinical carrier state or mild intestinal symptoms, with abdominal pains, flatulence, and mild diarrhea are the most common manifestations also in humans. A common symptom of chronic infection is infrequent urticaria of skin. Also in humans, the autoinfection can cause the infection becoming chronic. Indeed, *S. stercoralis* infections that have manifested 40–50 years after the exposure to the parasite have been described in humans. A chronic or sometimes even a recently acquired infection may develop into a life-threatening hyperinfection syndrome, in which the number of migrating larvae suddenly increases as the result of recurrent autoinfection, and larvae are found in organs that are not involved in the normal life cycle of the parasite. Defects in immunity caused by, for instance, malnutrition, tumor treatment, immunosuppressive treatment, or AIDS make hyperinfection possible.

PELODERA (SYN. *RHABDITIS*) *STRONGYLOIDES*

- A free-living nematode capable of invading hair follicles of several mammal species.
- Clinical cases are caused by contact with decaying detritus, such as moist stray bedding. Infection manifests as alopecic and crusting dermatitis.
- Diagnosis is made by detecting larvae in skin scrapings or biopsy.
- Correcting the living conditions of the dog is essential. Macrocyclic lactones and antibiotics can be used for therapy.

Identification

P. strongyloides is a small, saprophytic nematode living free in the environment. It is common in the decaying organic material, where it completes all stages of the life cycle. Within the species, the strain *P. strongyloides dermatica* has L3 larvae that can invade the hair follicles of several mammal species and cause dermatitis. For the correct diagnosis of the infection, it is important to be able to recognize the L3 and L4 larval stages. L3 and L4 are typical, worm-like nematode larvae with a thin anterior and posterior end. The length varies between 600 and 700 μm and the thickness in the middle 30–40 μm. The larvae are transparent in light microscopy. The exact diagnosis is based on the morphology of the rhabditiformic esophagus that has an elongated corpus, followed by a distinct swelling midway down the esophagus and narrow isthmus, ending aborally with a clearly defined valvulated bulb (Fig. 5.19). The worms that have invaded the skin are at the dead-end of their life cycle, since adult stages are not found in the skin.

Life Cycle

The entire life cycle of *P. strongyloides* takes place in the environment and the cycle does not require parasitic stages. The larvae that invade the skin are in L3 stage and cannot develop further than the L4 in the skin (Fig. 5.20). It is possible that the dermal larval stages may contribute to the survival of the worm population, when the environmental conditions are unfavorable, or to transferring worms to new locations.

Distribution

P. strongyloides infections have been reported in the United States, especially in the Midwest, and in central and northern Europe.

Morphology of *Pelodera strongyloides*

Only larval forms are detected in the diagnosis of *Pelodera* infection. If the skin scraping sample containing larvae is spread on blood agar, for instance, new worm generations and subsequently adult *Pelodera* rapidly develop on the medium. Adult worms have several features useful for species-specific diagnosis. The male has a well-developed copulatory bursa, in which 20 elongated papillary structures can be seen in microscopy (Fig. 5.21). Two papilla pairs are located bilaterally in the anterior side of the cloaca and eight on the posterior side. The papillae in the posterior side are further grouped laterally into groups of five at the anterior and groups of three at the posterior side. The spicule is seen in light microscopy as a light-brown, Y-shaped structure, as two of the most distal thirds of the spicules are conjoined (Fig. 5.21). The posterior end of the female worm is blunt, but it ends with a spiky appendage, about 20 μm long (Fig. 5.21).

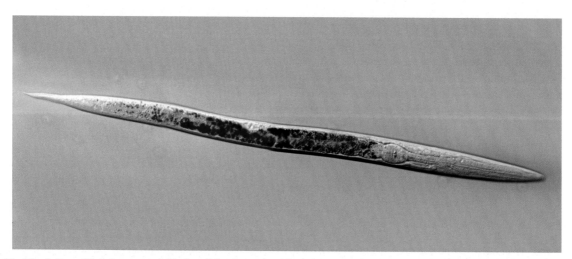

FIG. 5.19 Morphology of *Pelodera strongyloides* from light microscopy. A larva as seen in a skin scraping. The rhabditiform esophagus characterized by an elongated corpus, followed by a distinct swelling midway down the esophagus and narrow isthmus, ending aborally with a clearly defined valvulated bulb, is the most important morphological feature to differentiate *P. strongyloides* larvae from other nematode larvae. *(Reproduced with permission from Saari S, Nikander S: Case study: Pelodera (syn. Rhabditis) strongyloides as a cause of dermatitis—a report of 11 dogs from Finland, Acta Vet Scand 48:18, 2006, https://doi.org/10.1186/1751-0147-48-18.)*

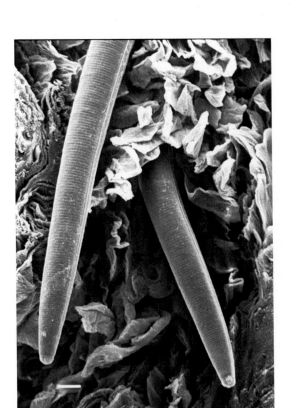

FIG. 5.20 A SEM micrograph showing two *P. strongyloides* larvae within a hair follicle with clearly discernible lateral alae and a striated cuticle can be observed intermingling with keratin. Scale bar = 20 μm. *(Reproduced with permission from Saari S, Nikander S: Case study: Pelodera (syn. Rhabditis) strongyloides as a cause of dermatitis—a report of 11 dogs from Finland, Acta Vet Scand 48:18, 2006, https://doi.org/10.1186/1751-0147-48-18.)*

Importance to Canine Health

Since this worm species lives in decaying detritus, canine clinical cases are almost always associated with a stay in this sort of environment. The disease history often tells about the dog being housed outside and the use of straw or other plant material as the bedding of the kennel or cage. Dermatitis lesions are often manifested in the skin areas that are in direct contact with rotting bedding straw, e.g., on the skin of legs and on the ventral surface (Fig. 5.22). Itchy, erythematous, and often crusting skin lesions are clinically observed on the contact surfaces. Alopecia is common. If the larvae or the inflammatory reaction they cause damage the follicular epithelium, the dermatitis is aggravated and often complicated by a secondary superficial or deep pyoderma with furunculosis (Fig. 5.23). Ectoparasitic differential diagnoses include demodicosis or sarcoptic mange, together with forms of contact dermatitis. A dog with *Pelodera* infection does not pose a serious infection risk to other dogs, and it is more important to correct the husbandry and make the conditions unfavorable for *Pelodera* than to treat the infection with anthelmintics. A case has been reported where a girl who had contact with a dog with *Pelodera* infection became ill with *Pelodera* dermatitis.

Diagnosis

The diagnosis is based on the typical case history (dog lives outside, straw bedding), characteristic dermal lesions (crusted and pruritic dermatitis and alopecia on contact surfaces) and the detection of *Pelodera* larvae in a sample taken with skin scraping or adhesive tape (Fig. 5.19). A skin biopsy can be used to diagnose *Pelodera* infection. A histopathological analysis reveals longitudinal and transverse sections of *Pelodera* larvae in the skin follicles. There is an inflammatory reaction in the follicles and the dermis (Fig. 5.24). The most important differential diagnosis is demodicosis, because the cross-sections of the worm and the inflammation are reminiscent of the histopathological changes in that disease.

Treatment and Prevention

Since the *Pelodera* live in decaying plant material, the essential procedure is to fix the living conditions of the dog. The bedding must be clean and dry. Correcting the circumstance alone usually is sufficient to affect a spontaneous cure. According to the literature, organophosphates, ivermectin, and selamectin have been used to treat *Pelodera* dermatitis. Antibiotics may be needed to treat secondary pyoderma.

UNCINARIA STENOCEPHALA, Northern Hookworm

- A hookworm up to 12 mm in length; endemic in temperate and cold climates.
- Infection is usually oral and acquired by ingesting L3 larvae or paratenic hosts from the environment.
- Mild anemia and gastrointestinal signs affect especially puppies.
- The larvae may pass through the interdigital skin of the dog and cause dermatitis.
- Detection of the eggs in a fecal sample and clinical signs lead to diagnosis.

Identification

U. stenocephala is a hookworm belonging to the nematodes. The female *Uncinaria* is 7–12 mm and the male 5–8.5 mm long (Fig. 5.25). The male has a well-developed copulation bursa. The buccal cavity is large and the chitin of the cuticle forms disk-shaped structures at the sides of the mouth (Figs. 5.26 and 5.27). The worm uses them to attach itself to the gut surface. The size of recently hatched L1-stage larvae is about 290–360 μm in the environment. When the larva is found in the skin, it is about 570 μm long and 28 μm wide. The esophagus of the larva develops from rhabditiform to filariform during the development from L1-stage

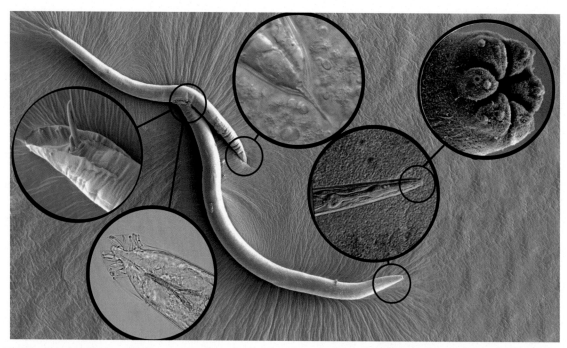

FIG. 5.21 Morphological details of adult *P. strongyloides*. A SEM micrograph showing a male and female worm in copulation. The round figures on the left display the posterior end of a male. The male has an open well-defined copulatory bursa with 10 pairs of elongated papillae. Two pairs are located precloacally, and the remaining eight pairs posterior to the cloaca. The anterior group of postcloacal papillae consists of five papillae and the posterior group with three papillae. Spicules form Y-shaped copulatory structure. The round figure up in the middle shows the posterior end of female *P. strongyloides*. The tail possesses a clear spine-like extension. Two additional round figures depict the anterior end of an adult *P. strongyloides*. The light micrograph reveals a deep buccal capsule and a rhabditiform esophagus, consisting of an elongated corpus, followed by a distinct swelling midway through the esophagus and the narrow isthmus, ending aborally with a clearly defined valvulated bulb. The SEM micrograph shows the oral opening *P. strongyloides*. Oral opening is surrounded by six well-defined lips. Distinct papillae are present on the lips. *(Reproduced and modified with permission from Saari S, Nikander S: Case study: Pelodera (syn. Rhabditis) strongyloides as a cause of dermatitis—a report of 11 dogs from Finland, Acta Vet Scand 48:18, 2006, https://doi.org/10.1186/1751-0147-48-18.)*

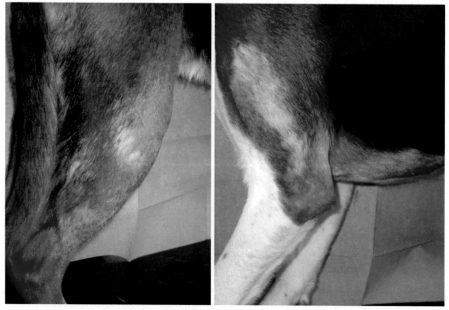

FIG. 5.22 A Finnish Hound with *Pelodera* dermatitis. Note alopecia and mild popular dermatitis with contact distribution affecting the extremities and ventral trunk. *(Courtesy of Pentti Tapio; Reproduced with permission from Saari S, Nikander S: Case study: Pelodera (syn. Rhabditis) strongyloides as a cause of dermatitis—a report of 11 dogs from Finland, Acta Vet Scand 48:18, 2006, https://doi.org/10.1186/1751-0147-48-18.)*

FIG. 5.23 A German shepherd puppy with *Pelodera* dermatitis and deep secondary pyoderma. Severe ulcerative dermatitis and deep pyoderma are observed. Affected areas have been clipped to show the extent of the disease. *(Reproduced with permission from Saari S, Nikander S: Case study: Pelodera (syn. Rhabditis) strongyloides as a cause of dermatitis—a report of 11 dogs from Finland, Acta Vet Scand 48:18, 2006, https://doi.org/10.1186/1751-0147-48-18.)*

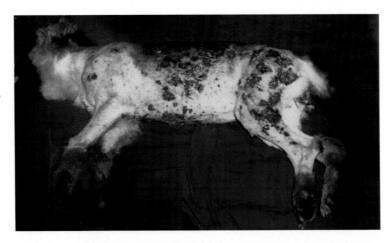

to L3. Two vacuoles may be seen cranially in the larva representing the precursors of the adult worm's buccal cavity. The size of eggs is about 68–80 × 40–50 μm. They are typical for the suborder Strongylida: oval and thin-walled, and they contain two to eight blastomers when secreted into the fecal mass (Fig. 5.28).

Life Cycle

The life cycle is direct. The infection is usually oral and acquired from L3 larval stages that have hatched from eggs in the environment. The development of the larvae is strongly dependent on the environmental conditions. Similar seasonality has been detected as in nematodes of ruminants. The larvae do not migrate, but instead stay in the alimentary tract, attached to the gut wall with the cutting plates. Similar to their distant relative *Ancylostoma*, the larval forms can penetrate the skin, but the larvae of *Uncinaria* acquired this way do not develop into adulthood. A paratenic host may also act as an infection source. Infection is not passed on through the placenta or in milk.

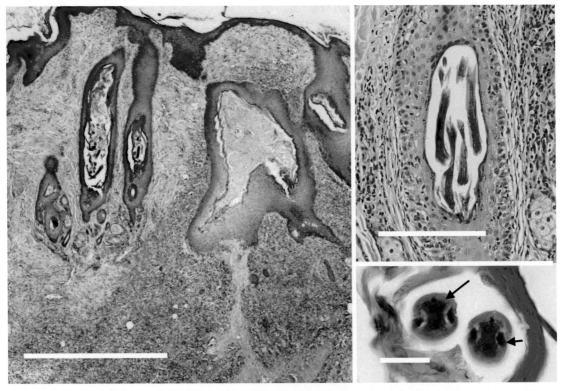

FIG. 5.24 Histopathological findings associated with *Pelodera strongyloides* infection. The left-hand figure shows histopathological findings from the dog depicted in Fig. 5.23. The epidermis is severely acanthotic. Hyperkeratosis is present in the epidermis and hair follicles. Numerous *Pelodera* larvae can be observed within the hair follicles. Severe folliculitis, furunculosis, and suppurative to pyogranulomatous cellulitis are observed. The upper right figure shows a superficial hair follicle distended with elongated larvae of *Pelodera strongyloides*. Lymphocytic mural folliculitis and perifolliculitis are present. The lower right figure shows a close-up of *P. strongyloides* from a hair follicle. Cross-sections of larvae demonstrate paired lateral alae (*short arrow*) and platymyrian musculature (*longer arrow*). *(Reproduced with permission from Saari S, Nikander S: Case study: Pelodera (syn. Rhabditis) strongyloides as a cause of dermatitis—a report of 11 dogs from Finland, Acta Vet Scand 48:18, 2006, https://doi.org/10.1186/1751-0147-48-18.)*

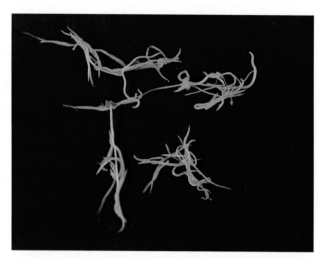

FIG. 5.25 Hookworms are Nematodes of up to 12 mm in length. They are endemic in temperate and cold climates.

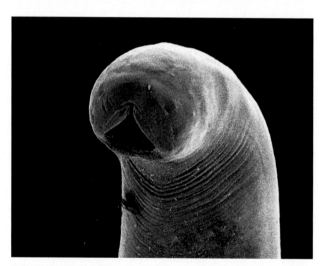

FIG. 5.26 Head of *Uncinaria stenocephala* hookworm in scanning electron microscopy. The cuticle discs surrounding the oral part are seen. The larger ones are located ventrally and the smaller dorso-laterally.

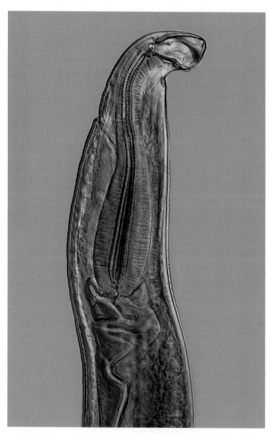

FIG. 5.27 *Uncinaria stenocephala* in light microscopy. The hooked appearance of the anterior part of the worm is clearly visible, as well as the large and funnel-like thinning buccal cavity and a well-developed, muscular esophagus.

FIG. 5.28 The egg of *U. stenocephala* is about 68–90 × 30–55 μm and is typical for Strongylida order: oval, thin-walled, and containing 2–8 blastomers.

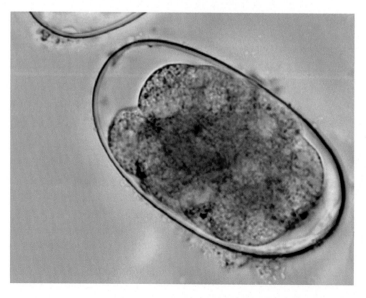

Distribution

U. stenocephala is endemic in temperate and cold climates, North America, and northern Europe. In addition to dogs, cats, foxes, and other wild canids and felids act as the definitive hosts of the parasite, although feline infections are not very common. In humans, larva migrans cases caused by *Uncinaria* are exceptional.

Importance to Canine Health

Uncinaria worms are not ferocious blood-suckers and therefore they cause only mild signs of anemia. The attached worms might damage the intestinal villi, which may lead to protein leakage into the gut. Hypoalbunemia may manifest. Diarrhea, anorexia, and lethargy are common in heavily infected puppies. The inflammation of interdigital and ventral abdominal skin is seen especially in dogs that have been previously exposed to larval invasion attempts. *Uncinaria* larvae

Morphology of *U. stenocephala*

The female *Uncinaria* is 7–12 mm and the male 5–8.5 mm long. Typically for hookworms, the anterior end is bent dorsally, causing the hook-like appearance of the worm (Figs. 5.26 and 5.27). The buccal cavity is large and funnel-shaped (Fig. 5.27). When the worm is made transparent, for instance, with lactophenol treatment, the groove-like dorsal gutter can be seen dorsally in the buccal cavity. The round mouth is surrounded by the disk-shaped structures of the cuticle, formed of chitin. The two most pronounced disks are located ventrally and the two smaller ones dorso-laterally (Fig. 5.26). The males have a distinct copulatory bursa (Figs. 5.29 and 5.30) with well-developed lateral lobes and a shorter dorsal lobe, partly divided from the lateral ones. The ventral branches of the bursa have a common stem and they are close to each other. The lateral bursa branches also share a common stem and they branch only in the distal part of the branch. Long and thin spicules that resemble

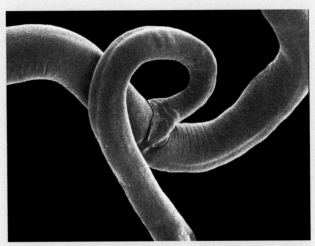

FIG. 5.29 Copulating hookworms. The male copulatory bursa clings around the female genital pore.

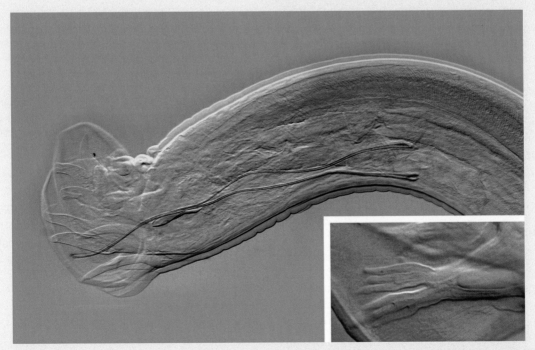

FIG. 5.30 The well-developed copulatory bursa of *Uncinaria stenocephala* male. The finger-like branches and the light-brown spicules can be seen. The spicules are long, thin, and similar to each other. The rectangle figure displays a detail of the dorsal ray of the copulatory bursa, which splits into two side branches, both of which divide into three processes.

Continued

Morphology of *U. stenocephala*—cont'd

each other are attached to the bursa. Their length varies between 0.6 and 0.8mm. The female genital pore is located somewhat posterior from the midline. The female distal end has a hook-like appendage. The size of egg is about 68–90 × 30–55 μm and the eggs are typical for Strongylida suborder: oval, thin-walled, and containing two to eight blastomers when the eggs are secreted into feces (Figs. 5.28 and 5.31).

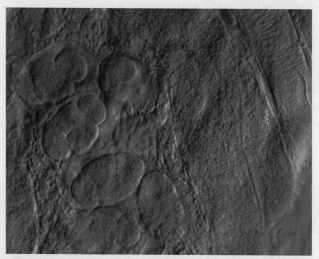

FIG. 5.31 Close-up of a hookworm female. Part of the uterus containing Strongylida-type eggs.

can cause skin infections also in humans, albeit much more infrequently than the *Ancylostoma*.

Diagnosis

Finding many hookworm eggs in feces with the flotation method suggests of an infection. If needed, the infection can be differentiated from that of *Ancylostoma* with larval culture and morphological examination. In puppies, the signs can manifest as early as the prepatent period, when eggs are not yet secreted in feces. When analyzing stool samples, it should be kept in mind that canine sample may contain other Strongylidia-type eggs, eaten by the dog in the stools of other animals, such as the horse, ruminants, or lagomorphs, and treatment is not required in these cases. The involvement of *Uncinaria* in skin lesions is suspected if the skin biopsy contains nematode larvae and the lesions are located in sites that have been in contact with soil.

Treatment and Prevention

Benzimidazoles, macrocyclic lactones, pyrantel, milbemycin oxime, piperazine, and nitroscanate can be used in the management of hookworm infection. The interdigital dermatitis is resistant to treatment, but heals spontaneously with time, if reinfections are prevented. The infective larvae in the environment are sensitive to drought and sunlight, which can be considered when choosing the material for the base of the pens in a kennel. Keeping a dog's

environment clean and dry is essential for the prevention of hookworm infestations.

ANCYLOSTOMA CANINUM, Hookworm

- A hookworm up to 22mm long, endemic in warm climates.
- The dog gets the infection by swallowing the larva, or the larva penetrates the skin. Puppies may be infected by eating a paratenic host or through the bitch's milk.
- Adult worms suck blood and may cause severe anemia and gastro-intestinal signs, especially in puppies.
- Transcutaneous infections cause dermatitis, which resolves about a week after onset o the infection.
- Several anthelmintics have been used, along with supportive therapy. Anthelmintic resistance has been reported.

Identification

A. caninum hookworm is endemic in warm climates. It is usually light-grayish (Fig. 5.32). After eating, there is a red tinge due to the blood visible through the cuticle. The female is 15–22mm and the male about 12mm long. The male has a clearly visible copulatory bursa (Fig. 5.33). Characteristically for hookworms, the posture of the worm is bent at the oral end. The buccal cavity is large and the extensions of the cuticle form tooth-like structures to its side (Fig. 5.34). The size of eggs is about 40–65 μm and they are typical for Strongylida suborder: oval, thin-walled, and containing two to eight blastomers when the eggs are secreted into feces.

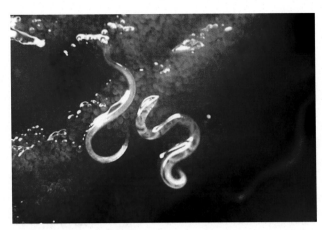

FIG. 5.32 Adult hookworms attached to a dog's small intestine. *(Photo by CDC, reproduced with permission from Science Source Images.)*

Life Cycle

Ancylostoma has a direct life cycle. The eggs secreted in feces into the environment hatch and develop through molting into infective L3-stage larvae. In suitable conditions this takes 5 days. The dog gets the infection by swallowing the larva, or the larva penetrates the skin, usually between the toes. A paratenic host can also serve as the infection source, or puppies may be infected from the bitch's milk, once the dormant hypobiotic larva stages have become active. The infection is not passed transplacentally.

In transcutaneous infection, the larva migrates in circulation into the lungs and molts there, reaching the L4 state. Having arrived in the pharynx through the trachea, the larvae are swallowed into the alimentary tract, where the last molting and the maturation take place. Part of the larval stages reaching the lung do not continue development

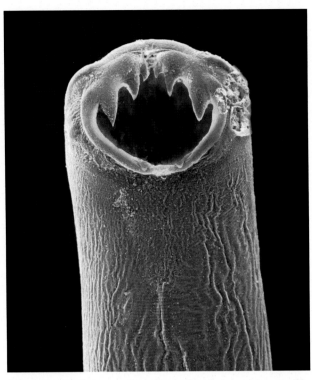

FIG. 5.34 *Ancylostoma caninum* in scanning electron microscopy. The large buccal cavity and the triangular tooth-like structures surrounding the mouth are visible. Three most strongly developed pairs are located ventrally. Dorsally, there is more weakly developed "teeth."

immediately, but instead are passed by circulation into the muscles, where they descend into the hypobiotic state. One infection of a bitch can be passed to three subsequent litters, when the hypobiotic larvae have become active at the end of the pregnancy and migrated to the mammary gland.

FIG. 5.33 Copulatory bursa of male *Ancylostoma caninum* in scanning electron microscopy.

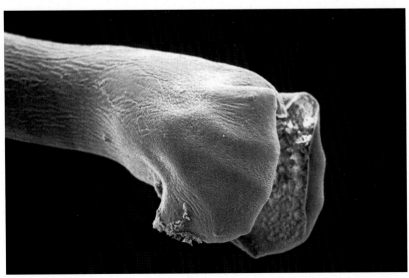

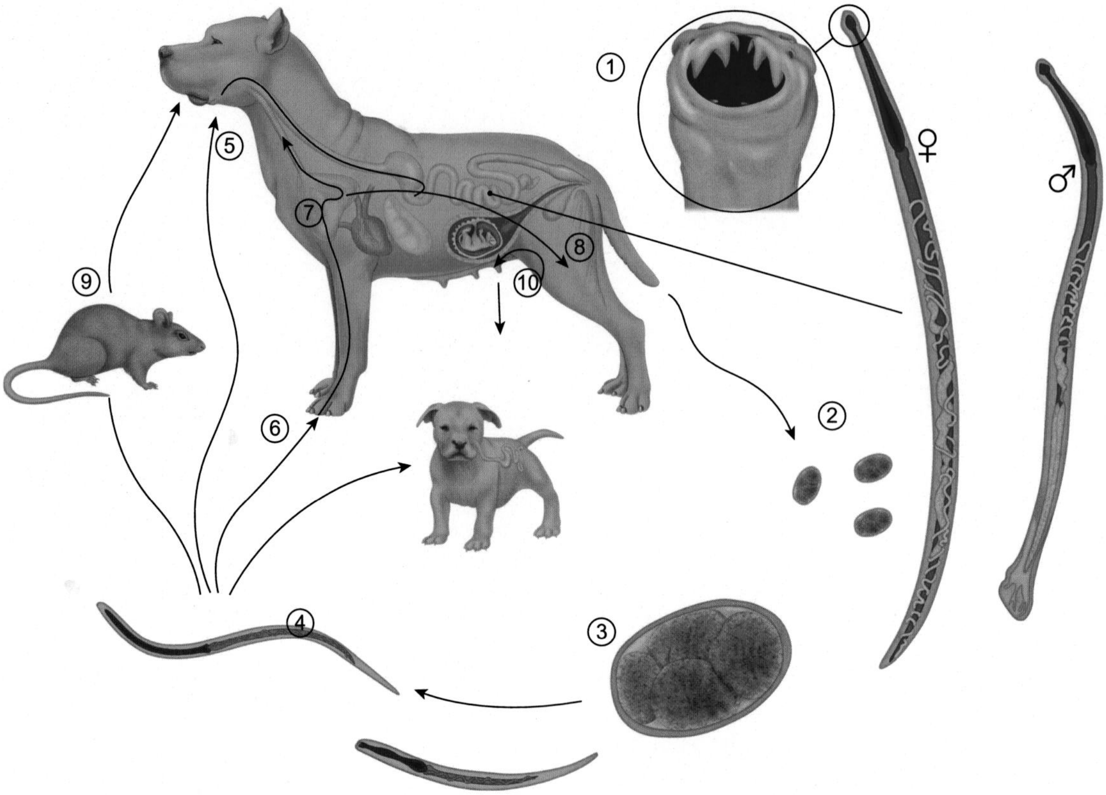

FIG. 5.35 Life cycle of *Ancylostoma caninum*: (1) adult hookworms live attached into the mucosa of the canine intestine and suck blood; (2) as a result of sexual reproduction, eggs are secreted into the environment in canine feces; (3) a larval stage develops inside the egg, and it hatches in the environment; (4) the life cycle in the environment consists of the development of the larva from stage L1 to infectious L3; (5) in orally acquired infection, the larva may penetrate the oral mucosa and migrate in a similar manner as in transcutaneous infection, or it can travel directly into the intestine; (6) larvae living free in the soil may penetrate the dog's skin, typically through the interdigital skin, and cause an infection; (7) the larvae end up in the lungs, and they are coughed to the pharynx and swallowed in the alimentary tract to mature; (8) part of the larval stages are passed by circulation into the muscles, where they descend into the hypobiotic state; (9) a paratenic host can also serve as the infection source; and (10) puppies may be infected from the bitch's milk, once the dormant hypobiotic larva stages have become active.

In oral infection, the larva may penetrate the oral mucosa and migrate in a similar manner as in transcutaneous infection, or it can go directly into the alimentary tract, where maturation takes place after a brief period of staying in the gut wall after the development stage.

Hookworms are blood-suckers. They grasp the intestinal mucosa with their oral parts, when the dental structures have grown to maturing hookworms in about 8 days after infection. The worms switch sucking site at a few hours' interval. The prepatent period is 2–3 weeks, after which millions of eggs are secreted into the feces daily during several weeks. An illustrated life cycle of A. caninum is presented in Fig. 5.35.

at the skin of the foot or the shin (areas in contact with soil), from where the larva begins to migrate forming winding, erythematous, pruritic lesions in the skin, the so-called creeping eruption (Fig. 5.36). The lesions recover usually without treatment in a few months. In some rare cases, the canine *Ancylostoma* may succeed to migrate into the human gut and to induce eosinophilic enteritis. The canine hookworm is, however, incapable of producing reproductive worms in the human intestine. The human has its own hookworm species.

A. caninum Infection Is a Zoonosis

Canine *Ancylostoma* can be pathogenic for humans. The transcutaneously passed L3 larvae may cause a condition called cutaneous larva migrans (CLM). In the early stages, a small, reddish, and protruding lesion is seen most common

Distribution

A. caninum is endemic in tropics and in temperate regions. In cooler climates, it is detected in imported dogs. Foxes can also act as definitive hosts for the parasite. Humans can be infected accidentally with cutaneous larva migrans, although they cannot be definitive hosts.

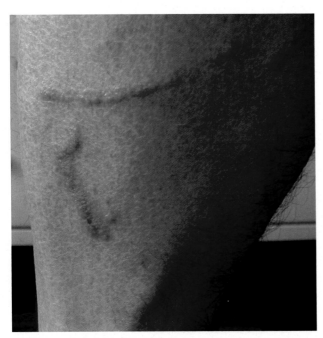

FIG. 5.36 Larva migrans lesions caused by migrating hookworm larvae in the skin. *(Reproduced with permission from Christel Sivula.)*

Importance to Canine Health

Puppies are most severely affected due to acute or chronic blood loss and anemia. Since one worm sucks about 0.1 mL blood daily, a severe infection can quickly lead to anemia. In addition, A. caninum secretes anticoagulants, which exacerbates the blood loss. The worms change frequently the sucking site. Due to anticoagulants, bleeding continues although the worm has left the site. A single worm can consume up to 0.1 mL blood within 24 h. One hundred worms consume up to 10 mL just in 1 day and leave about 600 injuries that continue bleeding. A few worms in healthy adult animals may remain asymptomatic. However, heavy infections cause hemorrhage and anemia due to blood loss that can be substantial, and even fatal. Dark and bloody diarrhea and vomiting are often observed, as well as pale mucosae (mucous membranes, e.g., the gums), weakness, apathy, and dull dry fur. In adult dogs, the infection is usually less severe and the bone marrow is able to compensate the blood loss for a long time. In the end, iron deficiency and corresponding anemia may manifest.

Small puppies are prone for diarrhea, which can be bloody. The pulmonary signs are caused by migrating larvae in the lung or the lack of oxygen caused by anemia. In transcutaneous infection, the skin areas exposed to larval migration may be infected and undergo ulceration, especially if the dog has earlier been sensitized to the parasite. In chronic infection, the general condition of the dog and the fur coat deteriorate, the weight diminishes, and the appetite is poor. Pica (eating unusual objects) can manifest.

Transcutaneously passed larval forms may cause erythema, pruritus, and papules especially in the skin between toes. The signs usually resolve spontaneously about 5 days after they have appeared.

Diagnosis

Finding many hookworm eggs (Fig. 5.28) in feces with the flotation method suggests of an infection. It should be noted that the signs may manifest during the prepatent period in a puppy. Canine stool samples may contain Strongylida-type eggs, eaten by the dog in the stools of other animals, which may lead to a false-positive diagnosis. No treatment is indicated in these cases.

Treatment and Prevention

Benzimidazoles, macrocyclic lactones, emodepsid, pyrantel, or nitroscanate can be used in the treatment. Pyrantel resistance has been reported. Supportive treatment can include iron and vitamin B12 supplementation to correct anemia. A diet rich in protein may be necessary. Anemic puppies may need a blood transfusion.

The infective larval stages survive in the environment of moist and shady sites for weeks, but they are sensitive to drought and sunlight. The material for the base of an outside yard should be chosen so that it does not maintain moisture. If a yard contaminated with *Ancylostoma* needs to be disinfected, sodium borate can be used, although this kills off the vegetation too. Infection foci may hide inside kennels. Moisture may persist in damaged surfaces, and the cleaning is difficult. Maintaining a clean and dry environment is essential for prevention of hookworm infestation. The dogs should not be allowed to defecate in children's play areas. In endemic areas, it is advisable to wear shoes and gloves, and to use a waterproof seat or mattress to prevent direct contact with the earth.

> **Morphology of *Ancylostoma caninum***
>
> The *Ancylostoma* female is 15–22 mm and the male about 12 mm long. Typically for hookworms, the anterior end is bent dorsally, causing the hook-like appearance of the worm. The buccal cavity is large and ball-shaped. The extensions of the cuticle form triangular tooth-like structures around the oral opening. There are three pairs of them ventrally and one smaller pair dorsally (Fig. 5.34). The male has a distinct copulatory bursa with well-developed lateral lobes and a shorter dorsal lobe (Fig. 5.33). The ventral rays of the bursa have a common stem and they are close to each other. The lateral bursal rays also share a common stem and they branch only in the distal part of the branch. The externo-dorsal bursal ray diverges with the dorsal branch from the common stem.

Continued

Morphology of *Ancylostoma caninum*—cont'd

Each dorsal bursal ray is further divided into three branches. Long, thin, and thread-like spicules that resemble each other are attached to the bursa. Their length varies between 0.73 and 0.96 mm. The female vulva is located in the junction between the middle third and the posterior third of the worm. There is a hooked appendage in the distal end of the female. The size of eggs is 65–40 μm and they are typical for the Strongylida suborder: oval, thin-walled, and containing two to eight blastomers when the eggs are secreted into feces.

ANCYLOSTOMA BRAZILIENSE

A. braziliense is endemic in dogs and cats in subtropical regions around the world. In contrast to *A. caninum*, it is not an important as a blood-sucking parasite—as its clinical significance arises from the intestinal signs, diarrhea, and protein-losing enteropathy. The larvae can penetrate the human skin, but they do not invade it very deeply. The infection passes in a few weeks and the larvae are destroyed in the skin.

OSLERUS (SYN. *FILAROIDES*) OSLERI

- Canine respiratory tract parasite; resides in nodules at the lower end and bifurcation of the trachea and bronchi.
- A kennel problem with low prevalence all over the world.
- Larvae in bitch's saliva or (less frequently) in feces infect puppies.
- Exercise intolerance and respiratory signs such as persistent, dry, and hacking cough are associated with the infection.
- Bronchoscopy is the recommended diagnostic technique, as it allows the visual location of the nodules. Sputum can be analyzed for the presence of larvae.

Identification

Oslerus osleri (former *Filaroides osleri*) is the canine lungworm, a Metastrongyloidea nematode living in the pulmonary tract, usually in the bifurcation of the trachea and the bronchi (Figs. 5.37 and 5.38). The males are about half a centimeter long and the female 9–15 mm. The tip of the tail of the male worm is round and it has no copulatory bursa. Instead, it has a bilateral row of a few papillae. The spicules are short and slightly curved. They are not totally identical. The tail tip of the female is round as well. Both the anus and the genital pore are located subterminally close to the end of the tail. The size of the egg is 50 × 80 μm.

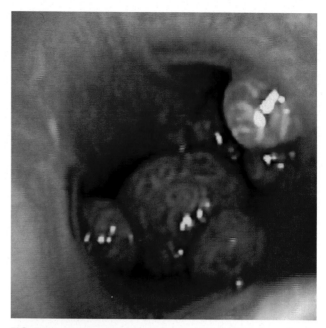

FIG. 5.37 Nodules typical for *Oslerus osleri* infection, obstructing the airways, seen in endoscopy. The worms are faintly visible through the thinning epithelium. *(Reproduced with permission from Thomas Spillmann.)*

It contains a larva immediately after having been secreted. The length of the first stage larva is about 350 μm and it has an S-bend in the tail.

Life Cycle

In contrast to most other canine lungworms, the life cycle of *Oslerus* is probably direct. The worms live in the dog's alveoli and the bronchi, and the predilection site for adults is the bifurcation of the trachea. A pinkish nodule, consisting of the worms, fibro-vascular stroma, and inflammatory reaction, grows protruding on the surface of the trachea. The size of the worm nodules varies between 2 and 20 mm, and the first ones, with their maturing larval stages, can be seen about 2 months after the infection. Inside the largest nodules, there is a knot of adult worms, faintly visible through the thin nodule wall. They can contain up to over 100 worms. The nodules may be lined side-by-side at the tracheal bifurcation. The female worms reach out of the nodules partly and produce eggs that hatch already in the trachea. The hatched L1-stage larva is infectious and it appears that some of them are capable of causing the auto-infection, which means that they mature directly in their canine host. The larvae are coughed up or they migrate in mucus from the trachea to the pharynx, where they are swallowed into the alimentary tract. Having passed through the intestine, the larvae come to the environment and can infect the next dog via feco-oral route. Larvae secreted in this manner, however, are slowly moving and the more common

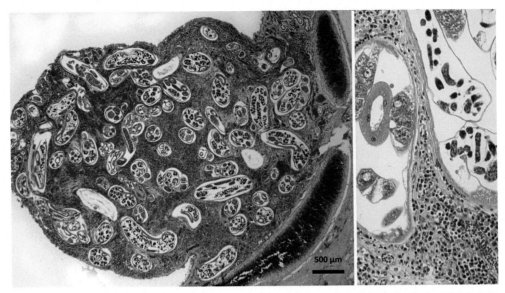

FIG. 5.38 *Oslerus* nodules in a histological section stained with HE. A cross section of the nodule that obstructing the bronchus is visible. Lots of sections through the worms and the accompanying inflammatory reaction are visible. The figure on the right displays a detail of a cross sectioned female worm and plasma cell rich inflammatory reaction.

infection takes place from the bitch to the puppies, when she licks the offspring. The sputum, together with the L1-stage larvae, end up in the puppy's mouth. The mother can also regurgitate food, and larvae with it, for the puppies. The larvae migrate from the intestine via the lymph and blood circulation into the lungs. The prepatent period is 10–21 weeks. For most other Metastrongyloidea lungworms the infectious larval stage is L3. This has not been shown in *Oslerus*. It is, however, possible that the L1 larvae coming to the environment in feces end up in invertebrates, where the development to L3 takes place. An illustrated life cycle of *O. osleri* is presented in Fig. 5.39.

Distribution

O. osleri is found infrequently but widely spread all over the world in dogs and wild canids. The prevalence in dogs is not high, and typically *Oslerus* is noticed as a kennel problem.

Importance to Canine Health

There are not necessarily any clinical signs. The signs usually manifest slowly and get gradually aggravated. Dyspnea and persistent, dry, and hacking cough, especially during exercise, may follow the infection. Exercise intolerance affects especially working dogs. The worsening cough can at worst lead to dyspnea, pulmonary emphysema, and pneumothorax. The number and size of the tracheal nodules does not always match with the severity of the signs. The dog may be suffering from a severe cough, while in the trachea there are only few parasite nodules of a few millimeters of diameter. Most clinical cases are diagnosed in young dogs aged 6–24 months.

Diagnosis

Bronchoscopy of the respiratory tract is the optimal diagnostic method, since it allows the examiner to take a sputum sample as well as to assess the location, number and size of the worm nodules (Figs. 5.37 and 5.38). The diagnosis of *O. osleri* infection is confirmed by finding pathognomonic worm nodules in the tracheal bifurcation. Sputum and pharyngeal mucus can be obtained as a smear without having to anesthetize the dog; however, false negative findings are common and the confirmation may necessitate several samplings. The largest nodules can be seen in radiography.

The larvae are secreted in the stools, from where they can be isolated with the Baermann method. However, there are fewer larvae in feces than in sputum, and they are not very lively. This makes the fecal analysis less sensitive. When larvae are found, the species-specific diagnosis can be done based on the morphology of the tail. The S-bend in the tail of *Oslerus* contrasts with the straight tail of *Crenosoma* and the wavy tail with a dorsal appendage of *Angiostrongylus*. The mouth of the *Oslerus* larva opens symmetrically in middle on anterior end. The histopathological analysis of worm nodules reveals that they are covered with respiratory epithelium, which is usually intact but stretched thin. The histological image is dominated by worm sections cut longitudinally and obliquely. Eggs and larvae of different developmental stages are commonly seen inside the female worms. The worm nodule is mixed with an inflammatory reaction consisting of lymphocytes and eosinophilic granulocytes. The nodules are usually equipped with connective tissue and blood vessels.

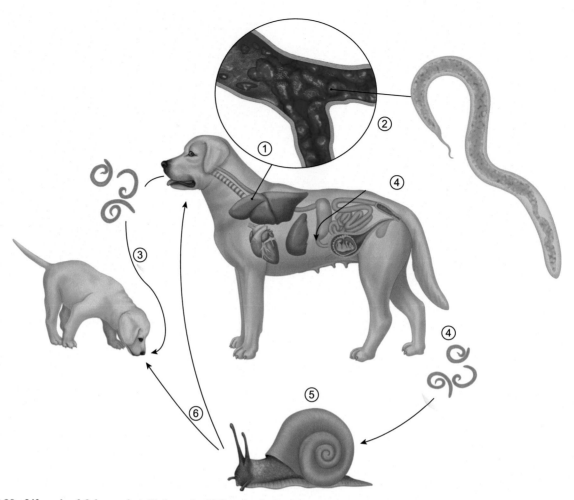

FIG. 5.39 Life cycle of *Oslerus osleri*: (1) the tracheal bifurcation is the predilection site of *Oslerus* lungworms. A nodule develops on the tracheal surface to protect the worms. Inside the largest nodules, there is a knot of adult worms, which can be faintly seen through the nodule wall; (2) females worms stretch out partly from the nodule and produce eggs, which hatch already in the trachea. The hatched L1 larva is infectious; (3) the most common infection method is when the bitch licks the puppies and passes sputum with L1-stage larvae into the puppy's mouth; (4) the larvae are also swallowed into the alimentary tract. Having passed through it, they end up in the environment and are to infect the next dog via the feco-oral route; (5) it is also possible that the L1 larvae coming to the environment in feces end up in snails or slugs, where the development to L3 takes place; and (6) through that route, the infection of the final host takes place while the host ingests the infected intermediate host.

Treatment and Prevention

Fenbendazole, oxfendaxole, thiabendazole, levamisole, doramectin and ivermectin are cited as some of the possible treatments against *Oslerus*. The nodules cause fewer signs, if the dog is not stressed and exercise is limited. Dogs living at home can usually manage the infection well. Preventive measures should be directed to kennel dogs, because the infection route between the bitch and the puppy is common. Treating the bitch before whelping can prevent the infection in puppies. According to the literature, it is possible to give the puppies to an infection-free foster mother immediately after the birth, but this method is neither practical nor in harmony with the welfare of the mother. The infection may also be passed between puppies kept in a same space via the feco-oral route.

FILAROIDES HIRTHI and *FILAROIDES MILKSI*

- Canine lungworms residing in lung parenchyma.
- Larvae in the bitch's saliva or regurgitate infect the puppy. Environmental larval forms may also be infectious.
- Infection is often subclinical, but respiratory signs may appear especially in immunosuppressed dogs.
- Diagnosis is by detecting larvae in a fecal sample.

Identification

Two *Filaroides* species are found in canine lung tissue. The adult worms are hair-like, small and about 0.4–1.3 cm long. Females are longer than males. A female

F. milksi is 116–174 µm and the male 50–101 µm thick. The difference of size, especially thickness, can be used to identify the species. L1-stage larvae are about 200 µm long and threaded, and their tail has a cleft before the thinner, hook-formed end.

Life Cycle

Adult *Filaroides* worms live in the lungs. They are ovoviparic. The females give birth to larvae or eggs, which hatch very quickly into larvae. The larvae travel with sputum into the pharynx and are either coughed out or swallowed to the alimentary tract. The most important infection route is the transfer from the bitch to the puppy with saliva or when the puppies eat food regurgitated by the bitch. It is also possible to receive the infection from larval forms found in the environment. The prepatent period is about 5 weeks.

Distribution

F. hirthi and *F. milksi* are endemic in canids in Europe, Japan, and North America. *F. hirthi* has also been diagnosed in Australian dogs.

Importance to Canine Health

In typical cases, the infection is subclinical. A severe infection may lead to dyspnea, cough, and other respiratory signs. An immunosuppressive state, such as powerful glucocorticoid treatment, cortisol-secreting tumor or another serious disease aggravates the signs of *Filaroides* infection. Autopsy findings such as small, grayish nodules under the pleura or focally in lung tissue suggest of *Filaroides* infection.

Diagnosis

L1 larvae can be searched in the feces with the Baermann method, but the zinc sulfate flotation is more effective in the diagnosis or this parasite. The species-specific diagnosis is done based on the tail morphology. The tail is conical and pointed and the mouth opens symmetrically in middle of the anterior end. The hair-like worms may be difficult to find in the lung tissue in autopsy. Squeezing the cut surface may facilitate finding eggs and larvae for microscopy.

Treatment and Prevention

Infections are assumed to be prevalent especially in kennel conditions. Since clinical signs are rarely displayed, treatment reports are scarce in the literature. However, the use of ivermectin, albendazole, and fenbendazole has been described.

ANGIOSTRONGYLUS VASORUM, French Heartworm

- "French heartworm," up to 2.5 cm in length, living in the pulmonary arteries and less often in the right cardiac ventricle.
- Infection from eating the intermediate host, a snail.
- The infection usually manifests with respiratory signs but also with bleeding.
- Diagnosis from the detection of the larvae in fecal sample. The tail of the larvae has a small dorsal thumb-like appendage before the bend.
- Macrocyclic lactones are commonly used for treatment, as well as prophylaxis.

Identification

A. vasorum, also known as the French heartworm, is a thread-like nematode living in the pulmonary arteries and in the right cardiac ventricle of dog and many wild canids. The female worm can grow up to 2.5 cm long, while the male is much shorter. The female resembles a barber pole with a helix of reddish and whitish stripes: the light ovaries and uterus form a helical structure with the red intestine. The species-specific identification of the male worm is based on the typical structural details of the copulatory bursa. Angiostrongylosis is most commonly diagnosed by identifying the L1-phase larval forms, typical of the species. The length of L1 larvae is 300–400 µm, while the width is about 15 µm. Other typical features of the larva are the bent tail and the adjacent small, dorsal appendage. The L1 larva of *O. osleri* has a similar bent tail.

Life Cycle

The eggs laid by the female *A. vasorum* are transferred in circulation to the pulmonary capillaries, where they usually hatch. The L1-stage larvae penetrate the walls of the capillaries and alveoli to the airways, from where they ascend with the sputum into the pharynx, further to the alimentary tract, and in the feces into the environment. The life cycle includes a gastropod intermediate host, in which *A. vasorum* larvae develop through the L2 stage and into the L3 stage, which is infectious for canids. The development takes 10–21 days. In cold conditions, it is slower than in warmth. The dog is infected by eating an infected gastropod or snail. In the dog, it takes about 1–3 months or more for the worms to become reproductive. Wild foxes have an important role as the source of *Angiostrongylus* infections. Apart from canids, other species may contribute to the epidemiology of *A. vasorum* infections. An illustrated life cycle of *A. vasorum* is presented in Fig. 5.40.

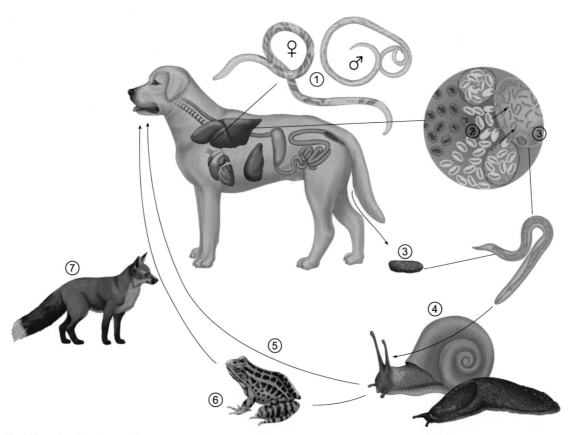

FIG. 5.40 Life cycle of *Angiostrongylus vasorum*: (1) adult *Angiostrongylus* live and multiply in large pulmonary vessels; (2) eggs laid by the female travel in the circulation into the pulmonary capillaries, where hatching usually occurs; (3) L1-stage larvae penetrate the walls of the capillaries and alveoli to the airways, from where they ascend with sputum into the pharynx, further to the alimentary tract and in the feces into the environment; (4) the life cycle includes a gastropod intermediate host, in which *A. vasorum* larvae develop through the L2 stage and onto the L3 stage, infectious for canids; (5) the dog is infected by eating an infected gastropod or a paratenic host (6) that has ingested the gastropod earlier. Shedding of *Angiostrongylus* larvae in the mucus of infected slugs and snails may enable and result in other routes of infection. For the worms to become fertile lasts from about a month up to 3 months in the dog; and (7) foxes serve as an important wildlife reservoir for canine *Angiostrongylus* infection.

Distribution

A. vasorum was first detected in a dog in the mid-1800s in Toulouse, southern France. This is why it is sometimes called the French heartworm. Today the parasite is found in different parts of the world, but especially in Europe.

Importance to Canine Health

Most dogs with clinical signs are young. Usually the clinical signs manifest only when the infection has been become chronic after months, sometimes years, of incubation. Tiredness, exercise intolerance and poor appetite are often seen in sick dogs. The most common signs of angiostrongylosis are cough, dyspnea, and tachypnea. The respiratory signs are primarily a result of an inflammatory reaction of the body, initiated by parasite eggs and the penetration of the pulmonary alveoli wall by larvae. The Cavalier King Charles Spaniel is a breed suspected to be more sensitive to clinical angiostrongylosis than other breeds. About one-third of dogs display different types of bleeding disorders.

Sometimes hemorrhage is the only visible sign. The pathogenesis of the bleeding disorders is not known for certain. It was previously assumed that the larvae cause an immune-dependent thrombocytopenia, but a more probable mechanism for bleeding tendencies associated with angiostrongylosis is the chronic intravascular coagulation syndrome (DIC). It is the state, in which a certain factor triggers exaggerated bleeding, exhausting the supplies of coagulation factors that are used for clotting, while simultaneously the lysis of clots through fibrinolysis accelerates. In addition, hemorrhage has been suggested to be caused by anticoagulant substances secreted by the parasite. The other theory is that the parasite stimulates the host animal to produce anticoagulants.

Various central nervous system signs have been found in connection with brain hemorrhage. At worst, sudden death may be the manifestation of angiostrongylosis. The cause is assumed to be the penetration of the parasite into heart muscle, or hypocalcemia, which has been suggested to be connected with granuloma growth stimulated by the parasite.

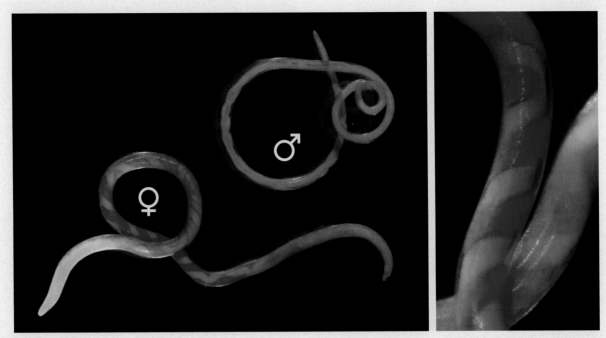

FIG. 5.41 Adult stages of the French heartworm (*A. vasorum*). The detail on the right shows clearly the helical structure formed by the female genital ducts and the intestine and resembling a barber pole.

Morphology of *A. vasorum*

Angiostrongylus is a nematode with long and slender body with tapering extremities. The orla opening is small and circular. The male is smaller and slenderer than the female (the average male is 12.9 mm long and 0.24 mm wide; the average female is 15.6 mm long and 0.27 mm wide) (Fig. 5.41). In fresh samples of female worms, the white genital ducts can be seen intertwined helicoidally around the red intestine through the fine and transparent cuticle. The male's copulatory bursa (Fig. 5.42) is well developed and short. Bursal rays are well developed: ventral rays originate from the common stem. In addition, lateral rays are originating from a common stem with the exception of an antero-lateral ray, separate from the other lateral rays. Dorsal ray is reduced and possess two digitations at distal tip. Spicules are long (approximately 0.47 mm in length), subequal, and strong. The female's posterior end is rounded. The genital opening is locating about 0.2 mm and anus about 0.07 mm from the terminal end. The length of L1 larvae is 300–400 μm, while the width is about 15 μm. Other typical features of the larva are the bent tail and the adjacent small, dorsal appendage (Fig. 5.42). The L1 larva of *O. osleri* has a similar bent tail.

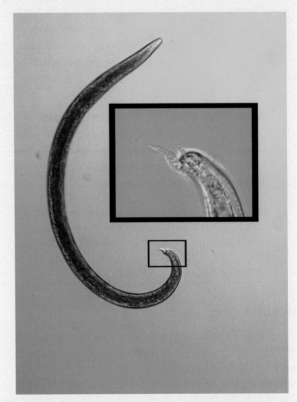

FIG. 5.42 L1 larva of *Angiostrongylus vasorum* in a fecal sample analyzed with the Baermann method. Features typical for the species are the bent tail and the small dorsal spine next to the tail bend.

Diagnosis

At present, the confirmation of the infection is based on finding larvae typical for the species in fecal samples or broncho-alveolar lavage. L1 larvae cannot easily be isolated from feces with flotation techniques. Instead, the sample must be analyzed by the Baermann method. The mouth of *Angiostrongylus* L1 opens symmetrically in middle of the anterior end. Other features typical for the species are the bent S-shaped tail and the small dorsal thumb-like appendage next to the tail bend. Other diagnostic options include analyzing antibodies against the larva or methods based on PCR techniques. As a nonspecific finding, eosinophilia of the blood is detected in about 50% of angiostrongylosis patients. Results of coagulation analyses vary between patients, and they can be totally normal. Radiography findings can also be nonspecific. A typical finding is a mixed image, with interstitial, bronchial, and alveolar densities of varying severity (Fig. 5.43).

Treatment and Prevention

Macrocyclic lactones, such as milbemycin oxime and moxidectin, are used to treat angiostrongylosis. The efficacy of fenbendazole has also been shown. In endemic areas, macrocyclic lactones are used prophylactically. Adult worms are long-lived. Without deworming, dogs can secrete *Angiostrongylus* larvae to the environment for the rest of their lives.

CRENOSOMA VULPIS, Fox Lungworm

- Fox lungworm up to 1.5 cm in length.
- Dogs may be infected by eating snails.
- Causes respiratory signs in dogs.
- Diagnosis is by detecting larvae in feces. The larval tail is conical, without specific morphological features.
- Several effective medications are available. The signs may worsen at the beginning of the treatment, due to dying worms.

Identification

C. vulpis is a Metastrongyloid nematode that reproduces in the lungs of the definitive host and may cause respiratory signs. Adult worms are about 1.5 cm long (Fig. 5.44). A folded cuticle is prominent in the anterior part of the body (Fig. 5.45). The fox lungworm is reddish and the alimentary tract and, in females, the uterus is faintly visible inside the worm. The L1 larvae are seen in sputum and feces is thinning, and it has no bend, spike, or protrusions, except for a small dimple close to the tip (Fig. 5.46). The mouth

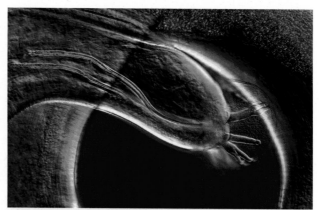

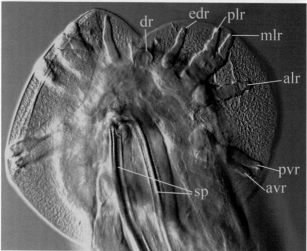

FIG. 5.43 The well-developed copulation bursa of a male *Angiostrongylus vasorum* as seen in lateral (upper figure) and frontal (lower figure) view. Characteristics typical for the species include the incision at the end of the bursa. The ventral bursal branches (avr, antero-ventral branch; pvr, postero-ventral branch) originate from a long, common stem. The antero-lateral branch (alr) is separated from other lateral branches (mlr, medio-lateral branch; plr, postero-lateral branch). The externo-dorsal ray (edr) is well developed and clearly longer than the dorsal ray. The dorsal ray (dr) is small and divided at the tip. The long and slender spicules (sp) are also visible.

opens obliquely at anterior end. The larvae are colorless, transparent, about 300 μm long, 20 μm wide, and are easily seen in light microscopy.

Life Cycle

Crenosoma has an indirect life cycle. Canids, most often the fox, are the definitive hosts, and the intermediate hosts include snails and gastropods. The definitive host is infected by eating the intermediate hosts. The infectious L3-stage larvae that develop inside the gastropods are released in the alimentary tract of the definitive host and migrate via lymph and in the hepatic and cardiac circulation into the lungs, where the *Crenosoma* larva develops, having molted twice, into a sexually mature adult. After copulation, the females begin to produce L1 larvae.

The prepatent period is about 3 weeks. Adult worms live about 10 months. The larvae migrate in the mucus of the airways via the pharynx to the intestine and further to feces and the environment. In the nature, the larvae reach the intermediate host by penetrating the foot of the gastropod, feeding on feces. Thereafter they mature during 3 weeks into L3 larvae, infectious for the definitive host.

Distribution

The fox lungworm is endemic all over the world in canids and several other carnivores.

Importance to Canine Health

Crenosoma cause respiratory signs. The infected dog coughs because of the irritation of lungs and bronchi caused by the parasite. The cough reflex can be provoked by pressing the bronchus from outside. Sometimes the dog sneezes and has nasal discharge and an increased respiratory rate. Fever and deaths are not common, as the signs of the infection are usually mild. It is common that a dog has received numerous antimicrobial treatments for a chronic cough before the possibility of parasites causing the signs is considered.

Diagnosis

The *Crenosoma* diagnosis is carried out with the Baermann method from a stool sample. In this method, the larvae in feces actively move though gauze or another type of filter into surrounding water and sink into the bottom of the vessel, wherefrom they are easily taken for microscopy. The L1 larvae move in a lively fashion and they can be seen clearly with an ordinary light microscope. The species can be determined based on the tail morphology. Since the method requires that the larvae are actively mobile, transporting and storing the sample must be done with care: freezing or otherwise causing the larvae to be killed leads to an erroneously negative result. The *Crenosoma* infection can also be detected with flotation methods, if the flotation solution is dense enough. However, the morphology of the larvae does suffer in hyperosmotic solution. Since larvae are infrequent present in stools, analyzing several samples can reduce the number of erroneously negative results. Sometimes bronchoalveolar lavage (BAL), carried out to investigate the cough, is diagnostic. L1 larvae and often eosinophilia is seen in a BAL sample, in which some of the larvae may be covered by a thin, membranous eggshell. Some dogs may display eosinophilia also in their blood. The radiological finding can be pronounced an broncho-interstitial pattern.

Treatment and Prevention

Many anthelmintics that are effective against nematodes can be used to treat canine *Crenosoma* infection. For instance, fenbendazole, febantel, and milbemycin oxime are used, as well as macrocycline lactones, e.g., ivermectin and the combination of imidaclopride and moxidectin. The prognosis is very good with all medical treatments. The control of intermediate hosts, in the form of getting rid of snails in the yard or stopping the dog from eating gastropods, is a useful preventative method. Early diagnosis and effective medication may also slow down the expansion of the infection, when larvae are not secreted for long periods into the feces of infected dogs.

Morphology of *Crenosoma vulpis*
The adult female *C. vulpis* reaches a length of 12–16mm (Fig. 5.44). The length of males varies between 3.5 and 8mm. Especially in the anterior part of the worm, 12–18 transverse, ring-like folds are seen in light microscopy. They make the surface of the worm appear segmented (Fig. 5.45). The male copulatory bursa (Fig. 5.47) is well developed and the finger-like branches of the bursa are long. The dorsal branch is without bifurcations, although papillar protrusions can be seen close to the tip of the branch. The lateral lobe of the bursa is further divided into two lobes. The gubernaculum can be seen in light microscopy. The spicules are thin and mid-sized; they are about 0.3–0.4mm long. The female genital pore is located in the middle of the worm. It is pronounced thanks to the surrounding cuticular plates. The L1 larvae (Fig. 5.46) are diagnostically essential. Their length varies between 250 and 340μm and they are 16–22μm thick. In the front end of the larva, there is a cephalic button. The esophagus is nearly cylindrical, with a slight posterior swelling; mouth cavity is inconspicuous. The larva lacks a tail bend as well as the spiky protrusion of the tail.

THELAZIA CALLIPAEDA and THELAZIA CALIFORNIENSIS

- Adult *Thelazia* are up to 2cm in length and live in the conjunctival folds and periocular tissues.
- The larvae are produced in lacrimal fluid, where flies, acting as intermediate hosts, ingest them and then pass them to a new host.
- Canine ocular signs vary and are dependent on the number of worms. Conjunctivitis and increased lacrimation are the most common signs.
- Diagnosis is made by detecting adult worms in the conjunctival folds, conjunctiva, or by microscopy of the larvae in lacrimal fluid.
- For treatment, the worms are physically removed and systemic macrocyclic lactones are prescribed.

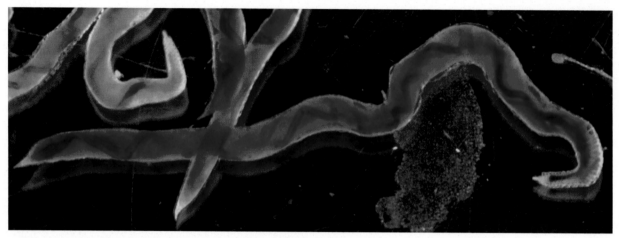

FIG. 5.44 Female *Crenosoma vulpis* is about 15 mm long. The figure shows the reddish color of the worm and the helix structure formed by the uterus and the intestine, faintly visible through the outer surface. The photo depicts also the cuticle folds of the worm's anterior end, giving the worm a segmented look. *(Photo by Antti Oksanen, FINPAR, reproduced with permission.)*

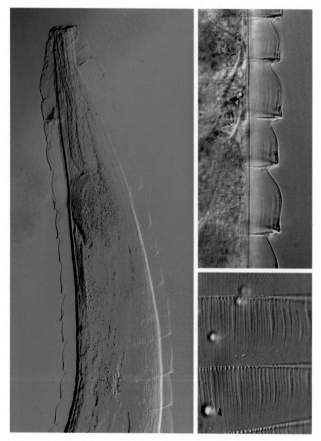

FIG. 5.45 The anterior end of *Crenosoma vulpis* lungworm in close up. The esophagus is quite short. The ring-like folds of the cuticle and the hem patters of their edges are clearly visible in the detail figures.

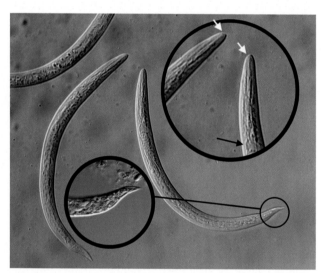

FIG. 5.46 The L1 larvae of *Crenosoma vulpis* lungworm. The larva is about 300 μm long. The tail gets abruptly thinner without bends, spikes, or protrusions. There is a small and slightly sloping dent close to the tail tip. The mouth opens obliquely at anterior end (*white arrows* in the round detail figure). *The black arrow* points to the nerve ring.

cavity and a rather short esophagus (Fig. 5.49). The lateral alae are missing from the male tail. The spicules are asymmetrical and they differ considerably in size and shape. One spicule is very short and sturdy and the other one is about 10 times longer and filamentous (Fig. 5.49). The genital opening of the female is located by the end of the esophagus.

Identification

The length of a male *Thelazia* varies between 5 and 10 mm and that of a female from slightly over 10 mm to almost 20 mm (Fig. 5.48). *Thelazia* have a well-developed buccal

Life Cycle

Thelaziae live in ocular tissues, such as under the nictitating membrane, in the folds of the conjunctiva or in the tear ducts between the eye and the nasal cavity. The eggs

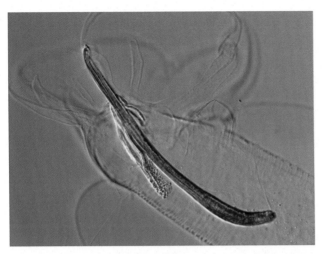

FIG. 5.47 The well-developed copulatory bursa of a male *Crenosoma vulpis* seen from the side. The very long finger-like bursa branches can be seen in the micrograph. Spicules, of which only one is visible here, are brown, similar in length, and medium sized. The lighter, stick-like, and partly granular structure below the spicule is the gubernaculum, which guides the spicules during copulation.

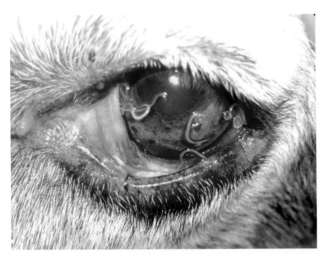

FIG. 5.48 Conjunctivitis and conjunctival edema in a *Thelazia callipaeda* infection. *(Reproduced with permission from Miró G, Montoya A, Hernández L, et al.: Thelazia callipaeda: infection in dogs: a new parasite for Spain, Parasit Vectors 4:148, 2011, https://doi.org/10.1186/1756-3305-4-148.)*

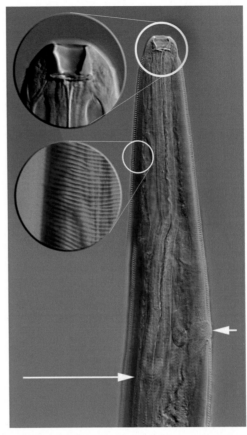

FIG. 5.49 Close-up of the anterior end of a female *Thelazia callipaeda*. The worm has a well-developed buccal cavity. The esophagus is rather short (*the long arrow shows the aboral end*). The genital pore is located close to the end of the esophagus (*short arrow*). The transversal striations of the cuticle are visible.

embryonate already in the uterus of the female worm, and the female gives birth to L1 larvae that are wrapped by the sock-like membrane formed from the eggshell. The larvae are born into the lacrimal fluid. Two-winged insects that use tear fluid as their food act as *Thelazia* vectors. Of these, the fruit fly *Phortica variegata* is most prominent in Europe. Larvae of *Thelazia* have also been found in *Fannia canicularis* and *F. benjamini*. The larva is released from the surrounding membrane in the fly and it penetrates the fly's gut wall and into the hemolymph of its body

cavity. The development continues up to the infectious L3 stage in the fly. The infective larva migrates further to the head of the fly. The larva infects a new host animal, when the fly seeks food in the vicinity of its eyes. Once the larva reaches the ocular tissues, it proceeds to develop into an adult worm. The maturation lasts about a month. *T. callipaeda* infects many wild animals, e.g., foxes, wolves, and martens, which can act reservoirs for parasitic invasions in nature. An illustrated life cycle of *T. callipaeda* is presented in Fig. 5.50.

Distribution

T. callipaeda is endemic in southern Europe (cases have been reported in Italy, southern Switzerland, France, Portugal, and Spain), the former USSR, and the Far East. The *T. californiensis* nematode, infectious for dogs, is endemic in northern America. Both *Thelazia* species are zoonotic.

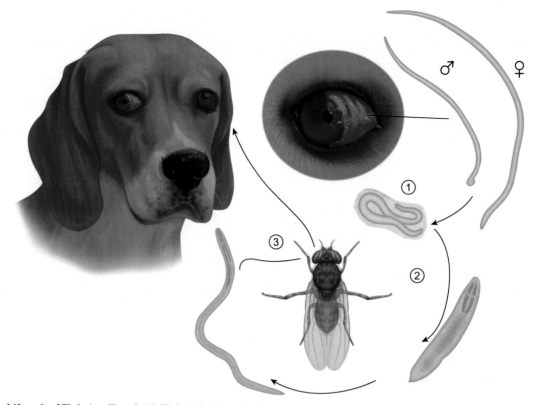

FIG. 5.50 Life cycle of *Thelazia callipaeda*: (1) *Thelazia* live in ocular tissues, such as under the nictitating membrane, in the folds of the conjunctiva or in the tear ducts between the eye and the nasal cavity. The female gives birth to L1 larvae into the tear fluid. The larvae are born wrapped by the sock-like membrane formed from the eggshell; (2) dipteran insects that use tear fluid as their food act as *Thelazia* vectors. The larva is released from the surrounding membrane in the fly and it penetrates the fly's gut wall and into the hemolymph of its body cavity, where it develops into the infectious L3 stage; and (3) the infective larva further migrates to the head of the fly. The larva infects a new host animal, when the fly seeks food in the vicinity of its eyes. Once the larva reaches the ocular tissues of the host, it proceeds to develop into an adult worm.

Importance to Canine Health

Many dogs do not exhibit clinical signs, but a variety of ocular signs may manifest. The severity of signs is not dependent on the number of worms. The most common signs are conjunctivitis and inflammation of eyelids, abnormal tear secretion, and ocular discharge that can be purulent (Fig. 5.48). Keratitis and corneal ulceration can also be seen. The worm-infested eye can be painful, which often manifests as squinting and photophobia.

Diagnosis

Since the ocular signs typical for thelaziosis can manifest in several other eye disorders and in trauma, for instance, the confirmation of the diagnosis requires the detection of morphologically typical nematodes in the clinical examination of the eyes. The parasites are often found in the folds of the conjunctiva, under the nictitating membrane and in lacrimal ducts. Finding nematodes in these particular sites

is highly suggestive for thelaziosis. In addition to the morphological features, the identification of the worm today often relies on molecular biological methods. Larvae or eggs can be detected in the microscopical examination of the tear fluid. Thelaziosis has also been reported in humans in endemic areas.

Treatment and Prevention

Adult worms are removed mechanically with forceps and saline flushing. Since worms may hide, for instance, in tear canals, medical treatment is also indicated. Macrocyclic lactones, such as the combination of imidaclopride and moxidectin, selamectin or milbemycin oxime are most commonly used. Because several fly species can act as vectors, traveling dogs and migrating wild animals may spread *Thelazia*. Some dogs in endemic areas are given constant preventative treatment with macrocyclic lactones.

Morphology of *Thelazia*

Adult worms are thin, thread-like, and creamy-white in color (Fig. 5.48). The cuticle is transversely striated (Fig. 5.49). The length of a male *Thelazia* varies between 5 and 12 mm and between 0.3 and 0.4 mm in width. The length of a female varies from slightly over 10 mm to almost 20 mm and 0.4 and 0.5 in width. In both sexes, the oral opening is hexagonal. *Thelazia* have a well-developed buccal cavity and a rather short esophagus (Fig. 5.49). The lateral alae are missing from the male tail (Fig. 5.51), which is blunt. The spicules are asymmetrical and they differ considerably in size and shape. The right spicule is very short and sturdy and the other one is about 10 times longer and filamentous. There are many (10 pairs in *T. callipaeda*) precloacal papillae and three or five pairs of postcloacal papillae. The genital opening of the female has a short flap and is located in the anterior region of the body anterior to the esophagus-intestinal junction (Fig. 5.49). Females are ovo-viviparous. Female's posterior end is rounded and blunt with subterminal pair of lateral papillae. The anal opening is close to the caudal end. The numbers of the male's pre and postcloacal papillae and the position of the female's vulva are used as a basis in differentiation of *Thelazia* species.

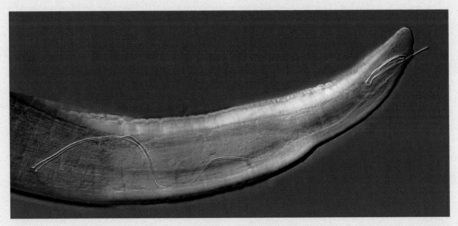

FIG. 5.51 The posterior end of male *Thelazia callipaeda*. The length and the form of the spicules, visible here, differ greatly. The left-hand filamentous spicule is about 10 times longer than the short and stubby spicule on the right.

SPIROCERCA LUPI, Eosophageal Worm

- A nematode up to 8 cm long, occurring in nodular lesions in the esophageal wall; damages the aorta as well.
- Coprophagic beetles act as intermediate hosts.
- Infection is acquired by eating beetles or paratenic hosts, such as poultry.
- Clinical signs vary; patent infection may be associated with poor appetite, swallowing difficulties, retching, and vomiting. Esophageal nodules may undergo carcinogenesis.
- Diagnosis is by imaging methods, endoscopy, or—during a short egg-producing period—by fecal examination.
- The infection has been treated with several drugs, especially with macrocylic lactones.

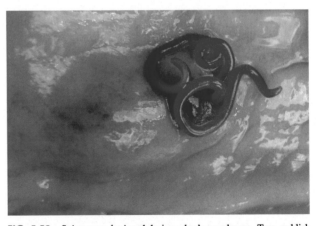

FIG. 5.52 *Spirocerca lupi* nodule in a dog's esophagus. Two reddish worms reach out from an orifice, through which the eggs, laid by the female, are released into the intestinal tract. (© *Bayer, reproduced with permission from Bayer and Dawie Kok.*)

Identification

S. lupi, a nematode of the order Spirurida, is prominent for causing fibrous parasitic nodules in the esophagus. The adult worms are coiled within the nodules and are bright red or pink (Fig. 5.52). The males are 30–55 mm and females 55–80 mm long. The mouth is hexagonal. The posterior end of the male is spiral with lateral alae and papillae. The spicules are of different length (about 2.5 and 0.75 µm). The female genital pore is located at the level of the caudal end of the esophagus. The eggs are of spiruroidea type, elongated 30–37 × 11–15 µm, and contain the larva in a U-shaped position (Fig. 5.53).

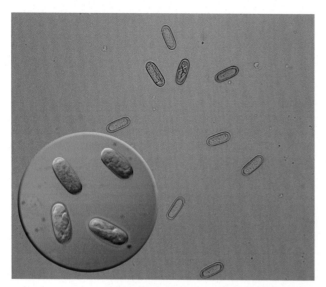

FIG. 5.53 Eggs of *Spirocerca lupi*. They are capsule-shaped. A larva in the shape of the letter U can often been seen within the egg. *(Background photo reproduced with permission from ClinVet/Dawie Kok.)*

Life Cycle

Canids act as definitive hosts of *Spirocerca*. Eggs, produced to the esophagus and containing a larva (Fig. 5.53) are secreted in feces or regurgitated. The larva hatches only after reaching the intermediate host, a dung-eating beetle. The development into the L3 phase, infectious for the dog, happens in the beetle in about 2 months (Fig. 5.54). The larva is encapsulated in the intermediate host and the definitive host gets the infection by eating an infected intermediate host. Many animals that use beetles for food, e.g., birds,

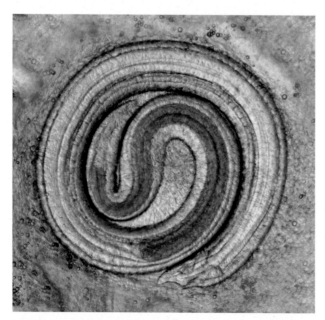

FIG. 5.54 Infective L3-stage larva of *Spirocerca lupi* found in a beetle, the intermediate host. *(Reproduced with permission from ClinVet/Dawie Kok.)*

reptiles, and insectivore mammals, can also infect dogs by acting as paratenic hosts. In a paratenic host that has eaten infected beetles, the larvae are released from the capsule, but they soon reencapsulate and remain waiting for access to the intestine of the definitive host. The larva penetrates the gut wall of the definitive host in about two hours after infection and it migrates along the stomach wall and the gastric arteries to the aorta. It takes about 10 days for the larva to make it there. In the aorta wall, the L3 stage develops into a L4 stage larva (Fig. 5.55). About 3 months later, most of the larvae migrate to the esophagus and mature. The worms live in the nodules, growing into the esophageal submucosa (Fig. 5.56). There are commonly one to four nodules in a dog. The number of worms within each nodule varies, but one can contain a colony consisting of several dozens of individual worms. The adult females

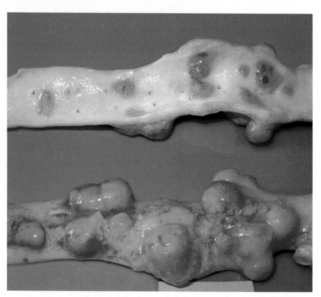

FIG. 5.55 Aortic lesions typical to *Spirocerca lupi* infection. The inner surface of the aorta above. The aorta seen from outside below. *(Reproduced with permission from Elanco Animal Health/ClinVet/Dawie Kok.)*

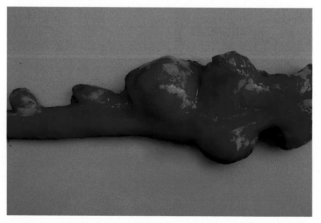

FIG. 5.56 Esophageal lesions, typical to *Spirocerca lupi* infection, seen from the outside. An autopsy finding of a dog that died as a result of aortic rupture. *(Reproduced with permission from ClinVet/Dawie Kok.)*

produce eggs to the esophagus thorough a hole made into the mucosa. They are further transferred to the alimentary tract and in feces or vomited into the environment. An illustrated life cycle of *S. lupi* is presented in Fig. 5.57.

Distribution

S. lupi is an internal parasite affecting dogs and other canids and infrequently cats in tropical and subtropical areas. *Spirocerca* infections are very common in certain regions. According to the literature, infections are especially prominent in Israel, Turkey, Greece, India, Pakistan, African countries, the southern United States, and Brazil. *Spirocerca arctica* is another *Spirocerca* species found in dogs and arctic foxes. It is endemic in northern Russian and Manchuria, and the patent infection manifests as pea-like nematode nodules in the stomach of the host.

Importance to Canine Health

The migrating larval stages cause hemorrhages in the stomach wall and hemorrhage and nodular scarring in the aorta. The lesions in the wall may weaken the aorta and even cause its rupture. The wall lesions are often associated with calcifications and sometimes even ossification. The aortic lesions are typical for this type of worms, sometimes even considered patognomonic (Fig. 5.55). The worm granulomas developing in the esophagus may have a circumference of several centimeters (Fig. 5.56). They may be associated with poor appetite, swallowing difficulties, retching, vomiting, and drooling as the result of the blockade and inflammatory reaction. If the granulomas are small, the dog may not have any signs. *Spirocerca* infection and chronic irritation and inflammation may result in carcinogenesis and some dogs develop a malignant mesenchymal tumor in the esophagus, usually fibrosarcoma or osteosarcoma. The esophagal sarcomas are very rare in dogs, but they often do have an association with *S. lupi* infection.

Since the canine *Spirocerca* infection is associated with the development of tumor-like neoplasms of the thoracic area, worm nodules and the tumors may lead to a secondary hypertrophic (pulmonary) osteoarthropathy (HPO). HPO most commonly manifests as clubbing, periostitis, and increased bone deposition manifested as the swellings and thickening of the distal part of the extremities.

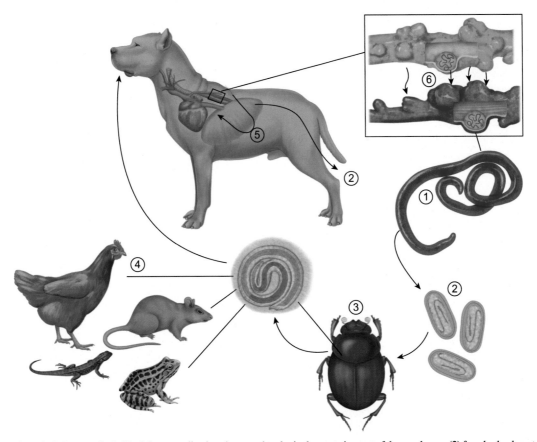

FIG. 5.57 Life cycle *Spirocerca lupi*: (1) adult worms live in submucosal nodes in the posterior part of the esophagus; (2) females lay larvated eggs that pass through an opening made into the mucosa to the esophagus and further to the intestine and in feces or with vomit into the environment; (3) the larva hatches only when it reaches the intermediate host, a coprophagic beetle. The development to the infective L3 phase lasts about 2 months; (4) the definitive host is infected by eating an infected intermediate host or a paratenic host; (5) the larva penetrates the stomach wall of the definitive host and migrates along the stomach wall and the gastric arteries to the aorta; and (6) the L3 stage develops into a L4-stage larva in the aortic wall. About 3 months later, most of the larvae migrate to the esophagus and mature.

Occasionally the migrating larvae stray from their ordinary route resulting in worm nodules in the subcutis, kidney, spinal cord, or parts of the intestine. About half of these cases involve anemia of some degree. Another typical or even pathognomonic lesion for spirocercosis is an inflammatory reaction of those thoracic vertebrae (spondylitis) that are close to the predilection areas of the worm. However, the pathogenesis of these lesions is poorly understood. In addition, inflammation and necrosis of salivary glands may be associated with the infection.

Diagnosis

Diagnosis can be carried out by detecting the large worm nodules radiographically with ordinary X-rays or computerized tomography or by endoscopy of the esophagus. In radiography, the nodules are best seen in dorso-ventral projection. In the flotation examination of the feces, spiruroid eggs (Fig. 5.53) can be detected. It should be noted that the egg-producing phase is relatively short in the life of the female. Hence, the fecal analysis is considered as an unreliable method of *Spirocerca* diagnosis and false negative analysis results are common.

Treatment and Prevention

Ivermectin, doramectin, bendzimidazoles, nitroscanate, and disophenol have been used to treat *Spirocerca* infection with mixed results. Doramectin has not only alleviated the clinical signs, but also cured the esophageal nodules and is the drug of choice in many endemic countries. However, in most of the countries, doramectin is not labeled for use in dogs. The nodules are surgically removed, especially in cases where it is suspected that the lesions are turning cancerous. Since the infection requires eating an intermediate or a paratenic host, an attempt can be made to prevent dogs from eating them in endemic regions. This may be difficult due to the large spectrum of host species. Uncooked offal of domestic or wild poultry should not be given to dogs in endemic areas.

PHYSALOPTERA SPP.

- Stomach worm up to 6 cm in length; consumes tissue fluids and blood from the gastric mucosa.
- Coprophagic arthropods (intermediate hosts) or paratenic hosts are a source of infection.
- Clinical signs include hemorrhages and inflammation of the stomach, vomiting, and melaena.
- Diagnosis is by detecting eggs in a fecal sample or worms in vomit or during gastroscopy.
- Anthelmintics have a varying efficacy; mechanical removal of worms is preferred.

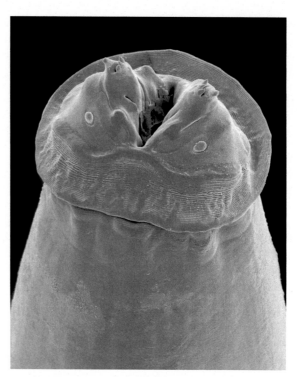

FIG. 5.58 The anterior end of *Physaloptera* sp. in scanning electron microscopy. *(Photo by Dennis Kunkel/Science Photo Library, reproduced with permission.)*

Identification

Dogs infrequently have stomach worms belonging to genus *Physaloptera* (Fig. 5.58) nematodes.

Male *Physaloptera praeputialis* are 1–4.5 cm and female 1.5–6 cm long. Male *Physaloptera rara* are 2.5 cm and females 3–6 cm long. The cuticle of *P. praeputialis* continues over the posterior end of the worm and forms—as the name indicates—a preputial protective sheath over the posterior part of the worm. *P. rara* has no such elongated cuticle. The vulva of both species is located anterior from the mid-point. The eggs voided to the ingesta and finally to the feces are oval, about $50 \times 30 \, \mu m$ in size, and have a thick shell. They are colorless and already contain a larva when being secreted.

Distribution

P. praeputialis is endemic in China, Africa, and the Americas. *P. rara* is known to be endemic only in northern America. Feline infections are frequently reported, but dogs are also sometimes infected.

Life Cycle

Adult worms live attached to the definitive host's stomach and the beginning of the small intestine and suck tissue fluid and blood from the mucosa. The eggs are secreted in feces to the environment and are eaten by intermediate hosts.

The *Physaloptera*, like other Spiruroidea nematodes, need an arthropod for their life cycle. For *Physaloptera*, these are typically coprophagic beetles, but cockroaches and crickets are as well suitable as intermediate hosts. The larva develops into an infective L3 larva in the intermediate host, and the infection is passed to the definitive host when it eats the arthropod. The infection may also reach the definitive host transmitted by numerous paratenic hosts, e.g., rodents and amphibians. The prepatent period is 8–10 weeks.

Pathogenesis and Clinical Features

The worms are tightly attached to the stomach mucosa and move about, causing erosions, hemorrhage and chronic inflammatory lesions. The signs may include vomiting (occasionally hemorrhagic) and dark melaena. Anorexia and weight loss are seen, especially in severe or chronic infections.

Diagnosis

The clinical signs are suggestive of the infection, but the diagnosis is confirmed by finding *Physaloptera* eggs in feces. Sodium chromate and magnesium sulfate are suitable for flotation. There are often few worms in the organism: only one to five at times. The produced egg number is therefore so small that the sensitivity of fecal analysis is not sufficient. In that case, the diagnosis can be made when the cause of emesis is being examined and endoscopy reveals worms in the stomach, or when worms are found in vomit.

Treatment and Prevention

Since an arthropod is necessary for the *Physaloptera* life cycle, there is no direct transmission of infection between dogs. As a preventative measure, the dog is restrained from eating intermediate or paratenic hosts, if possible. The worms can be mechanically removed in endoscopy. This is preferred, because anthelmintics have variable efficacy in different individuals. Fenbendazole or pyrantel given twice at a few weeks' interval have been used for medical treatment.

ONCHOCERCA LUPI

- Long and fragile filaroid nematodes, causing periocular helminthiasis.
- Blood-sucking insects serve as vectors. Black fly has been reported as a putative vector.
- A variety of ocular signs and asymptomatic infections have been reported. Typical infection is characterized by nodular lesions, usually on eyelids, conjunctiva, or sclera.
- Diagnosis is carried out by finding a nodular lesion with worms in periocular tissues.
- Treatment is the surgical removal of the mass, combined with antifilarial medication.

Identification

O. lupi is a filarial nematode originally detected in a wolf. The worm has a thick multilayered cuticle with fine striation and cuticular ridges on the outer surface. The male worm is 43–55 mm long but only 120–200 μm thick. The tail is spiral. The paired spicules are dissimilar: Left spicule is longer (about 200 ridges on the outer surface. The male worm is 43–55 mm long but only 120–200 μm thick. The tail is spiraThe female worms are also long and thin. The maximum length is unknown, but the longest measured parts have been 160–165 mm long, yet the worm is only 275–420 μm thick. The uterus fills about 70% of the body cavity and it has two long and parallel horns. The length of the microfilariae is 100–111 μm. They have a bent tail.

Distribution

O. lupi was first detected in a wolf in Russia. Canine infections have been diagnosed in North America and in central and southern Europe, but the true endemic area is unknown. In contrast to other *Onchocerca*, *O. lupi* parasitizes in canids but not artiodactyl species (hoofed animals). However, it can also infect humans. There have been about 10 reported human cases, and *O. lupi* should indeed be taken into account as a differential diagnosis in human ocular infections.

Life Cycle

The life cycle of *O. lupi* and its potential insect vectors are not completely known, but the parasite has been detected in Simulium black flies. The worms live in the tissue surrounding the canid eye, where the female produces microfilariae. The flying vector insects ingest the microfilariae, while they are eating. The larvae develop into the infectious L3 stage in the vector. When the insect again feeds, the infective L3 larva may be passed on to the next host. Since the black flies need waterways for their life cycle, infections are assumed to take place in wetlands.

Importance to Canine Health

The infection can cause a number of ocular signs, usually conjunctivitis, tear or exudate discharge, photophobia, exophthalmos, and edema of the ocular tissues. Ocular onchocercosis is characterized by ocular nodules that are often present on the eyelids, conjunctiva, or sclera. The nematodes may localize in the retrobulbar space of the eye. Microfilariae have been found also in the skin biopsies of healthy dogs, indicating that the infection is not always visibly harmful.

Diagnosis

When a mass containing worms is found in the periocular tissue, typically under the conjunctiva, the parasite is

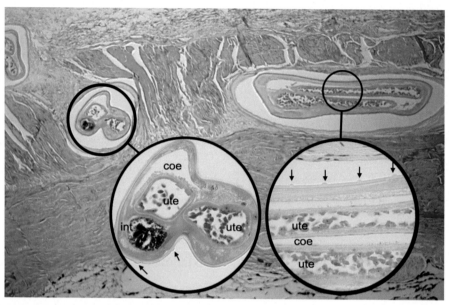

FIG. 5.59 Histopathology of ocular tissue of the dog with Onhocerca infection. In the sclera there are three cross and longitudinal sections of a coiled female of *Onchocerca lupi*. Note the double barrel uterus (ute) filled with remnants of eggs, an intestine (int), atrophied coelomyrian musculature, and pseudocoeloma (coe). The cuticle consists of two layers with an outer layer bearing ring-like ridges seen here as small knob-like protrusions (*arrows*). The infection is accompanied with chronic, mild fibrosing scleritis, and episcleritis. *(Photo by Veera Karkamo/Finnish Food Safety Authority Finland, reproduced with permission.)*

identified on the basis of morphology (Fig. 5.59) or using the PCR method. *O. lupi* is distinguished from other *Onchocerca* species based on body dimensions and the number of nuclei in the microfilarial head and the tail. The microfilariae are also much smaller than in other species. The infection and the *Onchocerca* can be diagnosed with PCR without the detection of worms in a biopsy.

Treatment and Prevention

A periocular mass is removed surgically. The surgical resection is combined with melarsomine treatment (possibly together with ivermectin), which almost invariably causes a transient eye edema and pruritus, lasting while the microfilariae remaining in the tissue die. The prognosis is good. Infections are prevented by managing the vectors, e.g., with insecticides. Drugs used in prevention of heartworms, such as milbemycin and selamectin, may act preventatively, but this has not been shown in studies.

DIROFILARIA IMMITIS, Heartworm

- Filaroid nematode up to 30 cm long, residing in the heart and pulmonary arteries.
- Vector-borne disease; various mosquito species serve as intermediate hosts.
- Clinical signs manifest with congestive right-sided heart disease and thrombo-embolism.

- Diagnosis is by identifying microfilariae in a blood sample or with antigen analysis.
- Eliminating the immature stages of the heartworm is the recommended prevention. Treatment of a patent infection is a health risk to the dog.

Identification

The adult heartworm resides in the right cardiac ventricle and in the pulmonary artery (Fig. 5.60). The female *D. immitis* is 25–30 cm and the male 12–16 cm long; both are white nematodes. The posterior end of the male (Fig. 5.61) is coiled into a spiral, and it has small lateral alae in the tail part. There are two spicules, and they differ in length and form. The posterior part of the male worm has many papillary structures on both the anterior and posterior side of the cloaca. Microfilariae, the larvae in circulation, are about 300 μm long and 6 μm wide. The head of the microfilaria is slightly conical and the tail straight, long, and thin (Fig. 5.62).

Life Cycle

The adult heartworm mostly lives in the right cardiac ventricle and in the pulmonary artery. The female is ovoviviparic and produces larvae (microfilariae) into the dog's circulation. The infection is spread by blood-sucking insects. Several genera of mosquitos, e.g., *Culex, Aedes,*

Malpighian within 1 day and, having molted twice, they penetrate into body cavity of the mosquito. From there they migrate to the oral parts of the mosquito and develop into the infective L3-stage larvae. The phase in the intermediate host usually lasts 15–17 days. In the tropics, the development is faster, and may be completed within 8–10 days. A constant temperature of over 14 °C and sufficient ambient moisture for over 2 weeks are necessary for the larval development in the mosquito. When the mosquito next time takes a blood meal from a suitable host animal, L3 larvae are released in hemolymph onto the skin surface, from where they push into the skin through the injection channel. The larvae develop and migrate in the submucosa and muscle tissue. It is assumed that L3 and L4 larvae migrate and develop in between the muscles and it takes months before young adult forms (L5) penetrate the blood veins to get to the heart and pulmonary arteries. By this stage, the larvae are several centimeters long. The final development into reproductive adult heartworms lasts another 2 months after this. Microfilariae can be found in the blood at the earliest about 6–7 months after infection. This prepatent period is often 9 months. If the dog and its pulmonary veins are not large enough, the worms favor pulmonary arteries as their living space. If there is not enough space left in the pulmonary arteries, worms are first found in the right cardiac ventricle then in the right atrium, and, in the worst case, in the vena cava. For instance, in a medium-sized dog, an infection with up

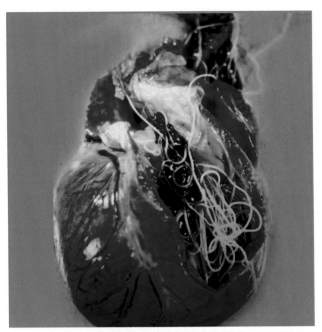

FIG. 5.60 Heartworms in the right heart ventricle. *(Reproduced with permission from Arlett Peréz.)*

Armigeres, Myzorhyncus, Taeniorhyncus, and *Anopheles,* have been shown to be able to act as vectors.

When the mosquito sucks blood from a dog, it gets heartworm microfilariae into its intestinal tract. They migrate from the gut through the hemocoele to the

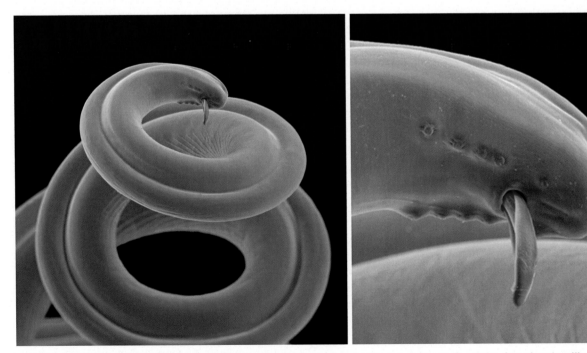

FIG. 5.61 Artificially colored SEM micrographs showing the coiled posterior end of the male *D. immitis.* Four pairs of pre-cloacal papillae, a small pair of papillae adjacent to the cloacal opening and postcloacal papillae are clearly visible in the detail micrograph. Cloacal opening and the channel-like structure formed by the smaller spicule are distinct. *(SEM micrograph by Dennis Kunkel/Science Photo Library, reproduced with permission.)*

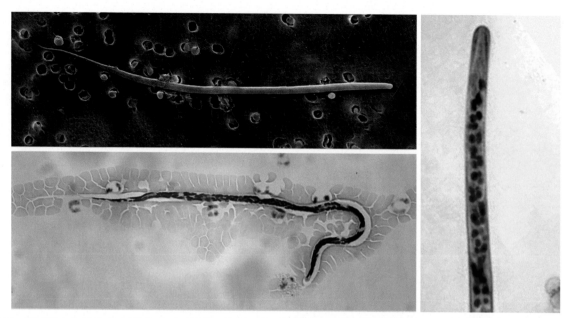

FIG. 5.62 *Dirofilaria immitis* microfilariae in the SEM and in May-Grünwald-Giemsa stained specimen. The microfilariae are about 300 µm long and 6 µm wide and unsheathed. The front end is slightly conical. The figure shows the nucleus-free cephalic space, which is much larger in *D. immitis* than in *D. repens*. *(A SEM mictograph (upper left) and a micrograph detail (on the right) by Emanuele Brianti and the micrograph (lower left) by Arlett Peréz, reproduced with permission.)*

to five adult heartworms does not occupy the heart at all. When in the heart or vena cava, the worms can interfere severely with the patency of heart valves. Adult worms live 5–7 years and microfilariae may stay viable up to 2 years. An illustrated life cycle of *D. immitis* is presented in Fig. 5.63.

Distribution

The canine heartworm is endemic almost everywhere in the world, where the climate is favorable for the worm's life cycle. In Europe, it is endemic in Mediterranean countries, but the worm is expected to benefit from climate change, and it is already evident that the endemic area is expanding toward the north.

Importance to Canine Health

Canine heartworm infection may be subclinical, but about 25 adult worms are enough to cause clinical signs. The thumb rule is that small dogs manifest signs due to fewer worms than larger dogs. The signs are the result of vascular lesions, disturbances in cardiac and pulmonary blood flow, and the rise of blood pressure in the pulmonary artery. Where worms live, the inner surface of the artery thickens, which causes the narrowing of the vessel. Inflammatory cells, platelets, and later connective tissue accumulate at the lesion.

At the first stage, reduced exercise tolerance and a cough are seen in the dog. Gradually the condition often

proceeds into congestive right-sided heart disease. The signs can be very varied. Typical signs include dyspnea and fluid accumulation (ascites) in the abdominal cavity. Dead worms travel in the circulation into lungs, where they cause blockages in blood vessels and a local inflammatory reaction. The signs of thrombo-embolism can be severe, especially if there are many dead worms. The worms occupying the right ventricle and vena cava may cause circulatory disturbances in the liver, leading to hepatic failure, which further causes hemolysis, hemoglobinuria, bilirubinemia, icterus, anorexia, and circulatory collapse. The infection may be associated with the formation of immuno-complexes, which may lead to glomerulitis and nephritis and further renal damage. Larvae loose in the peripheral circulation may migrate to different parts of the organism and cause inflammatory changes, especially when they die. Microfilariae are known to cause dermatitis, ocular infections, and problems caused by changes in ocular pressure.

D. immitis may infrequently infect humans. The infection may be subclinical and, if symptoms appear, they usually manifest as subcutaneous nodules containing worms. In very rare cases, worms may be detected in the pulmonary artery, but microfilaremia is exceptional.

Diagnosis

The disease can be diagnosed by analyzing a blood sample. The simplest way is to view a drop of fresh blood in microscopy. Although microfilariae are transparent, their wriggling movement is visible by observing the red blood

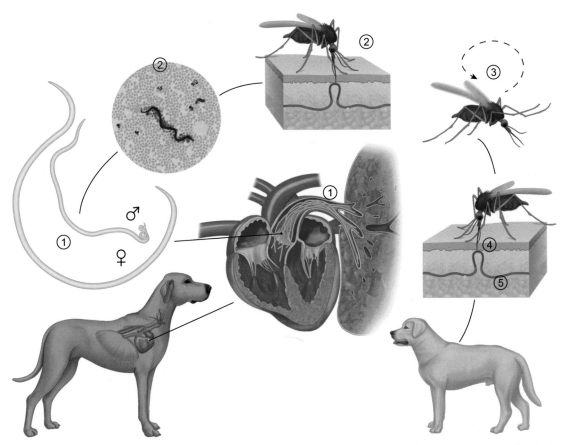

FIG. 5.63 Life cycle of *Dirofilaria immitis*: (1) the adult heartworm lives in the right cardiac ventricle and in the pulmonary artery. The female produces larvae (microfilariae) into the dog's circulation; (2) when the mosquito sucks blood from a dog, it gets heartworm microfilariae in its alimentary tract; (3) they migrate to the Malphigian tubules within 1 day and, having molted twice, they penetrate to the body cavity of the mosquito. From there they migrate into the oral parts of the mosquito and develop into the infective L3-stage larvae; (4) when the mosquito next time stings a suitable host animal, L3 larvae are released in the hemolymph onto the skin surface, from where they push into the skin through the injection channel. The larvae develop and migrate in the subcutis and muscle tissue for months; and (5) young adult forms of L5-stage penetrate the blood veins to get to the heart and pulmonary arteries. The final development into reproductive adult heartworms requires another 2 months.

cells that move together with the larvae. Despite the wriggling, the microfilariae stay usually stationary on the microscope slide. In a hematocrit tube, the microfilariae are located in the buffy coat, between the column of erythrocytes and the plasma, where the movement can often be seen even with the naked eye. Some laboratories employ filtering methods for concentrating microfilariae. To make microfilariae sufficiently visible for morphological analysis, Knott's method and staining of the smear is useful. With these methods, it is possible to distinguish *Dirofilaria* microfilariae from less harmless species (Fig. 5.62). About 30% of cases where adult heartworm live in the pulmonary arteries or heart are cases of occult dirofilariasis where microfilariae are absent. Many reasons may contribute to the absence of microfilariae: the worms may have not yet started reproduction, the adult worms are of one sex only, the dog has received antimicrofilarial medication, or the dog's immune defense is capable of eliminating the microfilariae. Today, antigenic

assays are more common in diagnostics. A test based on ELISA measures the concentration of protein originating in female worms in canine blood. The assay works only if there are sufficient numbers of adult females in the dog and if sufficient time has passed since infection happened, at least 6–8 months. If the dog has been treated with macrocyclic lactones, the period of negative antigen presence often extends to over 9 months after infection. In endemic heartworm regions, it is recommended that the dogs are tested annually. If the start of the heartworm prevention is not known or if the dog has not received adequate preventative treatment, three tests in half-year intervals are recommended at the beginning, followed by annual analyses.

In advanced cases of dirofilariasis, dilatation of pulmonary arteries is seen in radiography, and in severe cases, right-sided cardiac hypertrophy may develop. Other typical signs resulting from right-sided cardiac insufficiency include the accumulation of fluid in the thoracic and abdominal cavities. Valuable information on the severity of heartworm lesions in the thorax can thereby be obtained with radiography. Cardiac ultrasound examination is useful for analyzing the structural changes in the heart and blood vessels. Heartworms typically give a strong echo and are easily detected by an experienced radiologist.

Treatment and Prevention

Adult heartworms and microfilariae are controlled separately with different substances. The most common adulticide is melarsomine, which is effective against heartworms of over 4 months of age. Dead adults drift to pulmonary veins to be broken down by phagocytosis. This leads inevitably to blockages in pulmonary arteries. The results of stasis can be serious. All exercise and stress for the dog should be avoided during treatment and weeks after it. Adulticide treatment is often combined with supportive medication, such as nonsteroidal antiinflammatory drugs, glucocorticoids, and doxycycline, which can be started before the adulticide. In cases of serious dirofilariasis with severe signs, the worms must often be surgically removed. The worms are usually caught by fishing them out through the right-sided jugular vein. Treatment success is confirmed with the antigen assay done after one year, at the latest. Macrocyclic lactones are used for the elimination of microfilariae, usually together with ivermectin, selamectin, moxidectin, or milbemycin oxime.

In areas endemic for heartworm, dogs often receive permanent preventative medication.

The Symbiosis Between the Heartworm and *Wolbachia* Bacteria

The symbiosis between the heartworm and *Wolbachia* bacteria has been one of the most important findings of *Dirofilaria* research since the millennium. *Wolbachia* are gram-negative bacteria belonging to the groups of intercellular rickettsia. They are found as symbionts in many nematodes producing microfilariae. The *Wolbachia* symbiont of the canine heartworm is *Wolbachia pipiensis*. *Wolbachia* colonies live in the lateral cords that run under the outer surface of adult worms as well as in female genitalia. Female heartworms transfer the *Wolbachia* bacteria into their offspring. They are known to be essential for the heartworm, and killing the bacteria with antibiotics causes serious disturbances in the worm's embryogenesis, development of larval stages, and maturation into an adult. Giving doxycycline, an antibiotic that is effective for *Wolbachia*, to the dog during the 2 months following the infection causes the death of L3 and L4 larvae of the worms. Similarly, if the dog is carrying adult heartworms, doxycycline treatment will get rid of the microfilariae. If a mosquito sucks microfilariae with its blood meal, the development in the insect seems to proceed in a normal way, but once the L3-stage larvae reach the canine host, they do not mature into adult heartworms. *Wolbachia* is also known to play a role in the pathogenesis of dirofilariasis. A reaction by the immune defense of the heartworm takes place against *Wolbachia* surface proteins, leading to development of IgG antibodies. These antibodies are now known to have an important role in damaging the renal glomeruli and in inflammatory changes of lungs, associated with dirofilariasis. Research has shown that if nematode control is combined with doxycycline treatment, dead worms stuck in the pulmonary arteries cause significantly less damage in the lungs than when only melarsomine is used. Thus, *Wolbachia* apparently has an important role in the pathology of vascular clots that inevitably follow the killing of adult heartworms in particular.

Morphology of *Dirofilaria immitis*

Heartworms are long, white, slender nematodes (Fig. 5.60). The female is up to 25–30 cm and the male 12–16 cm long. The oral opening is circular and terminal. The esophagus is short, up to 1.5 mm long. The female genital opening is situated on the outer surface of the worm, immediately behind the esophagus. The posterior end of the male is coiled into a spiral (Fig. 5.61), and it has small lateral alae in the tail part. There are two spicules, and they differ in length and form. The longer is about 300 μm and the shorter about 200 μm long. The larger spicule lies in a channel formed by the small spicule. The posterior part of the male worm has many clearly protruding papillary structures on both the anterior and posterior side of the cloaca. There are four to six pairs of precloacal papillae, a small pair of papillae adjacent to the cloacal opening and 4 pairs of postcloacal papillae (Fig. 5.61). Microfilariae, the larvae in circulation, are about 300 μm long and 6 μm wide. They are unsheathed. The head of the microfilaria is slightly conical and the tail straight, long, and thin (Fig. 5.62). Microfilariae move actively.

D. immitis—Medical Adulticidic Treatment

In the nonendemic countries, the heartworm treatment is usually available only in the biggest animal hospitals. The dog should be observed carefully for any adverse reactions and its exercise should be restricted for the treatment period and for as long as 2 months after that. The adulticidic treatment starts with doxycylin, which is administered orally 10 mg/kg two times per day for 4 weeks to eliminate the symbiotic bacteria *Wolbachia*, before the actual killing of the worms. This reduces the side effects of the treatment and enhances the efficacy. Melarsomine dihydrochloride is an adulticide, which has not been shown to have a proper effect on juvenile heartworms under the age of 4 months. It is administered as intramuscular injections. A three-injection protocol is reported to kill as many as 98% of the worms. The first injection of melarsomine hydrochloride 2.5 mg/kg body weight is followed 1 month later by two injections, 24 h apart. Microfilarisidic macrocyclic lactones (ML) administered as

D. immitis—Medical Adulticidic Treatment—cont'd

much as 2 months before the actual adulticide treatment control the possible new infections, eliminate the existing ML-susceptible larvae, and allow the older worms to mature before the melarsomine administration to a point where they are susceptible to it. Preadulticide ML treatment should be used with caution to the patients with high microfilaremia. Any adjunct therapy depends on the clinical signs of the dog, but glucocorticosteroids and nonsteroidal antiinflammatories may be considered.

Source: Current canine guidelines for the prevention, diagnosis, and management of heartworm (*D. immitis*) infection in dogs, American Heartworm Society, Guidelines revised July 2014.

DIROFILARIA REPENS, Subcutaneous Worm

- A filaroid nematode of the subcutis; microfilariae are released into the circulation.
- Mosquitos serve as intermediate hosts and vectors.
- The parasite may cause subcutaneous nodules and an allergic reaction against microfilariae, but the infection is usually subclinical.
- Diagnosis is by identifying the microfilaria from blood sample or identifying an adult worm in a subcutaneous nodule.
- Nodules can be removed surgically; heartworm treatments can be attempted.

Identification

D. repens is a long, thin, and white or off-white nematode (Figs. 5.64 and 5.65). Adult females are about 15 cm long and males about 6–7 cm. The cuticle is longitudinally and prominently striated with less prominent transverse protrusions. The mouth is small and round and there are four pairs of small papillary structures around the oral opening. The esophagus has two parts: a muscular part and a glandular part with gland structures. The left-side spicule of the male worm is longer (about 530 μm) than the one on the right (about 180 μm). The tail of the male is spiral and the tip has numerous papillary protrusions that are important for morphological identification. The genital pore of the female is located about 15 mm from the head of the worm. Microfilariae are bigger than those of the heartworm, being about 370 μm long and 9 μm thick (Fig. 5.66). They are unsheathed. The head of the microfilaria is round and the tail has a sharp tip. In a Giemsa-stained blood smear, the nucleus-free cephalic space at the anterior end is shorter than that of heartworm. In this "empty" space, *D. repens* typically has a pair of nuclei, resembling eyes.

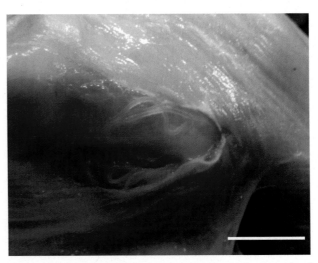

FIG. 5.64 Adult *Dirofilaria repens* on muscular fascia. *(Reproduced with permission from Emanuele Brianti.)*

Life Cycle

The adult worms live in the subcutis of the dog and the females produce microfilariae to the canine peripheral circulation. Mosquitoes act as vectors and intermediate hosts. Several genera of mosquitos, e.g., *Aedes, Anopheles, Culex,* and *Mansonia,* are known to act as intermediate hosts. They are infected while sucking blood. Once in the alimentary canal of the mosquito, the microfilariae penetrate the Malphigian ducts, where the larval stages develop. L3, the stage infectious for the dog, finds its way to the mouth parts of the mosquito. The development from a microfilaria into L3 takes at least 2 weeks. The L3 causes an infection in the dog when the mosquito sucks its blood. The larva penetrates the subcutaneous tissues and undergoes a series of two molts before maturation. The period between canine infection and the appearance of new generation microfilariae in the peripheral circulation usually takes more than 6 months. *D. repens* lives for a long time: up to 5–10 years. An illustrated life cycle of *D. repens* is presented in Fig. 5.67.

D. repens Is an Important Zoonotic Parasite

Although *D. repens* infection is usually harmless to dogs, it is worth remembering that this parasite is zoonotic. The human is an accidental host for it, since it is hardly ever able to mature to an adult, microfilaria-producing worm in a human. A typical human infection is manifested as a subcutaneous nodule, which grows close to the skin area where the infection-carrying mosquito sucked blood. The nodule may be sore. A young worm, encapsulated by the body's immune response, is inside the nodule. Apart from the skin and subcutaneous tissue, worm nodules have been described in different parts of the organism, such as the eye, mammary gland, testicles, and scrotum. A pulmonary nodule may resemble neoplasia.

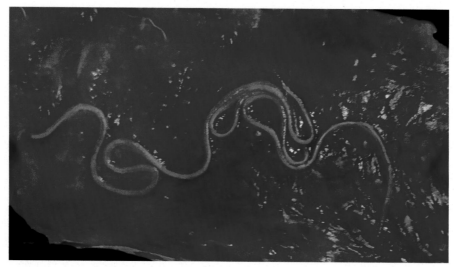

FIG. 5.65 Adult *Dirofilaria repens* in subcutaneous tissue. *(Photo by Hanna-Kaisa Sihvo, Finnish Food Safety Authority Finland, reproduced with permission.)*

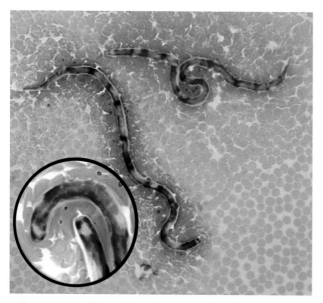

FIG. 5.66 Microfilariae of *Dirofilaria repens* in a Giemsa-stained blood smear. The microfilariae are larger than those of heartworm, *D. immitis*, about 370 μm long and 9 μm thick. They are unsheathed. The end of the microfilaria is round and the tip of the tail is sharp. In a Giemsa-stained blood smear, the cephalic space is seen in the anterior end. It is shorter in *D. repens* than in the heartworm. The parasite typically has a pair of nuclei, resembling eyes, in this "empty" space. It is clearly seen in the round, small image.

Distribution

D. repens is common in Mediterranean countries. Apart from dogs, it also infects wild canids and cats. It may cause symptoms in humans when it accidentally infects them. Recently, the endemic area of the parasite has expanded rapidly toward the north. It is now relatively common in central European and Baltic countries.

Importance to Canine Health

D. repens infection is usually subclinical in dogs. It likely depends on the immune response of each dog, whether the infection is limited to a nodule surrounded by a capsule of connective tissue or whether the worms live with fewer signs on the fascia of the subcutaneous tissue. The signs are nonspecific cutaneous lesions. The classical manifestation is a tumor-like nodule in the subcutaneous tissue. Skin reddening, pruritus, and edema can be associated with the infection. The affected area may be alopecic and hyperkeratotic with crusting of the epidermis. Since the worm lives for a long time, it must have efficient and functional protection against the dog's immune defense. The clinical signs may be associated with dead worms or *Wolbachia*, the worm's symbiotic bacteria (see also *D. immitis*). Microfilaremia may sometimes be combined with allergic reactions, especially when a large number of circulating microfilariae dies, for instance, as a result of anthelmintic treatment. The worm's zoonotic character increases the importance of *D. repens* as a pathogen.

Diagnosis

D. repens infection can be confirmed with a blood sample (Fig. 5.66). The presence of microfilariae can often be detected by examining a drop of fresh blood in microscopy. The wriggling movement of microfilariae is revealed when observing the red blood cells that move together with the larvae. Visualizing the microfilariae adequately for morphological examination requires the use of the Knott method or staining of a blood smear. The microfilariae can be morphologically distinguished from those of other canine microfilariae-producing parasite species. Diagnosis can often be reached when the parasitic skin nodule is excised surgically and sent for analysis (Fig. 5.68). A species-specific

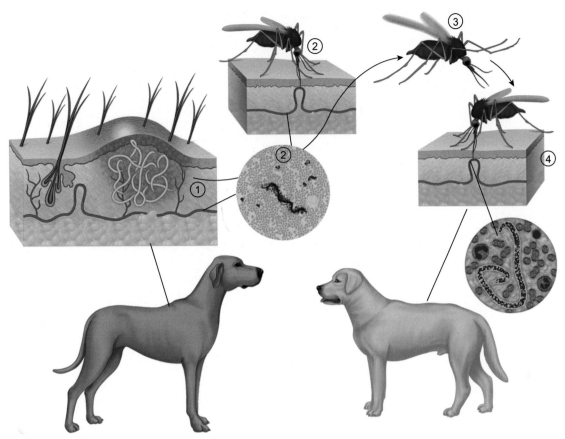

FIG. 5.67 Life cycle of *Dirofilaria repens*: (1) the adult worms live in the subcutis of the dog and the females produce microfilariae to the canine peripheral circulation; (2) mosquitoes act as vectors and intermediate hosts and are infected while sucking blood; (3) in the alimentary canal of the mosquito, the microfilariae penetrate the Malphigian ducts, where the larval stages develop L3, the stage infectious for the dog. The development from a microfilaria into L3 takes about 2 weeks at least; and (4) L3 finds its way to the mouth parts of the mosquito and the dog gets an infection when the mosquito sucks its blood. The larva penetrates the subcutaneous tissues and undergoes a series of two molts before maturation. The period between canine infection and the appearance of new generation microfilariae in the peripheral circulation usually takes more than 6 months. *Dirofilaria repens* lives for a long time: up to 5–10 years.

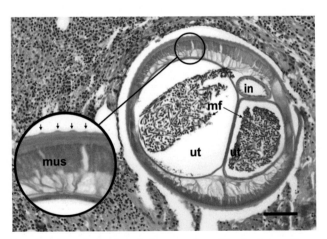

FIG. 5.68 Histopathology as seen in the subcutaneous lesion from the human patient with subcutaneous *D. repens* infection. A diffuse dermal inflammatory infiltrate composed of eosinophilic granulocytes and histiocytes surrounding an adult female filarioid nematode can be observed. A cuticle (*cut*) with evenly spaced external longitudinal cuticular ridges (*arrows*), a musculature of coelomyarian type (mus), a small intestine (in) and a paired uterus (ut) filled with microfilariae (mf) are considered typical of *Dirofilaria* spp. Hematoxylin-eosin stained histological section. Scale bars = 100 μm. *(Photo by Stig Nordling. Reproduced with permission from Pietikäinen R, Nordling S, Jokiranta S, et al.: Dirofilaria repens transmission in southeastern Finland, Parasit Vectors 10:561, 2017, https://doi.org/10.1186/s13071-017-2499-4.)*

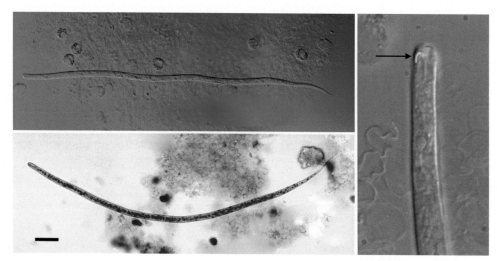

FIG. 5.69 *Acantoceilonema reconditum* microfilariae in unstained (above) and May-Grünwald-Giemsa-stained (below) specimen. Compared to *Dirofilaria* species, the microfilariae of *Acanthoceilonema* are both shorter and thinner. The microfilariae are about 270 μm long and about 4.5 μm thick in the widest part. In addition, the head of the *Acanthoceilonema* microfilaria has a short, hook-like structure (*arrow*). Scale bar = 20 μm.

diagnosis can be confirmed with PCR methods, done either from pieces of an adult worm or from microfilariae.

Treatment and Prevention

There is usually no need to treat routinely against adult worms. However, the infection risk to other dogs and humans may require an intervention aiming at the elimination of microfilariae produced by the female worms, if the infection is diagnosed. The treatment and prevention of *D. repens* infection can be carried out with the same substances that are used for heartworm control. It is probably best to remove an isolated nodule surgically.

ACANTHOCEILONEMA (SYN. DIPETALONEMA) RECONDITUM and A. DRACUNCULOIDES

- Microfilaria-producing nematode that lives in canine subcutis and on muscle fasciae.
- Adapted for living as a commensal in dogs; infection is usually subclinical.
- It is important to distinguish the microfilariae from those of more clinically important species.

Identification

A. reconditum is a microfilaria-producing (filaroid) nematode that lives in the canine subcutis and on muscle fasciae. The female worms are 21–25 mm and the males 9–17 mm long. The microfilariae are about 270 μm long and about 4.5 μm thick in the widest part (Fig. 5.69). The genera include other species, of which *A. dracunculoides* nematode is endemic in Europe. It usually lives in the abdominal cavity. The females of the species are 33–55 mm and males 15–31 mm long. The microfilariae are 121–218 μm long and 4.5–5.2 μm thick.

Life Cycle

Female *A. reconditum* produce microfilariae in the subcutis. They move into the peripheral circulation. Fleas are the parasite's vectors and intermediate hosts, taking the microfilariae into their system while sucking blood. It is also likely that the tropical chewing louse *Heterodoxus spiniger* and the sucking louse *Linognathus setosus* can act as vectors. Even though the older literature also cites many tick species as possible vectors, the present consensus is that they are not. The development from microfilaria into infective L3 takes about 2 weeks in the infected cat flea. The size and location of the L3 larva in experimentally infected cat fleas indicate that the infection may be transmitted not during sucking blood, but instead by the ingestion of the flea. The migration of the larvae and their entry to the subcutaneous tissue in the dog are poorly known. In addition, *A. dracunculoides*, resident of the abdominal cavity, produces microfilariae into the circulation. It has been suggested that its intermediate hosts include *Hippobosca longipennis* (louse fly), *Rhipicephalus sanguineus* (tick), and fleas.

Distribution

A. reconditum is a nematode widely prevalent in the world. In Europe, it is prominent in the Mediterranean, in similar areas to *A. dracunculoides*.

Importance to Canine Health

The *Acanthoceilonema* are very well adapted for living with dogs. Neither species is very harmful to canine health. The worms live long, and in death they lose their ability to avoid the immune defense of the host animal. The immune response against dead worms may be associated with clinical signs; however, these are limited to the worms' immediate vicinity.

Diagnosis

The diagnosis of *Acanthoceilonema* infection is commonly based on the detection of microfilariae in a blood sample. Since the clinical significance of the parasite is negligible, the primary goal of diagnosis is to distinguish the microfilariae from those of more clinically important worm species, such as heartworm. Compared to the *Dirofilaria* species, the microfilariae of *Acanthoceilonema* are both shorter and thinner. In addition, the head of the *Acanthoceilonema* microfilaria has a short, hook-like structure. Finding the cephalic hook, however, requires skillful microscopy. Fixing the sample in 2% formaldehyde turns the tail of the microfilaria into a hook, resembling an umbrella handle. When treated similarly, the tail of the heartworm remains straight. The diagnosis may be made more specific by staining with alkaline phosphatase or, as is increasingly the case, by using PCR methods.

Treatment and Prevention

There is no need to treat for acanthoceilonematosis.

CERCOPITHIFILARIA SPP.

- Females produce microfilariae in subcutis; larvae do not enter the circulation.
- *R. sanguineus* acts as the arthropod vector.
- Infection is usually subclinical but may be associated with dermatitis.
- Diagnosis is by a skin biopsy.
- Infection does not need to be treated.

Identification

Several *Cercopithifilaria* species are known to parasitize dogs. The best-known species are *Cercopithifilaria grassii* (former *Dipetalonema grassii*) and *D. bainae*. The female worms are 14–21 mm and the male 17–12 mm long. *C. grassii* microfilariae are quite long, (650 µm, thickness 15–17 µm). Many recognized *Cercopithifilaria* species,

such as *C. bainaella*, have very slender and short microfilariae (length about 180 µm, thickness 6–15 µm).

Life Cycle

The *Cercopithifilaria* live in the subcutis, where the females produce microfilariae. The microfilariae do not enter the canine circulation, but instead settle in the dog's dermal layer. The brown dog tick *R. sanguineus* acts as the arthropod vector for the infection. The castor bean tick, *Ixodes ricinus*, is known not to act as the intermediate host for *C. bainae* at least. The infection is transferred to the next developmental stage of the tick through transstadial transmission and the dog is infected when the brown dog tick sucks blood from the dog during its next development stage. The development to the infectious L3 stage lasts about a month. The stages of life cycle in the dog are poorly known. Microfilariae have been detected in dogs of about 6 months, indicating that the prepatent period is less than this.

Distribution

Cercopithifilaria species have been reported in different parts of the world. They are common in Europe, e.g., in Italy, Spain, and Greece. In some areas, over 20% of dogs carry the infection. Since the microfilariae are very rarely found in peripheral circulation, *Cercopithifilaria* infections are probably underdiagnosed.

Importance to Canine Health

Cercopithifilaria infections are usually subclinical. Moderate dermatitis signs may manifest as a reaction to dead worms. The inflammation may be caused not only by the worm's tissues but also by *Wolbachia* bacteria, symbiont to the worm.

Diagnosis

Microfilariae of Cercopthifilaria are hardly ever found in a blood sample. The microfilariae may be displayed by taking biopsies from the skin. They are soaked in saline in 37°C for about 10 min. A few drops of the sediment are viewed in a microscope for microfilariae. The sample may be stained, for instance, with methylene blue. Samples for microfilaria diagnosis should be taken especially from the skin of head, front legs, and the trunk. PCR is now often used for species diagnosis.

Treatment and Prevention

There is no need to treat for cercopithifilariosis.

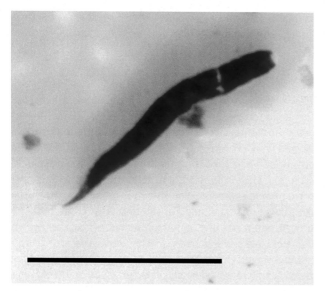

FIG. 5.70 A short and stubby microfilaria typical for *Microfilaria auquieri* observed in May-Grünwald-Giemsa stained blood smear of a dog from Ladakh, India. Scale bar = 50 μm. *(Megat Abd Rani PA, Irwin PJ, Gatne M, Coleman GT, MnInnes LM, Traub RJ: A survey of canine filarial diseases of veterinary and public health significance in India, Parasit Vectors 3:30, 2010, http://www.parasitesandvectors.com/content/3/1/30.)*

MICROFILARIA SPP.

Microfilaria auguieri is a Filaroidea nematode living in the lymph vessels. Its microfilariae can in rare cases be found in the dog's blood (Fig. 5.70). Infections have been diagnosed in dogs in India. The parasite is poorly known. Its insect vector intermediate host is reportedly the louse fly *H. longipennis*.

BRUGIA SPP.

Brugia species are important human parasites. Species infective to humans include *B. pahangi* and *B. malayi*. Mosquitos act as vector intermediate hosts, in which the

development to L3-stage larvae takes place. Adult parasites live in lymphatic vessels. Consequently, the typical signs are the enlargement of lymph nodes and edema as a result of lymphatic circulation impairment. Often one limb only becomes swollen. The diagnosis is based on the detection of microfilariae in peripheral circulation (Fig. 5.71), or on ELISA or PCR analysis.

DRACUNCULUS INSIGNIS

- Adult worms live in nodules in subcutaneous tissue, most commonly beneath the skin of the limbs.
- When fully matured, the nodule ruptures when the dog is in contact with water, and the female releases larvae to the environment.
- The larvae are eaten by freshwater copepods and the dog receives the infection by drinking water containing copepods harboring infective larvae.
- Infection is usually manifested as nodular cutaneous bruises.
- Dracunculosis is diagnosed by detecting skin nodules. Treatment is surgical.

Identification

D. insignis is one of the longest nematodes in the dog. The adult females are 17–25 cm long and 3–4 mm thick. Males are rarely seen, and they are substantially smaller than the females, with a maximum length of a few centimeters. The oral opening of the worm is small, triangular, and surrounded by a square cuticular plate. The esophagus has a spacious glandular part, while the muscular part is thin. In young female worms, the genital pore is seen in the mid-part of the worm. The genital pore atrophies with age and becomes poorly detectable. The uterus fills a large part of the female. It has an anterior and posterior branch,

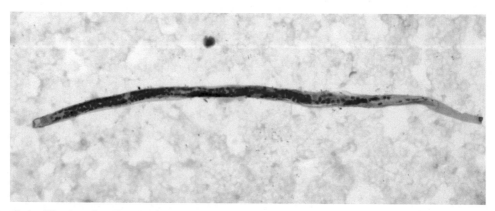

FIG. 5.71 Microfilaria of *Brugia malayi*. The microfilaria is sheathed, i.e., it can be seen inside a sock-like sheath. The nuclei are clustered together and oval. There are two separate nuclei close to the tail tip. The length varies between 180 and 230 μm.

and is filled with hundreds of thousands of worm embryos. Conflicting information is available on the morphology of the rarely encountered males. They have paired spicules of different lengths. The larvae are about 500 μm long and 50 μm thick, and they have a long and abruptly thinning tail.

Life Cycle

The adult worms live and develop larval nodules in the subcutis. The nodules are most commonly formed under the skin of the limbs. When the female worm is ready to give birth, it secretes substances into the nodule, causing tissue irritation, inflammation, hypersensitivity reaction, and itching. The skin covering the nodule gets thinner and a blister develops on the surface of the nodule. When the blister is in contact with water, e.g., when the dog wades or swims in waterways, the blister breaks down and masses of larvae are freed into the water from the female. The female does not give birth through the genital pore, but instead the enormously swollen uterus breaks the female cuticle. As a result, the folds of the uterus and larvae inside them are able to balloon out, giving the larvae access to the environment. The female dies soon thereafter. The male has died earlier after copulation. The larvae released in water have a few days to reach a Cyclops freshwater copepod and be eaten by it. Inside the copepod, the larva develops to L3 stage, infectious for the dog. The speed of the development in the copepod depends on the temperature; in +25° C the development takes a few weeks. In cooler conditions, it slows down or stops.

The dog usually gets the infection by drinking water containing infection-carrying crustaceans. It is also possible that copepods with their parasitic larvae end up in the body of a frog, for instance. In this sort of paratenic host, the infection survives, and the dog gets infected after having eaten an infection-carrying frog. Adult females, filled with larvae, appear in dogs 4–9 months after the infection. An illustrated life cycle of *D. insignis* is presented in Fig. 5.72.

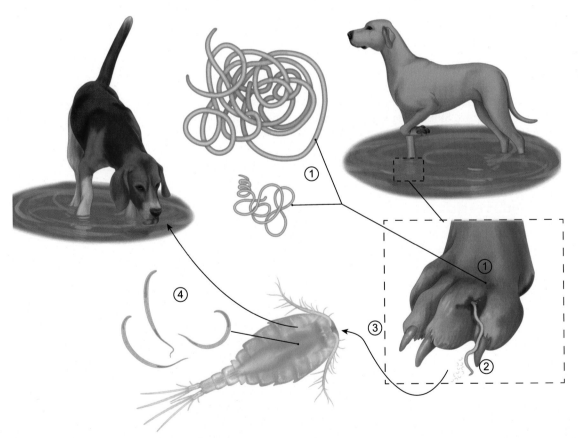

FIG. 5.72 Life cycle of *Dracunculus insignis*: (1) the adult worms live and develop larval nodules in the subcutis. The nodules are most commonly formed under the skin of the limbs. Female worm secretes substances into the nodule, causing a blister in the skin; (2) when the blister comes into contact with water, the blister breaks down and masses of larvae are freed into the water from the female; (3) the larvae released in water have a few days to reach a *Cyclops* freshwater copepod and be eaten by it; (4) inside the copepod, the larva develops to L3 stage, infectious for the dog; and (5) The dog usually gets the infection by drinking water containing infection-carrying crustaceans. The prepatent period is 4–9 months.

Distribution

D. insignis is endemic in North America. Apart from the dog, it is found in mammals such as minks, raccoons, and otters. The parasite favors host species that have a close connection with the water ecosystem. *Dracunculus medinensis*, a close relative, is more widely distributed than its cousin. It is an important human parasite. Reportedly, also the dog can be infected with *D. medinensis*.

Importance to Canine Health

An infected dog has nodules of a few centimeters in circumference. They are often located on limbs. When the female worm is ready to release its larvae, the nodule starts to show clinical signs, such as pruritus, burning sensation, urticaria-type dermatitis, and occasionally systemic signs such as fever and vomiting. General signs can manifest as early as the migration phase of the parasitic larvae. The parasite has probably been named after its Latin family, signifying a small dragon, as an inspiration from the associated pain and burning sensation.

Diagnosis

Dracunculosis is diagnosed on the basis of the skin nodules. In a smear sample taken from a nodule, inflammatory cells (macrophages, neutrophils, and eosinophilic granulocytes) can be seen. In addition, the sample may reveal larvae and sometimes adult worms. Stimulating the birth of larvae can be attempted by flushing the lesion with water. The worm is often revealed only when the lesions have been surgically removed and sent for analysis.

Treatment and Prevention

Isolated skin nodules should be surgically removed. The traditional treatment of human dracunculosis has been to catch the worm reaching out of the lesion and to roll it carefully, over several days, around a stick, until the whole worm has been removed. This method has reportedly been successfully used also for dogs. There are conflicting data regarding the efficacy of different medical treatments.

TRICHINELLA SPP.

- Intramuscular tiny nematodes. Life cycle begins with a short intestinal patent period resulting in female worms producing larvae, which are carried to striated muscles.
- Infection takes place by eating infected meat with larvae in the muscle tissue.
- During the acute phase, the clinical signs are gastrointestinal, later mostly muscle-related signs and fever.
- Diagnosis is serological and consequently usually delayed.
- Treatment is effective in the acute phase and a variety of anthelmintics can be used. Larvae in muscles are difficult to control with medications.

Identification

Trichinella worms are small nematodes. Adults living in the intestine are only 2–3 mm long. The *Trichinella* do not produce eggs. The eggs hatch inside the females, which thus gives birth to freely mobile larvae. These new-born *Trichinella* larvae are 100 µm long. They migrate into the muscles of the host animal, and some species form a connective tissue capsule around them. The capsule can be seen with the naked eye, if the infection is severe and the analyzed slice of muscle thin. Usually, however, a microscope is needed to detect the capsules. The larvae of the muscular phase are about 300 µm long.

Life Cycle

All stages of the parasite's life cycle take place in one host animal. There are no intermediate hosts or environmental forms in the cycle. *Trichinella* infections have traditionally been associated with the pig, but other meat-eating animals can be infected too, including other mammals, birds, and reptiles. Herbivores, such as horses, can be infected as well, if they have been fed meat with their feed.

The infection takes place by eating undercooked meat that contains *Trichinella* larvae. The larvae are released from the muscle by the action of hydrochloric acid and pepsin secreted by the stomach. The released larvae penetrate the epithelium of the small intestine, molt, and reproduce. The first larvae are born about 5 days after the infection. The larvae find their way inside the intestinal villi and migrate via lymph and blood circulation into striated muscle around the body. Once inside the muscle cell, the larva turns the cell into its nurse cell, which supplies nutrients and removes metabolic waste. Some species cooperate with the host to build a capsule of connective tissue around the larva. Some species lack this capsule. The capsule calcifies with time. The larvae remain infectious for years in the muscle, waiting to be eaten by the next host. In contrast, the intestinal phase ends spontaneously in about

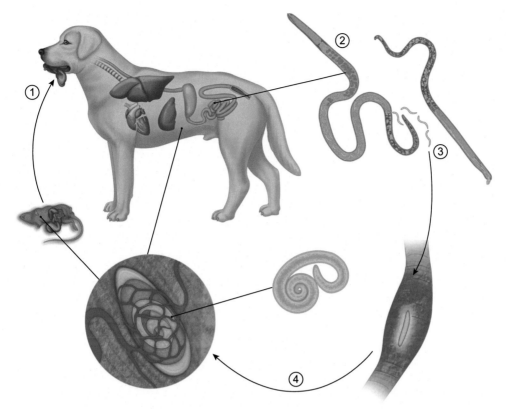

FIG. 5.73 Life cycle of *Trichinella* spp.: (1) the dog is infected by eating flesh containing *Trichinella* larvae. The larvae are released from the muscle in the stomach; (2) after several molts, the *Trichinella* reach maturity and reproduce sexually in the small intestine of the host animal; (3) the female worm gives birth to already hatched larvae (NBL) inside the intestinal villi. From there, the larvae quickly migrate via lymph and blood circulation to striated muscle. The larva penetrates a muscle cell and makes it its nurse cell; and (4) during the next weeks, the larva grows and curls up into a bundle inside the nurse cell. A capsule of connective tissue is formed around the larva of some *Trichinella* species. The larva remains infectious for years in the muscle waiting to be eaten by the next host. Morphological details redrawn based on the illustrations at www.trichinella.org. (*Reproduced with the permission from Dickson D. Despommier.*)

1.5 months. An illustrated life cycle of *Trichinella* spp. is presented in Fig. 5.73.

Distribution

Twelve *Trichinella* species or genotypes are currently recognized. *Trichinella spiralis* is probably the best known of all. *Trichinella* are endemic in all parts of the world, but the spectrum of species varies between regions.

Importance to Canine Health

Screening canine antibodies has revealed that infections are rather common in different countries, but clinical signs are rarely seen. However, nonspecific signs may be associated with other diseases, and since signs usually become subclinical with time, further investigations are not carried out. The possible signs during the intestinal stage are vomiting, diarrhea and fever, and during the muscular

phase mostly muscle pains. Unconsciousness and disturbances in heart function have been reported in association with canine trichinellosis.

Trichinella Is a Zoonotic Parasite

Man is infected with *Trichinella* in the same manner as other animals: by eating infected flesh. Typically, human infections are caused by eating pork or wild boar, but equine meat has also caused infections in Europe. The dog is not a source of human infection, unless dog meat is eaten. Meat of possible hosts, intended for human consumption, should be inspected for *Trichinella*. Different *Trichinella* species cause symptoms of varying severity to humans. *T. spiralis* is considered the most pathogenic of these. In the beginning of the infection, the symptoms are typically gastrointestinal. After the first week, the symptoms are gradually alleviated. When the parasites migrate to

Continued

muscles, the common manifestations are pain, capillary bleeding, and anaphylaxis, but it is possible that the function of many organs is disturbed. The symptoms and ultimately death may be caused for several reasons. Fatalities are, nevertheless, rare. The symptoms of the muscular phase may last several weeks.

Diagnosis

It is diagnostically noteworthy that female *Trichinella* do not produce eggs or larvae in the feces, but instead the larvae migrate from the intestinal tract to the muscles (Fig. 5.74). *Trichinella* is best detected by digesting the larvae artificially out of a piece of muscle—as large as possible—enriching the yield by sedimentation. The yield is analyzed with light microscopy. A species-specific diagnosis is reached with PCR analysis. Since it is not ethical to take large muscles samples from living humans or animals for diagnostic purposes, antitrichinella antibodies formed by the host can be analyzed serologically. The larvae in the muscle may also be revealed as an incidental finding if a histopathological analysis is done for any other reason. In practice, *Trichinella* examinations are very rarely necessary for dogs.

Treatment and Prevention

The course of *Trichinella* infection is best interrupted, if the treatment is given at the intestinal phase, when many antinematode substances are supposedly effective. Anthelmintics are rather poorly effective against the larvae settled in the muscles. There are no registered veterinary medicinal products for the treatment of canine trichinosis. Evidence is mostly available from the substances of the benzimidazole group. Anthelmintic treatment is combined with symptomatic treatment, e.g., antiemetics or rehydration during the intestinal phase, glucocorticoids for the alleviation of hypersensitivity, and antiinflammatory drugs to prevent muscle pains and fever.

Trichinella infections of humans and domestic animals are prevented by the analysis conducted during meat inspection and by rodent control in meat production facilities. Meat of potential *Trichinella* hosts should not be given uninspected or raw to dogs. In a typical case, Finnish hunting dogs were given offal from a killed wild boar. The wild boar was shown to be infected with *Trichinella* the next day. All exposed dogs were immediately treated with fenbendazole. Blood samples were taken at treatment and 2 weeks after this, for the analysis of antitrichinella antibodies. The treatment given at the intestinal phase was effective, and an increase of antibodies was not serologically detected.

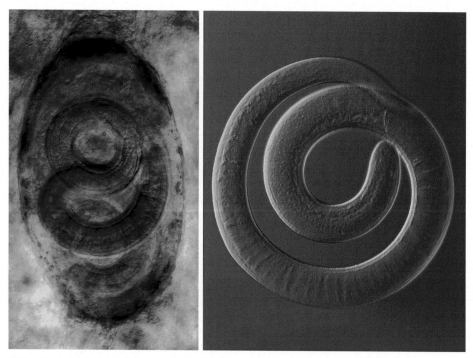

FIG. 5.74 *Trichinella* larva in muscular tissue (left) and separated from the muscle sample with digestion (right). This is an L1-phase larva, which does not molt until reaching a new host animal.

Morphology of *Trichinella*

The female *Trichinella* (Fig. 5.75) is 3–4 mm long and has a complete intestinal tract and uterus, inside which the larvae hatch. The ovary is located at the caudal end of the worm, and the fertilized eggs develop and hatch, moving progressively toward the anterior end, so that the larvae ready to be born wriggle close to the vulva orifice. The orifice is located very anteriorly behind stichosomes and esophagus. The male *Trichinella* is about 1.5 mm long. Its tail has two small, horn-like protrusions together with smaller papillae aiding with copulation (Fig. 5.76). This structure is often referred as a copulatory pseudobursa or copulatory appendage. The newborn larva (NBL) is in L1-stage and about 100 μm long. Specific structures are not yet distinguished and the sex of the larva cannot be morphologically identified. The muscle larva is about 300 μm long. It is still in the L1 stage, because the moltings do not happen until in the alimentary tract of the next host animal before maturation. All life stages of the *Trichinella* are covered with cuticle at the outer layer. Its most peripheral part is an acellular layer. The appearance of the muscle larva reveals whether it will be female or male. The dimensions of certain organs differ, and thickened cuticle can be seen close to the primordium of the female vulva.

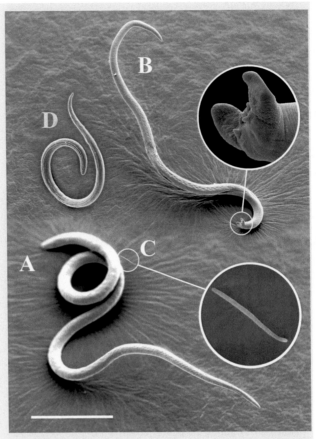

FIG. 5.76 Compilation of the developmental stages of *Trichinella* in scanning electron microscopy: (A) female; (B) male. The horn-like protrusions of the tail and the smaller nodules are visible in the round. (C) A new-born L1-stage larva. In the round detail, the same can be seen in close-up. (D) An infective L1-stage larva in muscle tissue. Scale bar = 200 μm.

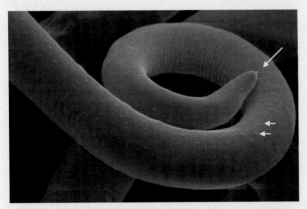

FIG. 5.75 SEM micrograph depicting female *Trichinella spiralis*. The row of small pimple-like structures (*small arrows*) on the cuticle are hypodermal gland cell openings. They are a typical feature of the adult of both sexes. The stylet (*longer arrow*) emerges from the oral opening.

The stichosome is a structure formed by 45–55 specialized cells, called stichocytes, at the anterior part of *Trichinella*. This produces granules, the components of which are found in the excretory-secretory (ES) substance of *Trichinella* that stimulates an immune response in the host animal. The stichosome is easily identified in many immunological stains.

TRICHURIS VULPIS, Whipworm

- Whipworms are up to 7.5 cm long. The worm is named after their distinct, whip-shaped appearance, with a thin anterior part and thick posterior part.
- Infection is acquired by eating eggs containing infective larva from the environment.
- Whipworms reside in the caecum and colon and may cause large-intestinal diarrhea, sometimes with blood.

- Diagnosis is by detecting lemon-shaped eggs in a fecal sample.
- The infection is treated with anthelmintics. May need repetition at 1-month intervals.

Identification

T. vulpis is a whipworm belonging to the nematodes. The name comes from the worm's general morphology, resembling a whip. The anterior end of whipworms comprises

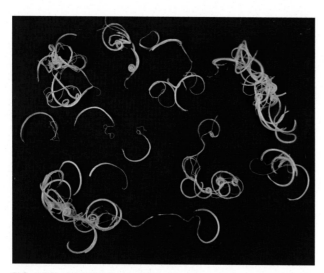

FIG. 5.77 Adult *Trichuris vulpis* worms.

three-quarters of the worm's full length, and it is long and thin (Fig. 5.77). The posterior end is thick and filled with genital organs and eggs. A structure called stichosome, consisting of a group of large glandular stichocyte cells, is in the posterior side of the esophagus. The female genital pore is close to the junction of the worm's thong of whip-like part and the thicker part. The male tail is a spiral, resembling a corkscrew, and it has one spicule covered with a spiked membranous structure. Adult *T. vulpis* worms are 4.5–7.5 cm long. The length of the egg is 70–90 μm and the width about 30–40 μm. The eggs are lemon shaped, yellowish brown, thick-walled, and smooth-surfaced, and they have a plug in both ends (Fig. 5.78). The plugs are

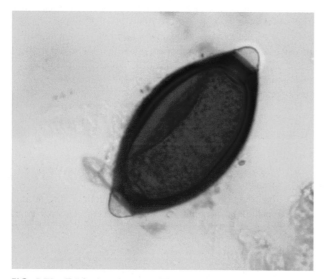

FIG. 5.78 *Trichuris vulpis* egg. The egg is *lemon shaped, yellow or brown*, and has a thick wall, smooth surface, and a plug in both ends. The plugs have ridge-like polar rings at their base.

surrounded by polar rings, which help to distinguish Trichurid eggs from very similar-looking *Eucoleus* eggs.

Life Cycle

Whipworms have a direct life cycle without any intermediate hosts. Before molting and maturation, the larvae that have hatched from the eggs ingested, penetrate the Lieberkühn glands of the canine small intestine for 2–10 days, before returning into the lumen. The worms live in the caecum and colon with their thin head buried in the intestinal mucosa, and the thicker part free in the lumen. The molting happens during the prepatent period lasting 69–114 days, after which eggs start to appear in the dog's feces. The eggs get to the environment along the feces. An infective L1-stage larva develops inside them in 1–2 months, if the conditions are suitably humid and warm. Whipworm eggs may survive in the soil for up to 5 years, but they do not withstand drought or direct sunlight. The dog is infected by eating infective eggs. An illustrated life cycle of *T. vulpis* is presented in Fig. 5.79.

Distribution

T. vulpis infections are common and ubiquitous in canids, although they appear to be uncommon in countries with cold climate. Whipworm seems to be particularly prevalent in kennels. Infections are less common in puppies than in adult dogs, since the prepatent period is long and the adults have had more time to be exposed to the infection. The worm is also usually more numerous in adults. *T. vulpis* and *A. caninum* are often found as mixed infections. A similar connection has been seen in human whipworm and hookworm infections. *T. vulpis* is not considered zoonotic, although suspected human infections have been reported in isolated cases.

Importance to Canine Health

Infections are most often subclinical, but severe infections cause intermittent, often mucous, sometimes hemorrhagic large-intestine diarrhea, typically with abnormally frequent evacuating of small fecal amounts. The condition may lead to electrolyte unbalance, hyponatremia, and hyperkalemia. The clinical signs of whipworm infection may resemble those of Addison's disease due to the disturbed electrolyte homeostasis. The risk of misdiagnosis is especially great, if the signs include general fatigue. Local inflammation and swelling of the gut wall may manifest as early as during the prepatent period. Later, when adult worms penetrate the mucosa, the damage may be more severe: the inflammation worsens and penetrates tissues deeper, and connective tissue increases in the lesions. The intestinal

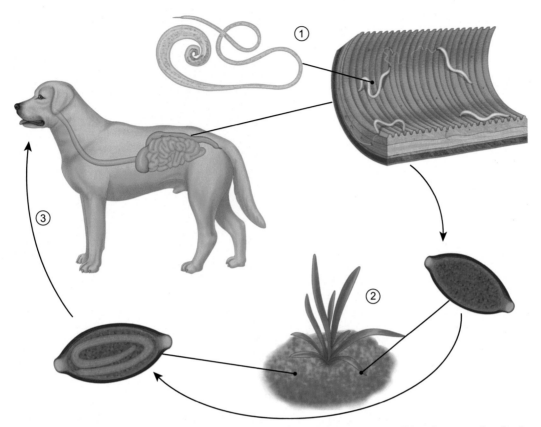

FIG. 5.79 Life cycle of *Trichuris vulpis*: (1) after infection, the hatched larva invades the glands of the small-intestine mucosa for a few days, then moves further in the intestine and molts four times before reaching maturity. Adult whipworms live in the canine caecum and colon; (2) the female lays lemon-shaped eggs with plugs in both ends. They end up in the environment with the feces. Depending on the conditions, the development of an infectious L1 larva inside the egg lasts 1–2 months; and (3) a dog is infected after swallowed the eggs. The plugs are released from the eggs and the L1-stage larva is freed.

serosa may become inflamed as well, leading to the development of adhesions. Anemia may result from a severe infection.

Diagnosis

For whipworm diagnosis, fecal samples must be taken frequently because of the intermittent egg production. The flotation solution must have a sufficient specific gravity, preferably over 1.3. Whipworm eggs found in feces need to be distinguished from similar eggs of *Capillaria aerophila (Eucoleus aerophilus)* and *Eucoleus boehmi*, based on symmetry, size, surface pattern, and the presence of polar rings at the lid bases. PCR techniques can also be used for identification. The sensitivity of the flotation techniques is not very good, especially when there are few eggs. An experimental fecal antigen ELISA has been found to improve sensitivity, and it allows for a diagnosis already during the prepatent period, 23 days after the infection. Whipworms can sometimes be visualized in the endoscopy

of the large intestine. Adult whipworms may be detected as high-echo bands, especially when the colon is filled with liquid, but the definitive diagnosis has to be done with other means.

Treatment and Prevention

According to the literature, *T. vulpis* infections have been treated with benzimidazoles, macrocyclic lactones, emodepside, and oxantel. It is recommended to repeat the treatment three times at 1-month intervals. Reinfections are common if the dog's environment is contaminated with worm eggs. The risk for kennel dogs is greater than for the general canine population. Infections can be controlled by keeping the environment dry and clean, because the eggs need moisture to survive. For instance, pen surface material should not absorb water, but instead let it through. Steam can be used for disinfection on contaminated structures. Canine stools should be removed daily to prevent the eggs from becoming infective.

EUCOLEUS (SYN. *CAPILLARIA*) SPP.

- *E. aerophilus* lives in canine lungs and airways and *E. boehmi* in the nasal cavity and sinuses. Both are long, thin, and hair-like nematodes.
- The life cycle is most probably direct, with earthworms having a role as paratenic hosts.
- May cause respiratory signs; mild infections are asymptomatic.
- Diagnosis is by detecting typical eggs with plugs and polar rings in both ends in a fecal sample.
- Several anthelmintics have been used for treatment, according to the literature.

Identification

Eucoleus nematodes are parasites of canine lungs and airways (*E. aerophilus*) or the nasal cavity and sinuses (*E. boehmi*). They are thin, thread-like worms of the family Trichuridae. The adult *Eucoleus* is about 1.5–4 cm long, and the males are slightly shorter than the females. The worms settle under the mucosa in tight folds. The egg of *E. aerophilus* is barrel-like and asymmetrical, and has a plug at both ends (Figs. 5.80 and 5.81). The size of eggs is 60–72 × 26–34 μm. The eggs of *E. boehmi* are similar but the dimensions are 54–60 × 30–35 μm, and the cellular part inside do not fill the entire egg. Eggs of *E. aerophilus* are covered with a net-like structure, with a wide mesh, whereas the surface of *E. boehmi* eggs is covered by a tight mesh.

Life Cycle

E. aerophilus is believed to have a direct life cycle. The eggs are transferred in sputum into the intestinal tract

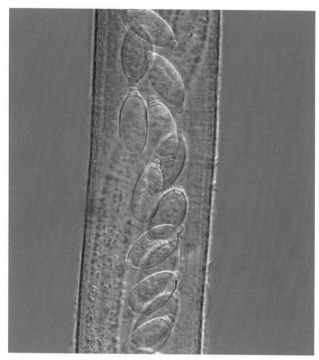

FIG. 5.80 A detail of a *Eucoleus aerophilus* female. Lots of eggs, typical for the species, are visible in the uterus.

and further with feces to the environment. The larva develops inside the egg in 30–50 days. When the dog receives embryonated eggs into its alimentary tract, either directly or via eating paratenic hosts, such as earthworms, the larva hatches from inside the egg. The larva penetrates the mucosa of the small intestine and migrates via circulation into the lungs within about a week after the moment of infection. The larva finds its way into the alveoli and ascends along the airways, meanwhile passing through developmental stages and finally maturing into an adult.

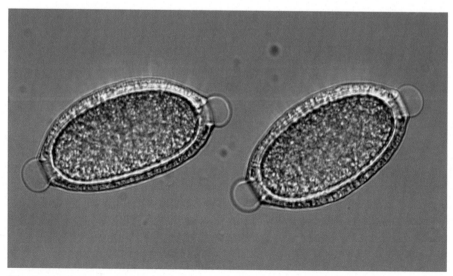

FIG. 5.81 The egg of *Eucoleus aerophilus* is barrel shaped and asymmetrical, and has a plug in both ends. The dimensions are about 65 × 30 μm and the internal cellular part fills the entire egg.

Adult worms live on the epithelium of bronchi and the trachea. The prepatent period lasts about 40 days. The life cycle of *E. boehmi* is unknown, but it is assumed to be direct. Reports about infections following coprophagic behavior support this assumption.

Distribution

E. aerophilus is a pulmonary parasite of wild and domestic carnivores. It is endemic at least in Europe, North and South America, and Australia, but the entire distribution is not known. The prevalence varies between regions. A dense population of foxes is favorable to the parasite. Infrequent human infections have been reported. *E. boehmi* infects carnivores as well, but its prevalence is also not thoroughly known. It is endemic at least in Europe and North America.

Importance to Canine Health

E. aerophilus causes respiratory infection, chronic dry or productive cough, wheezing, dyspnea and—in the worst cases—death. The respiratory damage, and consequently the signs, depends on the number of worms. Mild infections go undiagnosed. *E. boehmi* causes upper respiratory signs, including sniffling and mucous, purulent, and occasionally even hemorrhagic nasal discharge.

Diagnosis

The diagnosis of *Eucoleus* infection can be made with a fecal sample using flotation techniques. It is important to use a liquid of sufficient specific gravity, such as zinc or magnesium sulfate. The eggs are identified morphologically. They are distinguished from those of Trichuris on the basis of the pitted surface and the absence of polar rings at the base of the plugs. Since a single flotation test is good for diagnosing about half of the cases, it is preferable to analyze samples taken over several days. A sample of *E. boehmi* can be taken as a swab or lavage from the nasal mucosa. Lavage samples give a more reliable result. An eosinophilic inflammation is often visible in cytological samples. Adult worms may be seen in the endoscopy on the mucosa of the nasal cavity. A fecal sample should be taken for both flotation analysis as well as Baermann examination from patients with chronical respiratory signs and nasal discharge, to rule out parasite infection.

Treatment and Prevention

According to the literature, canine *Eucoleus* infections have been treated for example with ivermectin, fenbendazole, milbemycin oxime, or the combination of imidaclopride and moxidectin. Prevention consists of stopping the dog from eating stools and possible paratenic hosts.

Morphology of *E. aerophilus* and *E. boehmi*

Worms of the genus *Eucoleus* are thin, thread-like nematodes. The part of the worm consisting of the esophagus is shorter that the more caudal part. Glandular cells called stichocytes are located in the posterior part of the esophagus. Their number is an important feature in the species-level diagnosis. The male has wing-like cuticular alae in the tail and one sheathed spicule. The female genital pore is located at the caudal end of the esophagus, usually at the junction of the first and the second third of the worm. The anus is near the caudal end.

CAPILLARIA HEPATICA (SYN. *CALODIUM HEPATICUM*)

- A hepatic nematode of rodents and lagomorphs; can also infect dogs.
- The eggs are not secreted into the environment, but they encapsulate in the liver.
- Infection is transferred to a new host when the liver is eaten or when it decomposes in the environment and releases eggs.
- Infection may be associated with hepatitis and hepatic tissue damage and cirrhosis.
- Diagnosis is by analyzing liver biopsies or using immunological tests. There is no effective treatment.

Identification

C. hepatica is a thin, thread-like nematode of the family Trichuridae. It typically parasitizes rodents and lagomorphs, but occasionally also infects dogs. The anterior end of the worm is thinner than the tail end. Male worms are shorter than the female, and they have one long and thin spicule and a primitive bursal structure. The eggs are barrel-shaped, similar to other *Capillaria* and *Eucoleus*. Egg size is about $60 \times 30\,\mu m$ and there are plugs in both ends. The egg surface is thick and colorless apart from vague stripes.

Life Cycle

The life cycle of *Capillaria* is direct. No eggs are secreted into the environment. The adult worms reproduce in the liver and the eggs produced by the female stay in the hepatic tissue and encapsulate. An infective larval form develops inside the egg. The infection is transferred to the next host animal, when it eats the liver. When the host dies and decomposes in nature, the eggs are released into the environment from inside the liver and become accessible for the next host animals. When the host eats the eggs, the larvae are released into the intestinal tract; they penetrate the gut wall and migrate in lymph and blood circulation into the liver to mature.

Distribution

C. hepatica is endemic in rodents everywhere in the world. It is an incidental finding in dogs.

Importance to Canine Health

Since the worms live in the liver and the eggs are produced in the hepatic tissue as well, with no way out, the infection causes hepatic damage: hepatitis and cirrhosis. The eggs are produced in large clusters. Consequently, focal granulomas may be found in the sites of eggs in autopsy. Mild infections are usually subclinical.

Diagnosis

Since the eggs do not get into the alimentary tract, analysis of feces is not diagnostic. The infection is usually diagnosed in autopsy, but an exploratory abdominal surgery combined with taking liver biopsies in order to explore hepatic signs may lead to diagnosis as well. Immunological assays have been designed to analyze human and rodent serum samples.

Treatment and Prevention

Rodent control is necessary in the vicinity of homes and kennels. At the beginning of the infection, benzimidazole treatment lasting several days prevents the development of eggs, but the treatment is useless at a later stage. Since diagnosing the infection in live dogs is difficult, the treatment is seldom well timed.

PEARSONEMA (SYN. CAPILLARIA) PLICA

- Nematode parasite of the urinary tract.
- Earthworms are part of the life cycle; dogs are infected by eating them or paratenic hosts.
- Infection is often subclinical, but may lead to urinary tract infection and hematuria.
- Diagnosis is carried out by detecting eggs in urine sample or adult worms during the cystoscopy.
- The infection can be treated with benzimidazoles, levamisole, or ivermectin. Efficacy is poor.

Identification

P. plica is a small and hair-like parasite of the urinary tract (Fig. 5.83), belonging to the Trichuridae nematodes. The adult female is 30–60 mm and the male 13–30 mm long. The eggs are oval, surrounded by a thick capsule, and they have plugs at both ends (Fig. 5.82). The size of eggs is 63–68 × 24–27 μm.

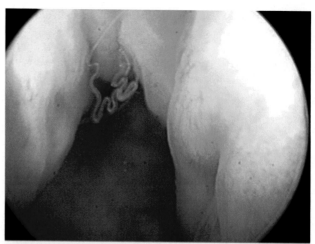
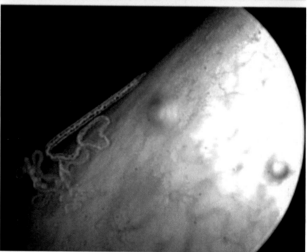

FIG. 5.82 Adult *Pearsonema plica* worms seen in bladder endoscopy. *(Reproduced with permission from Basso W, Spänhauer Z, Arnold S, Deplazes P: Capillaria plica (syn. Pearsonema plica) infection in a dog with chronic pollakiuria: challenges in the diagnosis and treatment, Parasitol Int. 63(1):140–142, 2014, https://doi.org/10.1016/j.parint.2013.09.002.)*

Life Cycle

The parasite is presumed to have an indirect life cycle. The earthworm acts as the intermediate host. It gets the parasite inside its body by eating eggs secreted in the urine of the definitive host. L1-stage larvae hatch from the eggs in the earthworm and settle in the worm's tissues. The definitive host is infected by eating the earthworm or a paratenic, e.g., a bird that has eaten the worm. L2 and L3 larvae develop in the definitive host through moltings, migrate into the kidneys via the circulation, and descend via the ureters into the bladder. The parasites mature in the bladder, penetrate the mucosa, and copulate. The females lay eggs that are secreted in the urine of the definitive host. The prepatent period is 2 months.

Distribution

The parasite is ubiquitous in dogs, cats, and wild carnivorous mammals. Foxes are an important reservoir host.

Importance to Canine Health

The infection often causes no signs at all, or only slight irritation of the mucosa lining the bladder, but it has also been reported occasionally to cause serious signs of urinary tract infection. The infection is usually self-limiting. In these cases, the secretion of eggs into urine gradually diminishes and then entirely ends. Reinfections are possible. If the disease is clinical, the signs are typical for urinary tract infection, such as frequent urination, breaking house-training, hematuria, and straining to urinate. Kidney failure, caused by the amyloidosis of the renal glomeruli, has also been reported. Signs of a bladder infection are the result of the parasite damaging the bladder mucosa or the mucosal lesions becoming secondarily infected with bacteria. *Pearsonema* infection is also on list of differential diagnoses in cases, where the urinary tract infection may have been already treated with antibiotics, but the signs continue despite the negative bacterial culture and the absence of crystals in the urine.

Diagnosis

Worms may be visualized in the cystoscopy of the urinary bladder (Fig. 5.82). The most common and easiest way of obtaining the diagnosis is detecting the *Capillaria*-type eggs (Fig. 5.83) in a urinary sample. When the urine is centrifuged, the eggs sediment and can be detected microscopically. The liquid phase of the centrifuged urine can be replaced with a flotation solution, which is then mixed with the sediment, enabling the concentration and recovery of floating eggs. Since the secretion of eggs into urine varies, a definite diagnosis may necessitate the analysis of urine samples taken on several consecutive days. It is important to ensure that the sample is clean. A fecal or soil contamination may cause a misdiagnosis, if eggs of other parasites are confused with those secreted in urine. If the progress of the treatment is monitored with urinary samples, they should be taken up to at least 2 weeks after the end of therapy.

Treatment and Prevention

There is no registered medical treatment for *P. plica* infection. Reported treatment options include benzimidazoles, levamisole, and macrocyclic lactones. The efficacy of the treatment was followed on the basis of egg secretion and cystoscopy in a case report. Fenbendazole and ivermectin were found to be ineffective in that study. In contrast, a 2-day treatment with levamisole killed the worms from the bladder. A preventive method in endemic areas is to choose the ground material of outside dog kennels to repel earthworms. Suitable materials include, for instance, a raised floor or gravel. Hunting is considered a risk factor, because the hunting dogs roam in the same areas as the major reservoir species, the fox.

> **Morphology of *Capillaria*, *Perasonema*, and *Eucoleus***
>
> *Capillaria*, *Pearsonema*, and *Eucoleus* are long, thin, hair-like nematodes. In microscopy, they have the stichosome structures around the esophagus, typical of the species in the same family (e.g., *Trichinella*, *Trichuris*, *Capillaria*). *Capillaria* has 20–60 stichosomes in three rows. The female genital pore is located very close to the worm's caudal end. The male has one spicule, protected by a sock-like sheath.

DIOCTOPHYMA RENALE, Giant Kidney Worm

- The largest nematode infecting dogs, up to 100 cm long. Adult worms are found in the kidneys.
- Life cycle includes a period in blackworms. Dogs are infected by eating them or paratenic hosts, mainly fish.
- Infection is associated with nephritis and renal insufficiency, and results in the destruction of the kidney.
- Diagnosis is based on finding eggs in urine or by detecting adult worms with the aid of imaging methods.
- The condition is treated by removing the kidney surgically.

Identification

D. renale is the largest of all canine nematodes (Fig. 5.84). Male worms are about 15–45 cm long and they can be 6 mm thick. The female may be up to 1 m (20–100 cm) long and 12 mm thick. The worms are red and

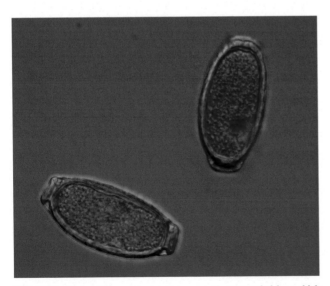

FIG. 5.83 Eggs of *Pearsonema plica* are oval, surrounded by a thick capsule, and have a plug in both ends. The size of the eggs is about 65 × 25 μm.

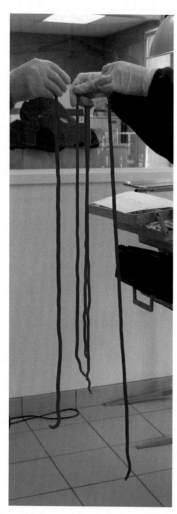

FIG. 5.84 *Dioctophyma renale* is the largest nematode parasite of the dog. The worms in the photo have been dissected from a hydronephrotic kidney surgically removed from a dog. *(Photo by Jennifer Vander Kooi, Thunder Bay Veterinary Hospital, reproduced with permission.)*

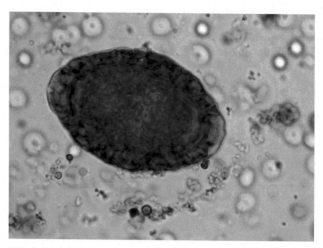

FIG. 5.85 The *Dioctophyma* egg in stained urine sample. When in an unstained sample, the egg is light, lemon-shaped, and thick-walled. The size of the egg is about 70 × 45 μm. Apart from the poles, the eggshell is uneven and prominently folded. *(Micrograph by Jennifer Vander Kooi, Thunder Bay Veterinary Hospital, reproduced with permission.)*

both ends are tapering but blunt. The male has a bell-shaped copulatory bursa at the tail end. The eggs of *Dioctophyma* are light and lemon-shaped, and have a thick shell. The size of the eggs is about 60–80 × 40–50 μm. Apart from the poles, the eggshell is uneven and prominently folded (Fig. 5.85).

Life Cycle

Adult worms live in the kidney and renal pelvis. The eggs laid by the female are passed via the urinary bladder in urine into the environment. In urine, the eggs are either in the monocellular or bicellular phase. The eggs must reach water, where their embryonation lasts from 2 weeks up to several months, depending on the temperature. The requirement for the continuation of the life cycle is that the

hatched larvae find their way to the alimentary tract of an intermediate host, an oligochaete annelid, blackworm, *Lumbriculus variegatus*, living in waterways. In the ventral vessel of the intermediate host, *Dioctophyma* develops via moltings into an infective L3 larva. The life cycle continues when a dog swallows an infection-carrying blackworm. However, the blackworm is more probably eaten by a fish or an amphibian than by the definitive host. Fish or amphibians can act as paratenic hosts, in which the parasite remains encapsulated, infective, and ready to infect the definitive host, when eaten. Raw fish is considered to be a major infection source for the dog. In the definitive host, the L3 larva penetrates the mucosa of the stomach and migrates further to the liver and, after more development, to the kidney. Adult worms are most often found in the right kidney and more seldom in the ureter or the bladder. In dogs, the worm often enters the abdominal cavity. The worm may remain reproductive for up to 5 years. An illustrated life cycle of *D. renale* is presented in Fig. 5.86.

Distribution

Apart from dogs, the infection is diagnosed in other carnivores, and it has in rare cases also been described in other than carnivore species, such as pigs, horses, and humans—the latter extremely rarely. The mink is considered to be the major definitive host and the reservoir. The distribution is considered worldwide (Europe, North and South America, Africa, and Asia).

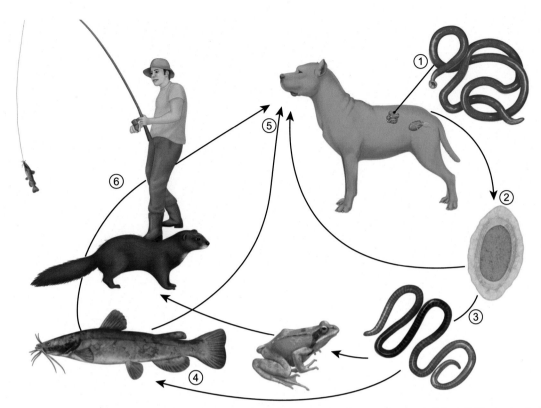

FIG. 5.86 Life cycle of *Dioctophyma renale*: (1) after the infection, the L3 larva penetrates the stomach mucosa of the definitive host and migrates from there to the liver and, having developed further, into the kidney. The adult worms live in the kidney and in the renal pelvis; (2) eggs laid by the female are transferred via the bladder in urine to the external environment. When in urine, the eggs are either in the monocellular or bicellular phase; (3) the eggs must reach water, where their embryonation lasts from 2 weeks to several months, depending on the temperature. The hatched larvae must be able to invade the intestinal tract of blackworms, annelids living in water, to develop into the L3 stage. The life cycle continues when a dog swallows a blackworm carrying the infection; (4) a fish or an amphibian will eat the parasite more probably than its proper definitive host. Hence, they may act as paratenic hosts, in which the parasite remains encapsulated and ready to infect a definitive host. Raw fish is considered to be the most important source of infection for the dog; (5) apart from dogs, the infection is diagnosed in other carnivores, and it has in rare cases also been described in humans (6), although extremely rarely. The mink is considered the major definitive host and the reservoir.

Morphology of *D. renale*

Confirming the diagnosis is not difficult even without knowledge of morphological details, if one finds in a dog's kidney or in the abdomen a worm that is 1 m long and over 1 cm thick. The mouth of the worm is simple. It has no lip structures. It is surrounded by a thin and smooth ring-like zone with six small, low papillae. Another ring structure, also consisting of six papillae, is located outside of that. The papillae of the outer ring are hemispherical and substantially larger than those of the inner zone. The esophagus is long and thin. The tail end of the male expands into a bell-like copulation bursa, which lacks the bursal branches. The bursa is adjoined with a single bristle-like spicule, the length of which varies between 5 and 6 mm. The female genital opening is located in the anterior part of the worm. The anus is terminally in the caudal end of the worm.

Importance to Canine Health

The massive worms cause pressure atrophy and necrosis in the adjacent kidney tissue. The end-result of the total kidney tissue destruction is that the worms are surrounded only by a stretched renal capsule and thin, adhesion-like, and calcified remains of the renal tissue. The situation is usually complicated by the inflammation of the renal tissue and pelvis. Generally, there are worms only in the right kidney, and the left kidney is able to compensate for the renal insufficiency, usually causing no signs of clinical kidney failure. The infection is often complicated by hematuria. If the renal insufficiency becomes manifest, it is combined with typical signs of uremia, such as weight loss and vomiting. A worm that invades the ureter may cause sudden, intense pain resembling a kidney stone attack. If worms invade the abdominal cavity, the common complications include

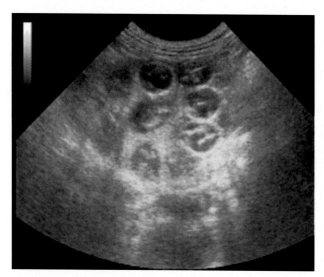

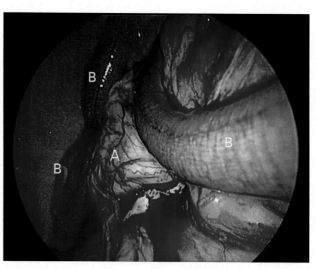

FIG. 5.87 Ultrasound findings from the dog with *Dioctophyma renale* infection. Kidney is atrophied and numerous transversal sections of a large worm can be seen. *(Photo by Jennifer Vander Kooi, Thunder Bay Veterinary Hospital, reproduced with permission.)*

FIG. 5.88 Laparoscopy findings from the same dog than in Fig. 5.87. Atrophied kidney (A) is distended by the intrarenal worms. Large worms (B) were even seen freely in the abdominal cavity. *(Photo by Jennifer Vander Kooi, Thunder Bay Veterinary Hospital, reproduced with permission.)*

peritonitis and adhesions. Eggs produced by a female worm maturing in the abdominal cavity will never reach outside world and an intermediate host. They will be targeted by the immune response of the dog, causing them to encapsulate as abdominal granulomas. It is common that the aberrant abdominal worms never reach full maturity.

Diagnosis

The diagnosis is based on detecting eggs, typical of the species, in a urine sample (Fig. 5.85). Thanks to the large size, ultrasound images (Fig. 5.87), X-ray, or laparoscopy

(Fig. 5.88) often suggest the presence of *D. renale*. Sometimes worms that have strayed into the abdominal cavity are found during abdominal surgery (Figs. 5.88 and 5.89).

FURTHER READING

Ajayi O, Omotainse S, Antia R, Antia F, Akande F, Olaniyi M: Hepatic histopathological changes in a dog with natural *Capillaria hepatica* infection in Nigeria, *Niger J Parasitol* 31:39–42, 2011.

American Heartworm Society: *Current canine guidelines for the diagnosis, prevention and management of heartworm (Dirofilaria immitis) infection in dogs,* 2016. www.heartwormsociety.org. (Accessed 16 January 2018).

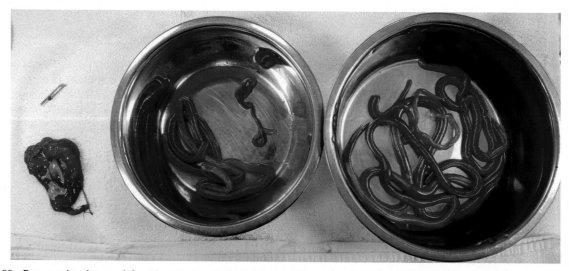

FIG. 5.89 Postoperative photograph from the same dog as in Figs. 5.87 and 5.88 showing right kidney remains (on the left), nematodes found inside the right kidney (the bowl in the middle), and nematodes located freely in the abdominal cavity. The size of the worms can be appreciated by comparing their size to a surgical blade on the left. *(Photo by Jennifer Vander Kooi, Thunder Bay Veterinary Hospital, reproduced with permission.)*

Azam D, Ukpai O, Said A, Abd-Allah G, Morgan E: Temperature and the development and survival of infective Toxocara canis larvae, *Parasitol Res* 110:649–656, 2012.

Baan M, Kidder A, Johnson S, Sherding R: Rhinoscopic diagnosis of *Eucoleus boehmi* infection in a dog, *J Am Anim Hosp Assoc* 47:60–63, 2011.

Bandi C, Trees A, Brattig N: *Wolbachia* in filarial nematodes: evolutionary aspects and implications for the pathogenesis and treatment of filarial diseases, *Vet Parasitol* 98:215–238, 2001.

Basso W, Spänhauer Z, Arnold S, Deplazes P: *Capillaria plica* (syn. *Pearsonema plica*) infection in a dog with chronic pollakiuria: challenges in the diagnosis and treatment, *Parasitol Int* 63:140–142, 2014.

Bauer C: Baylisascariosis—infections of animals and humans with 'unusual' roundworms, *Vet Parasitol* 193:404–412, 2013.

Bauer C, Bahnemann R: Control of Filaroides hirthi infections in Beagle dogs by ivermectin, *Vet Parasitol* 65:269–273, 1996.

Bazzocchi C, Mortarino M, Grandi G, et al: Combined ivermectin and doxycycline treatment has microfilaricidal and adulticidal activity against *Dirofilaria immitis* in experimentally infected dogs, *Int J Parasitol* 38:1401–1410, 2008.

Berry W: *Spirocerca lupi* esophageal granulomas in 7 dogs: resolution after treatment with doramectin, *J Vet Int Med* 14:609–612, 2000.

Bolt G, Monrad J, Frandsen F, Henriksen P, Dietz H: The common frog (*Rana temporaria*) as a potential and intermediate host for *Angiostrongylus vasorum*, *Parasitol Res* 79:428–430, 1993.

Bowman D, Darigrand R, Frongillo M, Barr S, Flanders J, Carbone L: Treatment of experimentally induced trichinosis in dogs and cats, *Am J Vet Res* 54:1303–1305, 1993.

Burke T, Roberson E: Fenbendazole treatment of pregnant bitches to reduce prenatal and lactogenic infections of Toxocara canis and *Ancylostoma caninum* in pups, *J Am Vet Med Assoc* 183:987–990, 1983.

Chalifoux L, Hunt R: Histochemical differentiation of *Dirofilaria immitis* and Dipetalonema reconditum, *J Am Vet Med Assoc* 158:601–605, 1971.

Chapman P, Boag K, Guitian J, Boswood A: *Angiostrongylus vasorum* infection in 23 dogs (1999–2002), *J Small Anim Pract* 45:435–440, 2004.

Chu S, Myers S, Wagner B, Snead E: Hookworm dermatitis due to *Uncinaria stenocephala* in a dog from Saskatchewan, *Can Vet J* 54:743–747, 2013.

Companion Animal Parasite Council: *Parasites of other systems—urinary tract nematodes*. Last updated: 2012-05-01. https://www.capcvet.org/guidelines/urinary-tract-nematodes. (Accessed 16 January 2018).

Conboy G: Helminth parasites of the canine and feline respiratory tract, *Vet Clin North Am Small Anim Pract* 39:1109–1126, 2009.

Cortes H, Cardoso L, Giannelli A, Latrofa M, Dantas-Torres F, Otranto D: Diversity of *Cercopithifilaria* species in dogs from Portugal, *Parasit Vectors* 7:261, 2014.

Costa JO, De Araujo Costa HM, Guimaraes MP: Redescription of *Angiostrongylus vasorum* (Baillet, 1866) and systemic revision of species assigned to the genera *Angiostrongylus* Kamensky, 1905 and *Angiocaulus* Schulz, 1951, *Revue Méd Vet* 154:9–16, 2003.

Devoy Keegan J, Holland C: A comparison of Toxocara canis embryonation under controlled conditions in soil and hair, *J Helminthol* 87:78–84, 2013.

Di Cesare A, Castagna G, Meloni S, Otranto D, Traversa D: Mixed trichuroid infestation in a dog from Italy, *Parasit Vectors* 5:128, 2012.

Dillard K, Saari S, Anttila M: Case report—*Strongyloides stercoralis* infection in a Finnish kennel, *Acta Vet Scand* 49:37, 2007, https://doi.org/10.1186/1751-0147-49-37.

Dryden M, Ridley R: Efficacy of fenbendazole granules and pyrantel pamoate suspension against Toxocara canis in greyhounds housed in contaminated runs, *Vet Parasitol* 82:311–315, 1999.

Du Plessis C, Keller N, Millward I: Aberrant extradural spinal migration of *Spirocerca lupi*: four dogs, *J Small An Pract* 48:275–278, 2007.

Egyed Z, Sréter T, Széll Z, et al: Morphologic and genetic characterization of *Onchocerca lupi* infecting dogs, *Vet Parasitol* 102:309–319, 2001.

Elsemore D, Geng J, Flynn L, Cruthers L, Lucio-Forster A, Bowman D: Enzyme-linked immunosorbent assay for coproantigen detection of *Trichuris vulpis* in dogs, *J Vet Diagn Invest* 26:404–411, 2014.

El-Tras W, Holt H, Tayel A: Risk of Toxocara canis eggs in stray and domestic dog hair in Egypt, *Vet Parasitol* 178:319–323, 2011.

Epe C: Intestinal nematodes: biology and control, *Vet Clin North Am Small Anim Pract* 39:1091–1107, 2009.

Fahrion A, Schnyder M, Wichert B, Deplazes P: Toxocara eggs shed by dogs and cats and their molecular and morphometric species-specific identification: Is the finding of T. cati eggs shed by dogs of epidemiological relevance? *Vet Parasitol* 177:186–189, 2011.

Fargo D: *Dracunculus insignis* (On-line), Animal Diversity Web, 2003. http://animaldiversity.org/accounts/Dracunculus_insignis/. (Accessed 12 September 2018).

Freeman RS: Helminth parasites of the red fox in Finland 1963–1964, In *First International Congress of Parasitology* (vol. 1), Rome, Italy, 1964.

Fuehrer H-P, Igel P, Auer H: *Capillaria hepatica* in man—an overview of hepatic capillariosis and spurious infections, *Parasitol Res* 109:969–979, 2011.

Furtado AP, Melo FTV, Giese EG, Santos JN: Morphological description of *Dirofilaria immitis*, *J Parasitol* 96:499–504, 2010.

Gabrielli S, Giannelli A, Brianti E, et al: Chronic polyarthritis associated to *Cercopithifilaria bainae* infection in a dog, *Vet Parasitol* 15:401–404, 2014.

Geary T, Bourguinat C, Prichard R: Evidence for macrocyclic lactone anthelmintic resistance in *Dirofilaria immitis*, *Topics Comp An Medic* 4:186–192, 2011.

Genta RM, Schad GA: Filaroides hirthi: hyperinfective lungworm infection in immunosuppressed dogs, *Vet Pathol* 21:349–354, 1984.

Georgi J, Georgi M: Patency and transmission of Filaroides hirthi infection, *Parasitol* 75:251–257, 1977.

Georgi J, Georgi M: Rhabditis (Pelodera). In Georgi J, Georgi M, editors: *Canine clinical parasitology*, Pennsylvania, USA, 1991a, Lea & Febiger, pp 165–166.

Georgi J, Georgi M: Strongyloides. In Georgi J, Georgi M, editors: *Canine clinical parasitology*, Pennsylvania, USA, 1991b, Lea & Febiger, pp 160–165.

Grove D: Human strogyloidiasis. In Baker JR, Muller R, Dollison R, editors: *Advances in parasitology* (vol. 38), 1996, Academic Press, pp 251–309.

Hassan K, Bolcen S, Kubofcik J, et al: Isolation of *Onchocerca lupi* in dogs and black flies, California, USA, *Emerg Inf Dis* 21:789–796, 2015.

Ionică A, D'Amico G, Mitková B, et al: First report of *Cercopithifilaria* spp. in dogs from Eastern Europe with an overview of their geographic distribution in Europe, *Parasitol Res* 113:2761–2764, 2014.

Karkamo V, Castren L, Näreaho A: Ketun keuhkomato, Crenosoma vulpis, koiralla—kirjallisuuskatsaus ja tapausselostus, *Suomen eläinlääkäril* 118:67–72, 2012 (in Finnish).

Komnenou A, Eberhard M, Kaldrymidou E, Tsalie E, Dessiris A: Subconjunctival filariasis due to *Onchocerca* sp. in dogs: report of 23 cases in Greece, *Vet Ophthalmol* 5:119–126, 2002.

Kopp S, Coleman G, McCarthy J, Kotze A: Application of in vitro anthelmintic sensitivity assays to canine parasitology: detecting resistance to pyrantel in *Ancylostoma caninum*, *Vet Parasitol* 152:284–293, 2008.

Lalosevic V, Lalosevic D, Capo I, Simin V, Galfi A, Traversa D: High infection rate of zoonotic *Eucoleus aerophilus* infection in foxes from Serbia, *Parasite* 20:3, 2013.

Lee A, Schantz P, Kazacos K, Montgomery S, Bowman D: Epidemiologic and zoonotic aspects of ascarid infections in dogs and cats, *Trends Parasitol* 26:155–161, 2010.

Lloyd S, Elwood C, Smith K: *Capillaria hepatica* (*Calodium hepaticum*) infection in a British dog, *Vet Rec* 151:419–420, 2002.

Mace T, Anderson R: Development of the giant kidney worm, Dioctophyma renale (Goeze, 1782) (Nematoda: Dictophymatoidea), *Can J Zool* 53:1552–1568, 1975.

Magi M, Guardone L, Prati M, Torracca B, Macchioni F: First report of *Eucoleus boehmi* (syn. *Capillaria boehmi*) in dogs in north-western Italy, with scanning electron microscopy of the eggs, *Parasite* 19:433–435, 2012.

McCall J, Genchi C, Kramer L, Guerrero J, Venco L: Heartworm disease in animals and humans, *Adv Parasitol* 66:193–285, 2008.

Megat Abd Rani P, Irwin P, Gatne M, Coleman G, McInnes L, Traub R: A survey of canine filarial diseases of veterinary and public health significance in India, *Parasit Vectors* 3:30, 2010.

Miró G, Montoya A, Hernández L, et al: *Thelazia callipaeda*: infection in dogs: a new parasite for Spain, *Parasit Vectors* 4:148, 2011.

Morgan E, Shaw S: Angiostrongylus vasorum infection in dogs: continuing spread and developments in diagnosis and treatment, *J Small An Pract* 51:616–621, 2010.

Morgan E, Shaw S, Brennan S, De Waal T, Jones B, Mulcahy G: Angiostrongylus vasorum: a real heartbreaker, *Trends Parasitol* 2:49–51, 2005.

Mutafchiev Y, Dantas-Torres F, Giannelli A, et al: Redescription of *Onchocerca lupi* (Spirurida: Onchocercidae) with histopathological observations, *Parasit Vectors* 6:309, 2013. https://doi.org/10.1186/1756-3305-6-309.

Mylonakis M, Rallis T, Koutinas A, et al: Clinical signs and clinicopathologic abnormalities in dogs with clinical spirocercosis: 39 cases (1996–2004), *J Am Vet Med Assoc* 228:1063–1067, 2006.

Naem S: *Thelazia* species and conjunctivitis. In Pelkan Z, editor: *Conjuctivitis—a complex and multifaceted disorder*, 2011, InTech. 978-953-307-750-5, http://www.Intechopen.com/books/conjuctivitis-a-complex-and-multifaceted-disorder/thelazia-species-and-conjuctivitis.

Napoli E, Brianti E, Falsone L, et al: Development of Acanthocheilonema reconditum (Spirurida, Onchocercidae) in the cat flea Ctenocephalides felis (Siphonaptera, Pulicidae), *Parasitology* 141:1718–1725, 2014.

Nevalainen M, Saari S, Nikander S: Toxocara canis ja Toxascaris leonina—koiran suolinkaiset, *Suom Elainlaakaril* 100:587–594, 1994 (in Finnish).

Nikander S: Sukkulamadon (*Spirocerca lupi*) aiheuttama osteosarkooma koiran ruokatorvessa, *Suom eläinlääkäril* 100:173–177, 1994 (in Finnish).

Olsen O: *Animal parasites: their life cycles and ecology,* ed 3, Baltimore, MD, 1974, University Park Press.

Otranto D, Dantas-Torres F: Transmission of the eyeworm *Thelazia callipaeda*: between fantasy and reality, *Parasit Vectors* 8:273, 2015.

Otranto D, Liu RP, Buono V, Traversa D, Giangaspero A: Biology of *Thelazia callipaeda* (Spirurida, Thelaziidae eyeworms in naturally infected definitive host), *Parasitology* 129:627–633, 2004.

Otranto D, Cantacessi C, Testini G, Lia LP: *Phortica variegata* is an intermediate host of *Thelazia callipaeda* under natural conditions: evidence for pathogen transmission by a male arthropod vector, *Int J Parasitol* 36:1167–1173, 2006.

Otranto D, Sakru N, Testini G, et al: Case report: first evidence of human zoonotic infection by *Onchocerca lupi* (Spirurida, Onchocercidae), *Am J Trop Med Hyg* 84:55–58, 2011.

Otranto D, Dantas-Torres F, Brianti E, et al: Vector-borne helminths of dogs and humans in Europe, *Parasit Vectors* 6:16, 2013.

Overgaauw P, van Knapen F: Dogs and nematode zoonoses. In Macpherson C, Meslin F, Wandeler A, editors: *Dogs, zoonoses and public health*, Wallingford, 2000, CABI Publishing, pp 213–256.

Panciera D, Stockham S: Dracunculus insignis infection in a dog, *J Am Vet Med Assoc* 192:76–78, 1988.

Pasyk K: Dermatitis rhabditiosa in an 11-year-old girl—a new cutaneous parasitic disease of man, *Br J Dermatol* 98:107–112, 1978.

Pinckney R, Studer A, Genta R: Filaroides hirthi infection in two related dogs, *J Am Vet Med Assoc* 193:1287–1288, 1988.

Pullola T, Vierimaa J, Saari S, Virtala A-M, Nikander S, Sukura A: Canine intestinal helminths in Finland: prevalence, risk factors and endoparasite control practices, *Vet Parasitol* 140:321–326, 2006.

Ramsey I, Littlewood J, Dunn J, Herrtage M: Role of chronic disseminated intravascular coagulation in a case of canine angiostrongylosis, *Vet Rec* 138:360–363, 1996.

Ravani M: *Dioctophyma renale* (On-line), Animal Diversity Web, 2003. http://animaldiversity.org/accounts/Dioctophyma_renale/. (Accessed 12 September 12 2018).

Ravindran R, Varghese S, Nair S, et al: Canine filarial infections in a human *Brugia* malayi endemic area of India, *Biomed Res Int*, 2014. https://doi.org/10.1155/2014/630160.

Reagan J, Aronsohn M: Acute onset of dyspnea associated with *Oslerus osleri* infection in a dog, *J Vet Emerg Crit Care* 22:267–272, 2012.

Roberts L, Janovy J: Nematodes: rhabditida, pioneering parasites. In Gerald D, Schmidt G, Larry S, editors: *Roberts' foundations of parasitology*, New York, 2005, McGraw-Hill, pp 411–416.

Roddiea G, Stafford P, Holland C, Alan Wolfe A: Contamination of dog hair with eggs of Toxocara canis, *Vet Parasitol* 152:85–93, 2008.

Saari S, Nikander S: *Pelodera* (syn. Rhabditis) *strongyloides* as a cause of dermatitis—a report of 11 dogs from Finland, *Acta Vet Scand* 48:18, 2006.

Saari S, Syrjälä P, Lappalainen A, Dahlqvist E, Nikander S: Filaroides osleri—madon aiheuttama trakeobronkiitti koiralla—kirjallisuuskatsaus ja kaksi tapausselostusta, *Suom Eläinlääkäril* 103:647–653, 1997 (in Finnish).

Schoning P, Dryden M, Gabbert N: Identification of a nasal nematode (*Eucoleus boehmi*) in greyhounds, *Vet Res Commun* 17:277–281, 1993.

Schrey C, Trautvetter E: Canine and feline heartworm disease—diagnosis and therapy, *Waltham Focus* 8:23–30, 1998.

Shoop W, Michael B, Eary C, Haines H: Transmammary transmission of *Strongyloides stercoralis* in dogs, *J Parasitol* 88:536–539, 2002.

Simonato G, Frangipane di Regalbono A, Cassini R, et al: Copromicroscopic and molecular investigations on intestinal parasites in kenneled dogs, *Parasitol Res* 114:1963–1970, 2015.

Söderblom A, Saari S, Järvinen A-K: Angiostrongylus vasorum infection in an imported dog—the first verified case in Finland. *Suomen eläinlääkäril* 114:199–208, 2008 (in Finnish).

Sorvillo F, Ash L, Berlin O, Yatabe J, Degiorgio C, Morse S: *Baylisascaris procyonis*: an emerging helminthic zoonosis, *Emerg Infect Diseases* 8:355–359, 2002.

Sudhaus W, Schulte F: Rhabditis (*Pelodera*) *strongyloides* (Nematoda) als Verursacher von Dermatitis, mit systematishen und biologishen bemerkungen über verwandte arten, *Zool Jb Syst* 115:187–205, 1988 (in German).

The Center for Food security and Public Health: *Zoonotic hookworms,* 2013, Iowa State University. http://www.cfsph.iastate.edu/Factsheets/pdfs/hookworms.pdf. (Accessed 16 January 2018).

Theisen S, LeGrange S, Johnson S, Sherding R, Willard M: *Physaloptera* infection in 18 dogs with intermittent vomiting, *J Am Anim Hosp Assoc* 34:74–78, 1998.

Traversa D: Are we paying too much attention to cardiopulmonary nematodes and neglecting oldfashioned worms like Trichuris vulpis? *Parasit Vectors* 4:32, 2011.

Vajner L, Vortel V, Brejcha A: Lung filaroidosis in the beagle dog breeding colony, *Veterinární medic* 45:25–30, 2000.

van der Merwe L, Kirberger R, Clift S, Williams M, Keller N, Naidoo V: *Spirocerca lupi* infection in the dog: a review, *Vet J* 176:294–309, 2008.

Venco L, Valenti V, Genchi M, Grandi G: A dog with Pseudo-Addison disease associated with Trichuris vulpis infection, *J Parasitol Res* 2011:682039, 2011.

Veronesi F, Morganti G, Di Cesare A, Schaper R, Traversa D: A pilot trial evaluating the efficacy of a 10% imidacloprid/2.5% moxidectin spot-on formulation in the treatment of natural nasal capillariosis in dogs, *Vet Parasitol* 200:133–138, 2014.

Wagner G, Seitz KA: SEM-Untersuchungen zur äußeren Morphologie von Rhabditis strongyloides (Nematoda, Rhabditidae), *Zool Jahrb Abt Anat Ontog Tiere* 103:62–72, 1980 (in German).

Willers WB: *Pelodera strongyloides* in association with canine dermatitis in Wisconsin, *J Am Vet Med Ass* 156:319–320, 1970.

Willesen J, Kristensen A, Jensen A, Heine J, Koch J: Efficacy and safety of imidacloprid/moxidectin spot-on solution and fenbendazole in the treatment of dogs naturally infected with Angiostrongylus vasorum (Baillet, 1866), *Vet Parasitol* 147:258–264, 2007.

Chapter 6

Acantocephala (Thorny-Headed Worms)

Acanthocephalan worms are not a very important group of canine parasites. They are pseudocoelomates and their body cavity is essentially filled with reproductive organs. As their name indicates, their head has a proboscis armed with numerous sclerotized hooks. By means of this proboscis the worm pierces the gut mucosa and attaches itself to the gut wall. The proboscis can be everted from or retracted into a well-developed, muscular diverticular sheath. Acanthocephalans lack mouth and alimentary tract, and nutrients are absorbed through the tegument. In addition, the tegument plays a role in osmoregulation and protection and inactivation of host's digestive enzymes. A paired fluid-filled lemniscus, hanging free from their distal ends and extending into the body cavity, is present at both sides of the diverticulum.

An acanthoephalan worm is either male or female. Males are usually smaller than females. The key structures of male reproductive organs are two testes, a small penis, cement glands, and copulatory bursa. The cement glands produce filler used for plugging the vagina of the female worm after copulation. By doing this, the male tries to prevent copulation and fertilization of the eggs by other males. To intensify these actions, males of some thorny-headed worm species use the cement substance directly on the genitals of competing males. The copulatory bursa is usually invaginated within the posterior part of the male and everted during copulation.

The female has fragmented rounded ovaries. The ovaries of the female fall apart early in the development to become cell masses that float freely in the body cavity liquid. The cells on the surface of these masses are fertilized after copulation, begin embryonal development, and disengage from the cell mass, exposing the deeper layers of cells for fertilization. As an end-result of fertilization, an embryo develops in the egg and further hatches into first stage larva: an acanthor. The free-floating eggs are caught from the body cavity by a bell- or funnel-shaped structure, referred to as a uterine bell. Through this uterine bell, the mature eggs are voided into the uterus. Between the uterine bell and uterus, there is an opening that sorts immature eggs from mature eggs. The eggs with incomplete development are smaller than the mature ones and they drift through the gaps of the uterine bell back to the body cavity, while the embryonated eggs are filtered into a route leading to the external environment through the oviduct. A basic morphology of a typical acanthocephalan worm is illustrated in Fig. 6.1. Acanthocephalan eggs are typically oval, brown, and thick celled. Three cell layers enclose a larval stage (acanthor).

The life cycle is indirect, involving suitable arthropod intermediate hosts, and may comprise paratenic hosts.

MACRACANTHORHYNCHUS SPP.

- Definitive hosts are pig and wild carnivores.
- Intermediate host is a beetle; paratenic hosts may have importance as a source of dog infections.
- Adult worms are large, ranging from a few centimeters to half a meter, depending on species.
- Most cases are subclinical; perforation of the small intestine might lead to peritonitis.
- Diagnosis is based on the detection of eggs in the fecal sample, but they are secreted only periodically.

Identification

Macracanthorhynchus hirudinaceus, *M. ingens*, and *M. catulinus* may infect dogs. They have a barbed, retractable, rather small rostrum, by means of which the worm penetrates into the intestinal wall, sometimes even perforating it. When retracted, the rostrum is in a proboscis sheath, or diverticulum, in the anterior part of the worm. *M. hirudinaceus* (Fig. 6.2) is a large worm, 10–40 cm long and 4–10 mm wide. The dimensions of *M. catulinus* are 4.5–12.5 cm. Females are larger than males. The color of the *Macracanthorhynchus* worms is pale reddish. They are flat and transversely wrinkled. They have a typically acanthocephalan basic morphology: they lack alimentary tract and are dioecious. The eggs (Fig. 6.3) of *Macracanthorhynchus* species are oval, thick celled, rough surfaced, and about $90-105 \times 46-54\,\mu m$ in size. The egg contains an acanthor larva.

Life Cycle

Wild carnivores such as foxes, skunks, minks, badgers, and especially pigs, are natural definitive hosts of

Canine Parasites and Parasitic Diseases. https://doi.org/10.1016/B978-0-12-814112-0.00006-4

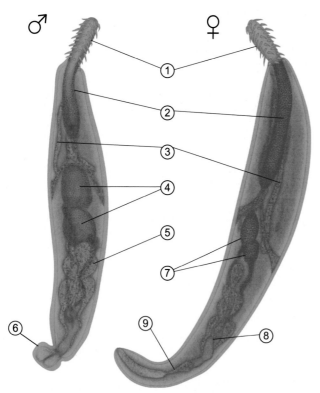

FIG. 6.1 Morphology of a typical thorny-headed worm. They are pseudocoelomates and lacking alimentary tract: (1) hold-fast organ, proboscis, armed with numerous hooks; (2) diverticular sheath; (3) lemnisci; (4) testes; (5) cement glands; (6) copulatory bursa; (7) ovaries; (8) uterine bell; and (9) oviduct.

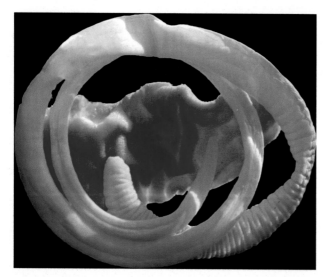

FIG. 6.2 *Macracanthorhynchus hirudinaceus* attached to the intestinal wall with the aid of its armed proboscis.

Macracanthorhynchus. In an endemic area, the dog may receive the infection by eating beetles or Myriopoda (millipedes and centipedes), which act as intermediate hosts for the parasite. Cystacanth, the infective larva, has developed

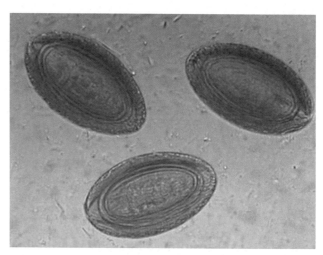

FIG. 6.3 The eggs of *Macracanthorhynchus hirudinaceus* are oval and 90–105 × 46–54 μm in size. A rough-coated, layered, thick cell envelopes the larval stage, called an acanthor. *(Reproduced with permission of Dr. Juan Antonio Figueroa Castillo, FMVZ-UNAM.)*

inside these hosts over 3 months, during the acanthella phase. If the infection-carrying intermediate host ends up in a host that is unsuitable for its life cycle (paratenic host), development is arrested, but the cystacanth remains infective. If the paratenic host, along with its cystacanth, is eaten by a definitive host, the life cycle can be completed. In the small intestine of a dog or another definitive host species, the worm pierces its thorny proboscis into the gut wall and attaches itself. The prepatent period is 2–3 months. *Macracanthorhynchus* worms are short-lived in the dog, and the patent period with egg production is short. In contrast, an adult female is fecund and can produce 260,000 eggs daily in the small intestine of a pig over several months. The eggs survive in a wide variety of environmental conditions, and the acanthor larva remains infective for years, until it reaches the intermediate host and is able to develop into the next stage. Some thorny-headed worms display postcyclic transfer to a new definitive host. In this case, an animal suitable for the host eats another animal that has thorny-headed worms in its gut. The worms capable of postcyclic transfer can avoid digestion by the new host and continue their life in the intestine of the new host.

Distribution

Macracanthorhynchus species are ubiquitous in the world, although some regions, for instance, in Europe, are almost free of them. *M. hirudinaceus* is the most widely spread species. *M. catulinus* is endemic especially in Asia and *M. ingens* in North and South America. The parasite can be rather common in endemic areas. The infectivity is season-dependent according to the prevalence of intermediate host beetles.

Importance to Canine Health

Mild infections are typically without any clinical signs. Diarrhea has been described in dogs as a result of *Macracanthorhynchus* infection. The penetration of the small intestine by the proboscis of the worm causes a typical strawberry mark and, if the penetration extends to full-thickness of the gut, even peritonitis. Isolated human infections have been reported. Humans obtain the infection by eating intermediate hosts; they do not catch it from the dog.

Diagnosis

Since the eggs of thorny-headed worms float, a patent infection can be diagnosed with standard flotation methods. However, in canine infections, eggs are produced only periodically. If the worm itself is isolated, the analysis starts by placing the worm in water, in which the rostral part and male genital protrude out for species diagnosis. After this, the worm can be preserved.

Treatment and Prevention

Ivermectin is cited in many case reports as a treatment for *Macracanthorhynchus* infection, likely based on evidence accrued from porcine infections as ivermectin is widely used as a parasiticide in swine husbandry. In endemic areas, dogs may be prevented from eating paratenic hosts or arthropods acting as intermediate hosts to prevent infection. However, this is neither easy nor practical.

Oncicola canis

Oncicola canis (Fig. 6.4) is a thorny-headed worm rarely seen in canids in North and South America. Compared to *Macracanthorhynchus* worms, it is small, at just over 1 cm long. The worm gets thinner towards the tail end and there is a distinct proboscis in the front end, a structure with backward-pointing thorns. The size of eggs that are secreted into feces is $43–50 \times 67–72\,\mu m$, and they can be detected with flotation techniques, for instance. The life cycle is not completely known, but arthropods act as intermediate hosts and the dog is typically infected by eating paratenic hosts, such as lizards, birds, and armadillos. The assumed life cycle is depicted in Fig. 6.5. Clinical signs are rare.

FURTHER READING

Aiello SE, Moses MA, editors: *The Merck veterinary manual*, Rahway, NJ, 2016, Merck & CO.

American Association of Veterinary Parasitologists: Heterophyes heterophyes. http://www.aavp.org/wiki/trematodes-2/trematodes-small-intestine/echinostomatidae/echinochasmus-perfoliatus/. (Accessed January 2018).

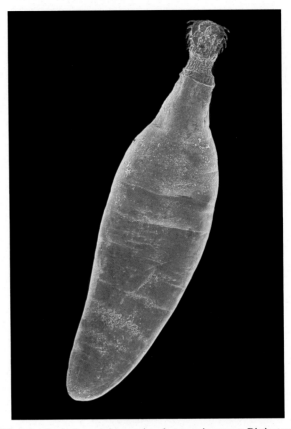

FIG. 6.4 *Oncicola canis* in scanning electron microscopy. Distinct proboscis and wrinkled appearance of the trunk are clearly seen. *(Reproduced with permission of Dennis Kunkel/Science Photo Library.)*

American Association of Veterinary Parasitologists: http://www.aavp.org/wiki/trematodes-2/trematodes-small-intestine/. (Accessed January 2018).

American Association of Veterinary Parasitologists: Mesostephanus milvi. http://www.aavp.org/wiki/trematodes-2/trematodes-small-intestine/cyathocotylidae/mesostephanus-milvi/. (Accessed January 2018).

Arrellano L: Paragonimus kellikotti, Animal Diversity Web, University of Michigan. http://animaldiversity.org/accounts/Paragonimus_kellicotti/. (Accessed January 2018).

Barr S, Bowman D: *Blackwell's five-minute veterinary consult clinical companion: canine and feline infectious diseases and parasitology,* ed 2, Oxford, 2012, Wiley-Blackwell.

Blair D, Xu ZB, Agatsuma T: Paragonimiasis and the genus Paragonimus, *Adv Parasitol* 42:113–222, 1999.

CABI, International Institute of Parasitology: *8th International training course on identification of Helminth parasites of economic importance,* UK, 1996.

Chai J, Darwin Murrell K, Lymbery A: Fish-borne parasitic zoonoses: status and issues, *Int J Parasitol* 35:1233–1254, 2005.

Conboy G: Helminth parasites of the canine and feline respiratory tract, *Vet Clin North Am Small Anim Pract* 39:1109–1126, 2009.

Doanh P, Yukifumi Nawa Y: Clonorchis sinensis and Opisthorchis spp. in Vietnam: current status and prospects, *Trans R Soc Trop Med Hyg* 110:13–20, 2016.

Dunn AM: *Veterinary helminthology,* ed 2, London, 1978, Heinemann.

El-Gayar A: Studies on some trematode parasites of stray dogs in Egypt with a key to the identification of intestinal trematodes of dogs, *Vet Parasitol* 144:360–365, 2007.

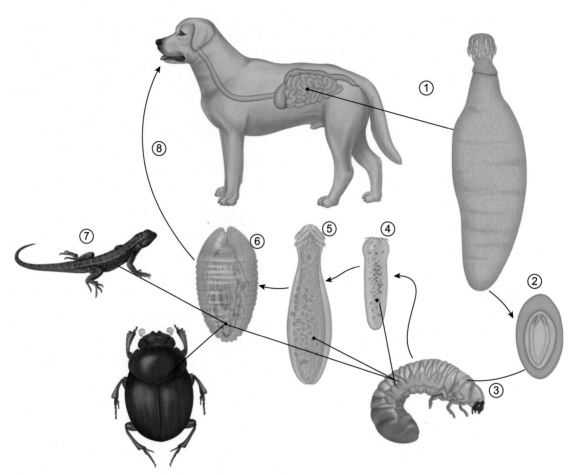

FIG. 6.5 Life cycle of *Oncicola canis*: (1) this is a small acanthocephalan worm residing in the small intestine; (2) female worms excrete embryonated eggs containing a larval stage, acanthor, within the feces of the host. Various species of dung beetles may act as intermediate hosts for the parasite; (3) they become infected when they or their larvae feed on egg-containing manure or soil; (4) inside the intestine, the acanthor is released; (5) it penetrates the body cavity and develops into the larval stage called acanthella; (6) acanthella continues its maturation into the infective stage, a cystacanth; (7) if the infection-carrying intermediate host ends up in a host that is unsuitable for its life cycle (paratenic host), the development is arrested, but the cystacanth remains infective; and (8) if the intermediate or paratenic host, along with its cystacanth, is eaten by a definitive host, the life cycle can be completed. In the small intestine of a dog or another definitive host species, the worm pierces its thorny proboscis into the gut wall and attaches itself.

Fang F, Li J, Huang T, Guillot J, Huang W: Zoonotic helminths parasites in the digestive tract of feral dogs and cats in Guangxi, China, *BMC Vet Res* 11:211, 2015. https://doi.org/10.1186/s12917-015-0521-7.

Flowers JR, Hammerberg B, Wood SL, et al: *Heterobilharzia americana* infection in a dog, *J Am Vet Med Assoc* 220:193–196, 2002.

Freeman R, Stuart P, Cullen J, et al: Fatal human infection with mesocercariae of trematode *Alaria americana*, *Am J Trop Med Hyg* 25:803–807, 1976.

Fürst T, Keiser J, Utzinger J: Global burden of human food-borne trematodiasis—a systematic review and meta-analysis, *Lancet Infect Dis* 12:210–221, 2012.

Guildal J, Clausen B: Endoparasites from one hundred Danish red foxes (Vulpes vulpes), *Norw J Zool* 21:329–330, 1973.

Gunn A, Pitt S: *Parasitology—an integrated approach,* ed 1, Oxford, 2012, Wiley-Blackwell.

Headley S, Scorpio D, Vidotto O, Dumler S: Neorickettsia helminthoeca and salmon poisoning disease: a review, *Vet J* 187:165–173, 2011.

Horák P, Kolarová L, Adema C: Biology of schistosome genus Trichobilharzia, *Adv Parasitol* 52:155–233, 2002.

Hung N, Madsen H, Fried B: Invited review: global status of fish-borne zoonotic trematodiasis in humans, *Acta Parasitol* 58:231–258, 2013.

Jacobs D, Fox M, Gibbons L, Hermosilla C: *Principles of veterinary parasitology,* Chichester, 2016, Wiley Blackwell.

Johnson E: Canine schistosomiasis in North America: an underdiagnosed disease with expanding distribution, *Comp Cont Ed Vet* 32:E1–E4, 2010.

Kumar V: *Trematode infections and diseases of man and animals,* Dordrecht, 1999, Springer.

Lemetayer J, Snead E, Starrak G, Wagner B: Multiple liver abscesses in a dog secondary to the liver fluke Metorchis conjunctus treated by percutaneous transhepatic drainage and alcoholization, *Can Vet J* 57:605–609, 2016.

Lin R, Tang J, Zhou D, et al: Prevalence of Clonorchis sinensis infection in dogs and cats in subtropical southern China, *Parasit Vectors* 4:180, 2011.

Mehlhorn H: *Encyclopedic reference of parasitology,* ed 2, Berlin/Heidelberg, 2001, Springer.

Millemann RE, Knapp SE: Biology of Nanophyetus salmincola and "salmon poisoning" disease, *Adv Parasitol* 8:1–41, 1970.

Nesvadba J: Dicrocoeliosis in cats and dogs, *Acta Vet Brno* 75:289–293, 2006.

Olsen O: *Animal parasites—their life cycles and ecology,* Baltimore, MD, 1974, University Park Press, pp 237–240.

Paulsen P, Forejtek P, Hutarova Z, Vodnansky M: Alaria alata mesocercariae in wild boar (Sus scrofa, Linnaeus, 1758) in south regions of the Czech Republic, *Vet Parasitol* 197:384–387, 2013.

Persson L, Christensson D: Endoparasiter hos rödräv i Sverige, *Zool Rev* 33:17–24, 1971 (in Swedish).

Roberts L, Janovy J: In Schmidt GD, Robert's LS, editors: *Foundations of parasitology,* 8 ed, New York, 2009, McGraw-Hill, pp 291–292.

Rodriguez JY, Camp JW, Lenz SD, Kazacos KR, Snowden KF: Identification of Heterobilharzia americana infection in a dog residing in Indiana with no history of travel, *J Am Vet Med Assoc* 248:827–830, 2016.

Saari S, Westerling B, Nikander S: Madot tappoivat suden Hämeessä: kuolemaan johtanut Alaria sp. -imumatoinfektio sudella, *Suom eläinlääkäril* 104:716–721, 1998 (in Finnish).

Schmidt G, Roberts L: *Foundations of parasitology,* St Louis, MO, 1989, Times Mirror/Mosby College Publishing, pp 260–264.

Schuster R, Heidrich J, Pauly A, Nöckler K: Liver flukes in dogs and treatment with praziquantel, *Vet Parasitol* 150:362–365, 2007.

Shoop W, Corkum K: Migration of Alaria marcianae (Trematoda) in domestic cats, *J Parasitol* 69:912–917, 1983.

Sitko J, Bizos J, Sherrard-Smith E, Stanton D, Komorová P, Heneberg P: Integrative taxonomy of European parasitic flatworms of the genus Metorchis Looss, 1899 (Trematoda: Opisthorchiidae), *Parasitol Int* 65:258–267, 2016.

Soulsby EJL: *Helminths, arthropods and protozoa of domesticated animals,* ed 7, London, 1982, Balliére Tindall.

Taylor M, Coop R, Wall R: *Veterinary parasitology,* ed 4, Oxford, 2016, Wiley Blackwell.

Willingham A, Ockens N, Kapel C, Monrad J: A helminthological survey of wild red foxes (*Vulpes vulpes*) from the metropolitan area of Copenhagen, *J Helminthol* 70:259–263, 1996.

Yamaguti S: *Synopsis of digenetic trematodes of vertebrates* (vol. 1), Tokyo, 1971, Keigaku Publishing Company, p 1074.

Ye C, Yang Z, Zheng H: Fatal multi-organ Clonorchis sinensis infection in dog: a case report, *Vet Parasitol* 195:173–176, 2013.

Zajac A, Conboy G: *Veterinary clinical parasitology,* ed 8, West Sussex, 2012, John Wiley & Sons.

Chapter 7

Annelida (Segmented Worms, Ringed Worms)

HIRUDO MEDICINALIS, European Medicinal Leech and Other Leeches

---

- Leeches are blood sucking segmented worms and have been historically used in medicine to remove "bad blood."
- Leeches are mostly aquatic and freshwater based, where they also attached to the host. Some species are of a land, usually rainforest, variety.
- Usually not a health problem to a dog; short-term bleeding and bruises may be seen.
- Treatment involves removing the leeches cautiously. It is important to avoid leaving the parts of the leech in the skin, as they can cause a slowly healing granulomatous inflammation, and to prevent the dog from swimming or drinking from waters and walking in rainforests inhabited by leeches.

Identification

Leeches belong to the phylum Annelida, segmented worms. The European medicinal leech, *Hirudo medicinalis,* is up to 20 cm long, dark brown, and has six brown or reddish stripes on the dorsal side longitudinally. The ventral side is spotted. The trunk is cylindrical and the dorso-ventral profile is somewhat flat. The outer surface is divided into 33–34 segments. Both the head and the tail have a sucker, but only the head's sucker has dental structures for cutting skin and sucking blood. The head segment has five pairs of eyes. Other leeches differ in their patterning.

H. medicinalis is hermaphrodite. It has several pairs of testes and one pair of ovaries. A ring-like thicker muff, clitellum, secreting mucous substance, can be seen in a sexually mature worm. Despite hermaphrodism, sexual reproduction is the normal method in species whose reproduction has been studied.

Life Cycle

In tropical areas, leeches are often terrestrial and a menace in rainforest areas. Aquatic leeches live in small and muddy, preferably rushy, lakes, and ponds. They swim fast and smoothly with moray-type movements; when still, they use their suckers to attach surfaces, such as pieces of wood at water's edge. When the water temperature rises, the sensitivity of the leech to the water waves rises as well, and it is ready to attach to a host in the water. The leech perforates the host's skin with its teeth and secretes local anesthetics and anticoagulants (hirudin) along its saliva. The blood-sucking is efficient: in about half an hour's feeding period the leech is able to suck about 10–15 mL of blood from the host. At the attachment site, a Y-shaped bite mark can be seen for some time. Reproduction happens onshore. The female lays egg packages of over 10 eggs in each on the moist ground, close to the water line. In 4–10 weeks, young leeches, about 1 cm in length, hatch and travel to water. They can live up to 100 days without feeding. Due to their delicate teeth, the young leeches usually feed on amphibians instead of mammals. Frogs existing in the habitat is essential to leeches. Reaching adulthood and to be able to reproduce takes 1–3 years and 3–5 blood meals.

Distribution

H. medicinalis is rare or endangered in the Northern Europe and Eurasia, whereas *Hirudo verbana* (Fig. 7.1) occurs in more southern areas, around the Mediterranean. Populations have been exported to outside the natural habitat. Other leeches found in human or animal hosts include *Limnatis nilotica, Myxobdella* spp., *Dinobdella ferox, Phytopdella catenifera,* and *Teromyzom tessulatom.*

Importance to Canine Health

Thanks to their rarity, leeches in nature do not pose a noticeable health risk to dogs. As efficient blood suckers, leeches may cause anemia in a small dog. The condition is healed by removing the worms. Leeches can be useful in veterinary care in the treatment of hemorrhagic bruises and chronic pain.

Canine Parasites and Parasitic Diseases. https://doi.org/10.1016/B978-0-12-814112-0.00007-6

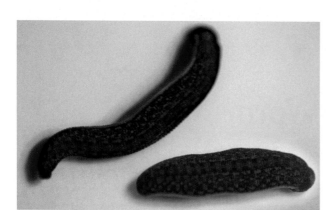

FIG. 7.1 *Hirudo verbana* leeches.

Diagnosis

A leech attached to the dog's skin or mucous membrane can be identified thanks to its large size and its morphological features.

Treatment and Prevention

Attached leeches are pulled away from the attachment site and reinfections are prevented. Fresh drinking water must be available in risky areas, because a dog drinking from a pond, or a lake can get leeches in its mouth.

Leeches in Medicine

Leeches have been used since the Middle Ages to evacuate disease-causing "bad blood" and to "balance humors," in a similar manner to bloodletting or cupping. Modern medicine has reinvented the use of leeches. Hirudotherapy is used in postsurgical care, to maintain circulation in tissues that are in risk for necrosis—for instance, in peripheral transplants. The efficacy is based on controlled hemorrhage and the effects of the leech's saliva on vascular dilation, local analgesia, and antiinflammation. In veterinary medicine, othematoma, and other hemorrhagic bruises have been treated with success. Leeches have also been used for treating chronic pain in canine locomotory organs. The origin of leeches used in any medical purposes must be confirmed. Many species are rare in nature and only cultured strains can be used. In addition, the risk of blood-transmitted diseases may rise when the origin is unknown.

Chapter 8

Insecta

Arthropoda consists of two major classes: Insecta (insects) and Arachnida, including subclass Acari (ticks and mites). Insects (Fig. 8.1) have three body parts—head, thorax, and abdomen—and six legs. Some of them have segmented antennae and/or wings; in others these features are lacking or are rudimentary. The process of transformation from an immature arthropod stage to an adult stage is referred as metamorphosis. It can be, depending on species, holometabolic (complete)—egg, larva, pupa, adult—or hemimetabolic (incomplete), with eggs, and nymphal stages resembling adults preceding the actual adulthood. Insects have a digestive tract which is a tube from mouth to anus divided to a foregut, midgut, and hindgut, possibly with some pouch-like caecae.

The Malpighian tubule system is an excretory and osmoregulatory system consisting of branching tubules extending from the alimentary tract. It absorbs dissolved matter, water, and nitrogen-containing waste from the surrounding hemolymph.

The nervous system consists of the supraesophageal ganglio (brain) connected to a ventral nerve cord. The eye may be a really complex compound eye enabling a very large view angle and the ability to detect fast movement, or just an aggregation of some sensory cells (ocelli) capable of sensing light but not forming images.

The gas exchange takes place through openings or spiracles on arthropod's exoskeleton. They allow air to enter the tracheal tubes or tracheoles, which deliver oxygen directly into the arthropod's tissues. There are no lungs present.

Arthropods have an open circulatory system. Blood or hemolymph mostly flows freely within body cavities with the direct contact with internal tissues and organs.

Dorsally, there is a large tube-like vessel that runs longitudinally along the inside of the dorsal body wall. This vessel serves as a primitive heart. It consists of chambers that are separated by valves and muscles contract and force the hemolymph to move from one chamber to another. Openings (ostia) allow hemolymph to flow into the heart.

Arthropods are dioecious species, meaning that each individual is of only one sex. There are distinct male and female individual arthropod organisms. The male's reproductive system contains a pair of testes. Mature sperm pass out of the testes through short ducts connected to the storage, called seminal vesicles. Similar ducts lead away from the seminal vesicles, and merge to form a single duct leading out through the male's copulatory organ (aedeagus). There are usually accessory glands connected to the male's reproductive system producing secretions that sustains and nourishes the sperm. These glands also produce pouch-like structures that protect the sperm and allow the delivery of the sperm in packages during copulation.

The female's reproductive system contains a pair of ovaries. A fertile and actively reproducing arthropod female can be recognized based on swollen ovaries filled with developing eggs and hence, occupying the majority of the abdominal cavity.

Mature eggs leave the ovaries via short oviducts, which merge to form a common oviduct leading into a chamber called the copulatory bursa. During copulation, the male deposits his spermatophore into the copulatory bursa. From there the spermatophore is pushed into the structure known as spermatheca, a storage pouch for the sperm in the female. With the aid of glandular secretions, sperm may stay alive for months, or even longer, in the spermatheca.

Fertilization takes place after ovulation. When the egg passes the opening of the spermatheca, a few sperm are unleashed on the egg surface. Fertilization occurs after a sperm has found its way into the egg through the small opening of the egg shell. After fertilization, eggs are ready for an oviposition and their embryonic development may begin.

Parasitic insects might spend their whole life in contact to the host, like lice do, or they might have part of the life cycle outside the host, which is the case with fleas. The nutrition of different ectoparasitic insects varies. Some suck blood and the others feed on epidermal material or tissue fluids, for example. Usually the clinical signs associated with the infestation by insect parasites are reactions to their bites resulting in itching and scratching, because of the irritating feeling when the insects move in the fur coat. Repeated insects bites, however, may trigger insect bite

Canine Parasites and Parasitic Diseases. https://doi.org/10.1016/B978-0-12-814112-0.00008-8

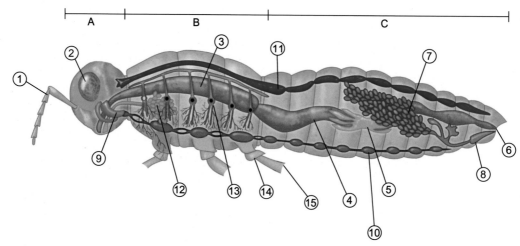

FIG. 8.1 A schematic illustration of a female insect: (A) head; (B) thorax; (C) abdomen. (1) antenna; (2) eye, behind the eye; supraesophageal ganglion; (3) foregut; (4) midgut; (5) Malphigian tubules; (6) anus; (7) ovary; (8) oviduct; (9) subesophageal ganglion; (10) ventral ganglion; (11) dorsal vessel; (12) salivary gland; (13) spiracles and tracheoles; (14) coxa; and (15) femur. *(Redrawn based on the illustration by Piotr Jaworski, https://en.wikipedia. org/wiki/Insect_morphology#/media/File:Insect_anatomy_diagram.svg.)*

hypersensitivity reaction and allergy, which are often associated with profound clinical signs. If the skin is damaged, secondary bacterial infections may complicate the clinical outcome. Insects play an important role as vectors for diseases too. Examples of these are mosquitos spreading dirofilariosis, sand flies transmitting leishmaniosis and fleas acting as an intermediate host for a *Dipylidium caninum* tapeworm.

Diagnostics of the insect ectoparasites is based on their morphological features. Sometimes the key structures are easy to spot, like the size, and shape of the head. There might be some chitinous extensions (stenidia) or "hairs" on the outer surface or legs, which are used in species diagnostics. It is wise to ask the owner to catch the macroscopic ectoparasite at home, before coming to the clinic, for two reasons: sometimes it is hard to find the ectoparasites if the infestation is not heavy; and it is also advisable to diagnose the parasitic disease based on the sample supplied rather than to allow the infested dog to come inside the clinic premises where it can infest other dogs.

A huge range of choice is available nowadays for the medical control and treatment of canine ectoparasitic infestations. The ever-lasting importance of fleas and an increased attention to ticks and tick-borne diseases have served as key drivers for research and development of veterinary ectoparasitic pharmaceuticals. Knowing the biology and life-cycles of the most important ectoparasites in important, as quite often the duration of the medication has to be long enough to ensure there will be no reinfection from the surroundings and that the life cycle of the parasite has been broken. Cleaning of the dog's bed and other in-contact places is part of ectoparasite control in cases of many infestations.

LINOGNATHUS SETOSUS, Dog Sucking Louse

- Ectoparasite of dogs in parts of Scandinavia and other colder countries, where flea and tick protection is not routine, elsewhere very uncommon.
- Dorso ventrally flattened body. Head narrower than thorax.
- Sucks blood and causes irritation of skin and hypersensitivity reaction. Sometimes heavy infestations found without clinical signs.
- As a constant parasite, easy to control with many insecticides.

Identification

Sucking lice (Figs. 8.2 and 8.3) are wingless, gray-to-brown, dorsoventrally flat insects, with a length of about 2 mm. The head of the louse is narrower than the trunk and specialized in sucking blood. It has hooked feet that for gripping hair. The egg, or nit (Fig. 8.4), is equipped with a lid and glued tightly to the hair from its other end with adhesive substance.

Life Cycle

The sucking lice are species specific. *Linognathus setosus* do not infest other animals beside canids. The louse spends all stages of its life cycle in canine hair coat. If it is separated from its host animal, it survives at most for a few days. At low temperatures, the slow-moving lice become even

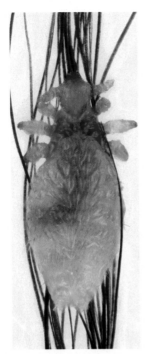

FIG. 8.2 Dog's sucking louse attached to hairs. *(Photo by Sami Karjalainen, reproduced with permission.)*

more passive and their chances of finding a new host animal are minimal. Transmission between dogs usually happens with direct contact, less often via contaminated grooming equipment. If the host's body temperature rises, for instance, because of fever, or drops for example because of death, the lice will try to flee and find a new host.

When preparing to suck blood, the louse pushes its piercing structure (Fig. 8.3) out of the oral cavity and anchors it to the skin. Oral cutting parts are used for penetrating the skin. The sucking lice copulate several times during their life, which lasts about 1 month. The female louse lays up to 200 eggs during its lifetime. It attaches the lid-equipped eggs or nits one by one to the hairs from their posterior part (Fig. 8.4). The egg is oval but the side, set against the hair, is straighter. After the incubation period lasting about 1 week, a nymph phase, resembling an adult louse, hatches from the egg. As for the human head louse, the optimal temperature for hatching nits is 29–32°C and ambient humidity about 75%. In these conditions, 70%–90% of the nits will hatch. A decline of only 5 degrees from the optimal temperature diminishes the hatching proportion to 10%. There are three nonreproductive nymphal stages before the adult stage. The transfer from one stage to another takes place through molting. The length of *Linoghathus setosus* life cycle is poorly known, but the nymph phases of the human head louse is known to last 8–9 days, while the total life cycle from a laid egg to a reproducing adult takes about 1 month.

Distribution

The dog sucking louse is rare. The louse, spending all phases of its life cycle in the dog's fur, is sensitive to different, even short-acting, ectoparasite treatments. Substances that are used to control flea and tick infestations have driven the sucking louse almost to the brink of extinction. It is distributed, but rare, everywhere in the world, particularly in places where many dogs converge and their husbandry is primitive. In regions where dogs are well cared for but tick and flea prevention is not routine, sucking louse infestations still occur. Surviving colonies of sucking lice are still found in Nordic countries that are almost free of pet fleas, and dogs do not receive ectoparasitic medication for long periods. However, the distribution of ticks continues to expand northwards in both Europe and North America. This means more treatments against ticks pushing dog sucking lice to extinction.

Importance to Canine Health

The term pediculosis is often used in the literature for sucking louse infections. The name is misleading, since it derives from the genus *Pediculus* of the human louse. It is more correct to use the term linognathosis for the canine infestation. Linognathosis is most commonly seen in autumn, winter, and early spring, when the inner coat is at its thickest. In many dogs, the infection is subclinical. If signs manifest, they are often associated with sensitization of the dog to recurrent blood sucking.

The most common sign of sucking louse infection is pruritus of variable severity. Some dogs react to the presence of a few lice with serious itch, some can have a massive infestation without clinical signs. A clinical examination can reveal dandruff and secondary trauma due to scratching. A severe louse infestation can lead to failure to thrive and anemia, especially in puppies or small dogs.

Diagnosis

Linognathosis is diagnosed easily by recognizing the parasites and their eggs in clinical examination of the skin and fur coat. They are especially numerous in areas of thick fur and around the eyes, ears, and body orifices. It should be noted that unhatched nits and the shells of hatched nits remain attached to the hair for a long time. Along the progression of the hair growth cycle, they rise progressively higher from the skin and may become more visible. Finding nits in hairs is a sign of louse infestation, but the efficacy of therapy should not be judged based on the presence or absence of nits.

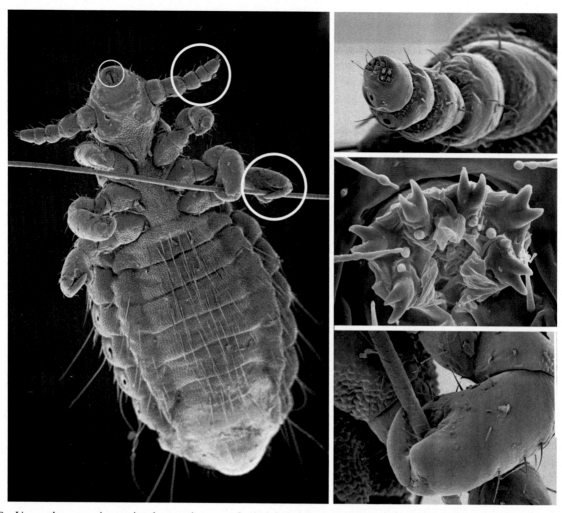

FIG. 8.3 *Linognathus setosus* in scanning electron microscopy. On the left, the louse is depicted from the ventral side. The head is clearly narrower than the trunk. The extremities, which end to claw structures, are attached to the central part (thorax) of the body. The chitinous exoskeleton in the rear of the body is divided into nine segments with breathing holes, or spiracles, at the lateral edges. A SEM micrograph at the upper right corner depicts a small antenna consisting of five segments. The antennae are equipped with chemoreceptors. A SEM micrograph in the middle is a close up of sucking louse's teeth-like oral structures specialized for piercing the skin. A SEM micrograph at lower right corners depicts the sucking louse's claw, present as one for each leg. Together, the claw and the thumb-like protrusion of the tibia form a grip that fits perfectly to the hairs of the canine inner coat.

The most important differential diagnosis is that of the canine chewing louse. These two are easy to distinguish based on the shape of the head, which is narrower than thorax in a sucking louse.

In rare cases, stray human lice (head louse, body louse, and pubic louse) can be found in a dog's fur. They do not, however, infest dogs, and neither do the dog's lice infest humans.

Treatment and Prevention

Since sucking dog lice are rare, there are few registered drugs for the treatment of linognathosis. Most products intended for controlling fleas and ticks or other ectoparasites are effective against adult lice. All dogs that are in direct contact should be treated, and the treatment should be of sufficient length to break the life cycle. During the treatment, it is advisable to clean mechanically the dog's bed and other areas, where the dog spends lots of time, even though the lice survive for only days in the surroundings.

Morphology of a Dog's Sucking Louse

Sucking lice are wingless, gray to brown, dorso ventrally flattened insects, with a length that varies between 1.7 and 2.5 mm (Figs. 8.2 and 8.3). The body has three parts: the head, thorax, and abdomen. Unlike some louse species, the dog's sucking louse lacks eyes. Typically for an insect, the louse has three pairs of jointed legs and small antennae, consisting of five segments. The antennae are equipped with chemoreceptors. The head is substantially narrower than the thorax. The sucking louse has oral structures specialized for skin penetration and sucking blood. They are located, except when the louse is feeding, in a retrograde oral cavity. The legs are

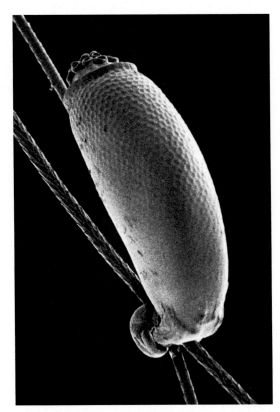

FIG. 8.4 The egg of a sucking louse is called a nit. Its lower edge is firmly glued to the hair. The nit surface has similar pattern as a golf ball and it is equipped with a lid.

Morphology of a Dog's Sucking Louse—cont'd

attached to the thorax and they end in claw structures that are typical for this group. Each leg has only one of them. Together, the claw and the thumb-like protrusion of the tibia form a gripping structure. Its diameter fits exactly with the hairs of the canine inner coat, and thus allows a firm grip of the hair. The chitin cuticle of the abdomen is divided into nine segments. The respiratory pores, or spiracles, are located at the lateral edges of the segments. In addition, the louse has two larger respiratory pores laterally, at the middle part of the thorax. The thorax and the abdomen are covered with a tightly packed cover of chitin scales. Several long hairs rise up from the chitinous cuticle. The rear edge of the abdomen of a male sucking louse is round, and sclerotinized genitals can be seen at the ventral surface of the abdomen. The rear edge of the female abdomen has two sections. At the ventral surface of the alimentary tract, there is a group of cells called the mycetome, an essentially important structure for the louse. The mycetome consists of mycetocytes, the specialized cells of the mid-part intestine of the louse, and of their intracellular symbiotic bacteria belonging to the proteobacteria group. Without the mycetomes the louse cannot break down red blood cells. The female louse passes this structure, and the ability to digest erythrocytes, to its offspring through the ovaries. Without the symbiotic bacteria, the female is sterile and the louse nymphs hatching from the eggs survive for only a few days.

Human's Lice May Stray to the Dog's Hair Coat

Linognathus setosus is an ectoparasite of dogs and other canids. It does not infect humans. Neither do man's lice infect dogs, but they do occasionally stray into canine fur coat. The most common human louse found in dogs is the pubic louse (*Phthirus pubis*) (Fig. 8.5). It is easily distinguished from other lice on the basis of its short and stubby appearance. Finding a pubic louse in the hairs of a dog is usually a sign of an infestation of the owner. The human body louse and head louse may also stray to dogs, albeit much more seldom than the pubic louse. Both subspecies have eyes and their morphology differs substantially from that of sucking louse in other ways too. Sometimes, in cases of persistent human louse infestations, it has been necessary to treat the dog as well, since a dog that sleeps with the human may offer shelter, warmth, and humidity to the human louse, enabling it to survive longer and to provide a source of reinfection. However, treating dogs for human louse infestations is by no means routine.

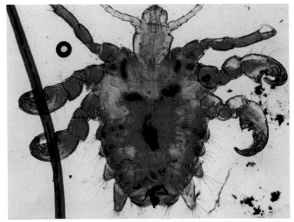

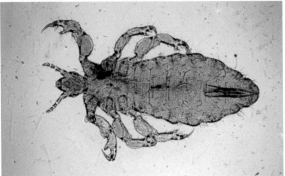

FIG. 8.5 Human lice may stray onto a dog. The upper figure depicts the most common human louse species found in dogs, the pubic louse (*Phthirus pubis*), which can easily be distinguished from other louse species thanks to its short and stubby appearance. The head louse (*Pediculus humanus capitis*), in the lower figure, can distinguished from the sucking louse on the basis of its claw structures. In contrast to *Linognathus setosus*, *Pediculus humanus* has eyes.

TRICHODECTES CANIS, Canine Chewing Louse

- Very rare in areas where constant flea and tick treatments are in use.
- Dorso-ventrally flattened body. Head broader than thorax.
- Chews organic material on skin. Causes irritation and pruritus while moving.
- Typically a kennel problem.
- As a constant parasite, easy to control with many insecticides.

Identification

Canine chewing lice are wingless, light yellow, dorso ventrally flattened insects. They are about 2 mm long (Figs. 8.6–8.8). The head is broader than long, and broader than the louse's middle body (thorax). The head is shaped like a rounded trapezoid and specialized for chewing and holding on to hair. The louse egg, or nit, has a lid and it has been glued firmly to the hair.

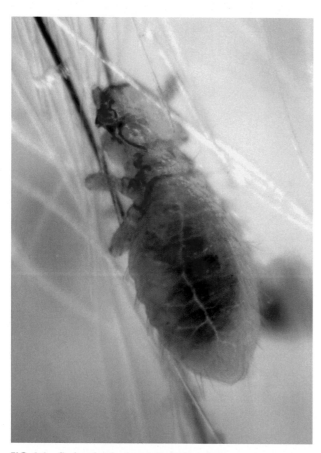

FIG. 8.6 Canine chewing louse attached to a hair.

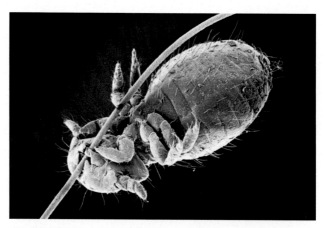

FIG. 8.7 Canine chewing louse in scanning electron microscopy. The lice are wingless, *light yellow*, dorso ventrally flattened insects. Their length is about 2 mm. The head of the louse is wider than the length and its middle body. The head is shaped like a rounded trapezoid. The well-developed mouthparts specialized for chewing and grasping hairs are located in the ventral side of the head.

Life Cycle

The chewing lice are host-specific, and the canine louse does not infest other species. The louse spends all stages of its life cycle in the dog's fur coat. When it is separated from the host, it survives up to a few days. Transmission between dogs happens through direct contact between animals or their grooming equipment. If the body temperature of the host animal rises, for instance, because of fever, or descends substantially, such as when the host has died, the chewing lice will try to exit the host. They use keratin and sebum that seep from the surface of skin for nutrition. Their mouthparts are incapable of penetrating the skin, but they evidently eat blood or tissue fluids in areas of traumatically damaged skin, when the opportunity arises.

The chewing lice copulate several times during their life span of about 1 month. The female glues the lid-equipped eggs, or nits, one by one to the hairs. After the incubation period of about 5–8 days, the eggs hatch and a nymph, resembling the adult louse, emerges from the nit by pushing the lid off through the perforated lid, producing a nymph that resembles an adult louse. The life cycle comprises of three nymph stages. The last molting produces the adult stages of the louse. The entire life cycle of the louse, from nit to adulthood, lasts 3–5 weeks.

Morphology of Canine Chewing Louse

Canine chewing lice (Figs. 8.6–8.8) are wingless, gray to brown, dorso ventrally flattened insects. They are about 1.6–1.8 mm long. Males are somewhat smaller than females. The body has three parts: head, thorax, and abdomen. Typically for an insect, the louse has three pairs of jointed legs and small antennae, consisting of three segments. The antennae are equipped with chemoreceptors. The head of the chewing

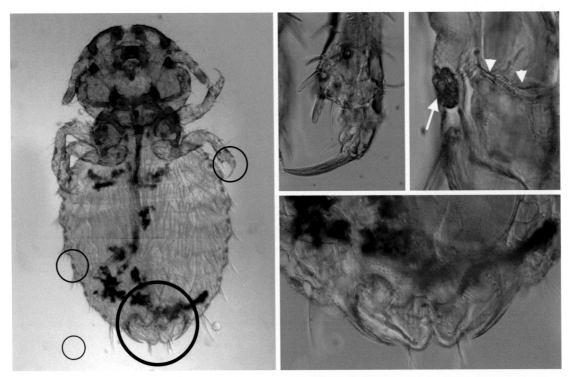

FIG. 8.8 Morphological details of canine chewing louse in light microscopy. Each leg (a micrograph up in the middle) has one claw, and each claw is matched by two stick-like structures. Respiratory pores, or spiracles, are located at the lateral edges, six on each side (micrograph at upper right corner). They allow air to enter the tracheal tubes or tracheoles, which deliver oxygen directly into the louse's tissues. A micrograph at the lower right corner depicts a detail of the rear end.

Morphology of Canine Chewing Louse—cont'd

louse is shaped like a rounded trapezoid and it is wider than the head's length and the middle of the body. Well-developed mouthparts specialized for chewing and grasping to hairs, are located on the ventral side of the head. The chitinous cuticle of the middle body consists of three segments. The two most caudal segments are partly conjoined. The extremities are attached to the middle of the body, and claw structures, typical for this group of parasites, are in the tip of the leg. Each leg has one claw, and each claw is matched by two stick-like structures that are protrusions of tibia. The chitinous cuticle is divided into distinct segments. An evenly spaced, sparse row of sensor hairs runs along the dorsal surface of each segment. Respiratory pores, or spiracles, are located at the lateral edges, with six on each side.

Distribution

Canine chewing louse is quite rare today. A louse that spends all stages of its life cycle in dog's hair is sensitive to many ectoparasitic treatments. Especially long-acting treatments against fleas and ticks have created havoc among populations of chewing lice. Chewing lice are found in rare cases everywhere in the world in places with a high canine population density and poor hygiene. They are an important

menace in areas where the climate is too cold for fleas and ticks. The chewing louse is, for instance, still the most significant ectoparasite in Nordic sled dog kennels.

Importance to Canine Health

Similar to canine sucking louse infestations, the term pediculosis is used for infestations of chewing lice. It would be more correct to call a canine chewing louse infestation trichodectosis. Cases of trichodectosis are at their most common in autumn, winter, and early spring, when the inner coat of dog fur is at its thickest. Spring shedding reduces the louse population substantially, because the majority of the lice and their nits that are attached to the hairs are removed permanently with the loose hair. Infection is often subclinical. Common clinical signs are pruritus, dandruff, hair loss, restlessness, and traumatic skin lesions as a result of scratching. The chewing louse may act as an intermediate host for the *D. caninum* flea tapeworm and *Acanthocheiloma reconditum* nematode.

Diagnosis

A chewing louse infection is diagnosed easily by recognizing the parasites and their eggs in the clinical examination of the skin and the fur coat. The lice can be found especially in the thick fur at the back, neck, and head.

The most important morphological differential diagnosis is the sucking louse, but it can easily be distinguished from the chewing louse on the basis of its narrower head.

Treatment and Prevention

There are many insecticides that can be used to manage chewing louse infestations. The treatment needs to be long enough, and all dogs in the household should be treated at the same time. The dog's bed and other places where it spends a lot of time should be mechanically cleaned, even though the chewing lice do not live for long outside the host.

Heterodoxus spiniger, a Tropical Canine Chewing Louse

The tropical canine chewing louse is *Heterodoxus spiniger*. It belongs to the suborder Amblycera of chewing lice. Other species of Amblycera are mostly ectoparasites of birds, marsupials, and certain mammalia originating in South America, such as guinea pigs. The color of *Heterodoxus* (Fig. 8.9) varies from resin to dark brown, and it stays close to the canine skin surface, most often at the lower back. Many morphological features typical for chewing louse, such as mouthparts suitable for gnawing, are found in the tropical chewing louse. There are differences as well. The antennae are protected in holes at the sides of the head, leaving only the tip visible. In contrast

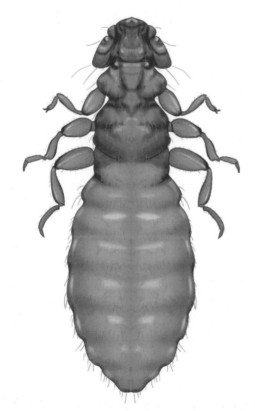

FIG. 8.9   *Heterodoxus spiniger*, the tropical chewing louse.

---

to the canine chewing louse, the tropical chewing louse has two claw-like structures in the tip of each leg. Eye rudiments are located at the sides of the head. The life cycle, from nit to adulthood, takes 3–4 weeks. The clinical importance of the tropical chewing louse is similar to that of *Trichodectes canis*. It also can act as an intermediate host for *D. caninum* flea tapeworm and *Acanthocheiloma reconditum* nematode.

CIMEX LECTULARIUS, Bed bug

- Nocturnal blood sucker that spends the most of the time hiding in the apartment.
- Emerging and reemerging ectoparasite due to traveling.
- Causes skin irritation and itching to humans, but also most likely to dogs living in infested environments.
- Eviction from the apartment is achieved by professional pest control.

Identification

Cimex species that suck blood from humans (bed bugs) include the tropical and subtropical *Cimex hemipterus* and its cosmopolitan cousin *Cimex lectularius*. Both are capable of sucking blood from several animal species. The bed bug (Fig. 8.10) is a dorso ventrally flattened and oval insect, usually 4–5 mm long. It is reddish brown and gets darker after a blood meal. The parasite has long antennae, consisting of four segments. Distinct,

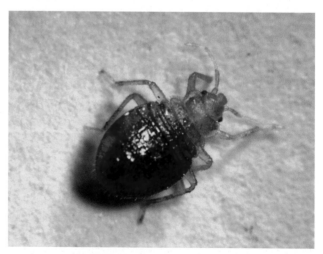

FIG. 8.10   *Cimex-lectularius* is a dorso ventrally flattened insect 4–5 mm long. It has long antennae, consisting of four segments. Raspberry-like compound eyes can be seen clearly on both sides of the head. The front of the middle part of the body is sunken in the middle, so that the louse's head is partly surrounded by the body.

raspberry-like compound eyes can be seen clearly on both sides of the head. The front of the middle part of the body appears sunken in the middle, so that the louse's head is partly surrounded by the thorax. Typical of insects, there are three pairs of legs.

Morphology of the Bed Bug

Bed bugs (Fig. 8.10) are oval shaped and flattened dorso-ventrally. The bug's color varies from pale brown to reddish brown depending on its feeding status. The average length of the adult bug is about 5.5 mm and the width 2.5 mm, respectively. Females are larger than males. The head is short, broad and pointed at the tip and had a pair of prominent red or black compound eyes resembling raspberries. The antenna consists of four segments; the first segment is shorter than other segments. The three segments closest to the antenna tip are thin and elongated. Mouthparts or labium are three-segmented and specialized in piercing and sucking and are located on the ventral side of the head. The tip of the labium extends to the level of the first pair of legs. The thorax also is three-segmented. *C. lectularius* can be morphologically differentiated from *C. hemipterus* based on the broader prothorax of *C. lectularius* compared with *C. hemipterus*. The front of the middle part of the body (prothorax) appears sunken in the middle, so that the louse's head is partly surrounded by the thorax. Wings seem to be absent but bed bugs are micropterous as the rudiments of forewings are still visible as small pads. Each thoracic segment contained a pair of jointed legs; there were thus three pairs of legs. Two claws are present at the tip of tarsus. The abdomen is 11-segmented and seven pairs of respiratory pores or spiracles are present ventro laterally on segments 2–8. The segments of the abdomen are separated by membranous and softer cuticle material, enabling the posterior body to expand when the bed bug feeds on blood. A small curved reproductive organ, the aedeagus or paramere, is located ventrally at the tip of the male abdomen. A small incision is present on the left side of the fourth abdominal segment of the female. This incision is the opening of a blind copulatory pouch referred as paragenital sinus or Berlese's organ. The life cycle of the bedbug consists of egg, five instars of nymphs, and adults.

Life Cycle

The bed bug is an obligate hematophagous (bloodsucking) insect. It feeds at night and is most active just before sunrise. During daylight hours, the bed bug hides in crevices, cracks and, for instance, in the seams of mattresses and furniture textiles. The body temperature and carbon dioxide released by the host animal signals to the bed bug about the feeding opportunity. Adult bed bugs usually feed twice weekly. A single blood meal takes only 5–10 min. The insects can remain without food for months and survive without blood for up to 2 years. They are known to be cannibals. Apart from eggs, all life stages are hematophagous. Copulation of bed bugs is a curious undertaking: the male perforates the female body cavity membranes with its external genitals through a special groove (ectospermalage) and emits the sperm into the body cavity. This is called traumatic insemination. The female genital pore has no role in the copulation; its role is limited to laying eggs. The female lays eggs on the rough surfaces of its hideaway. A nymph stage, resembling an adult bed bug, hatches from the egg. The life cycle continues through molts and involves a total of five nymph stages before adulthood. Feeding on blood is obligatory to move to each next stage.

Distribution

The advent of pesticide use reduced the importance of bed bugs substantially. The bed bug nuisance has reemerged lately and bugs have reinvaded many former and new living environments. Apart from limitations set for pesticide use, the factors facilitating the reemergence include tourism, dormitory living, and recycling, especially that of old furniture.

Importance to Canine Health

The reaction to a bed bug bite (cimicosis) varies individually in humans and animals. Some hardly react at all. Local erythematous swellings or lumps of different sizes are common, and some individuals may develop generalized allergic symptoms, even anaphylactic reactions. If bed bugs are abundant, affected small-sized animals may even show signs of anemia. The bed bug is not considered an important vector of contagious diseases.

Diagnosis

Recognizing a bed bug problem may be difficult. Nocturnally appearing skin lesions are a good reason for suspecting an invasion of unwanted visitors in a household. Lesions may be found in dogs as well as in humans. It is worth remembering that many other blood-sucking parasites are also active at night. Finding small and dark fecal stains in the bedding may be revealing. Bed bugs have a distinctive, sweet smell that they spread into their environment, especially when threatened. When this odor appears in a home, it is a sign of a severe bed bug problem. A captured individual is easily recognized as a bed bug based on its morphological features.

Treatment and Prevention

It appears that the ban of some pesticides, such as DDT, has led to the increase of the bed bug population. The life of bed bugs has also been made easier thanks to the resistance that they have developed against many insecticides, especially pyrethroids. Bed bugs are most commonly introduced to the household with luggage or recycled furniture. Consequently, meticulous hygiene is important in preventing the problem. It is wise to delegate the chemical treatment of affected premises to professionals. Bed bugs can survive temperatures of under −15°C for a few hours. The temperature must rise to more than 50°C to achieve the elimination of bed bugs.

The True Bugs

Several insects are called bugs, but the true bugs belong to Hemiptera order with tens of thousands of species; the bed bug is only one example. Most bug species feed on plant fluids, but in veterinary medicine the blood-sucking bug species are the most important. The saliva of feeding bugs contains proteins that may induce hypersensitivity and allergic reactions. In addition to the local reaction in the biting site or even more severe anaphylactic reaction, some species may transmit diseases. For example, the kissing bugs, Triatominae, which are notably larger (about 2.5 cm long) than bed bugs, can act as vectors for Trypanosoma protozoans (see Chapter 2, Protozoa). The infection happens via contamination of the bite wound or mucous membranes with the fecal, trypanosoma-containing material of the kissing bug. As many blood-sucking bugs, the kissing bugs are active at night. The common name comes from their habit to bite sleeping humans on the face, typically around the mouth. For bug prophylaxis, several kinds of insecticides and mechanical protection can be used, but the low host-specificity of bugs, with several possible hosts in wildlife, means that control of trimatomine bugs remains a challenge.

CTENOCEPHALIDES CANIS, Dog Flea, *CTENOCEPHALIDES FELIS*, Cat Flea, and Other Fleas Affecting Dogs

---

- Laterally flattened insects, about 1–6 mm long, the most posterior pair of the legs is for jumping. Comb-like chitin spines, ctenidiae, used for species identification.
- Only a small proportion of the flea population are adults and parasites.
- Eggs, larvae, and pupae are nonparasitic and live in the dog's environment.
- Adults suck blood and cause pruritus. Flea allergy dermatitis is the most important and common clinical manifestation.
- Fleas serve as vector for several infectious diseases and intermediate host for dog tapeworm.
- Adults are easy to kill or repel with various veterinary pharmaceuticals, but it is as important to break the life cycle of the flea by controlling the environmental stages or extend the treatment.

Identification

Fleas (Siphonaptera) are laterally flattened insects (Fig. 8.11). They are about 1–6 mm long, depending on the species. The females are bigger than the males. The flea has six legs. The most posterior pair is for jumping. The head of an adult flea has comb-like chitin spines, ctenidiae, which possess useful characters for distinguishing flea species. The eggs have a glossy surface and their size is about 0.3–0.5 mm. The larva is light and vermiform, and its size varies depending on the developmental stage between 4 and 10 mm. The size of the cocoon is about 3×1 mm.

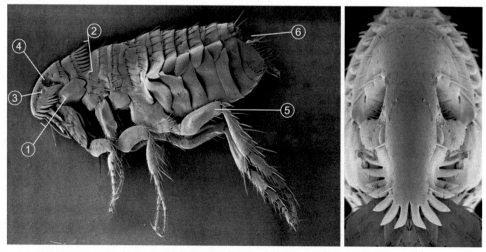

FIG. 8.11 Cat flea (*Ctenocephalides felis*) in scanning electron microscopy: (1) genal comb (genal stenidiae); (2) pronotal comb (pronotal stenidiae); (3) eye; (4) antenna; (5) the most posterior pair of legs, specialized for jumping; and (6) sensilium.

Morphology of the Flea

Fleas (Siphonaptera) are insects. They are dark brown and about 1–6 mm long, depending on the species. Their lateral flatness and glossy surface facilitate moving among thick fur (Figs. 8.11–8.14). The females are larger than males of the same species. Both the dorsal and ventral outline of the female are convex, while the dorsal surface of males is almost straight. Body is covered with backwards directed setae. Fleas lack compound eyes, but many species have large or small simple eyes.

The head of an adult flea has comb-like row of chitin spines, ctenidiae. The so-called genal comb is at the low edge of the head, and the pronotal comb at the neck on the posterior border of the first thoracic segment. The number of ctenidiae or the lack of them can be used for species identification (Fig. 8.13). The rather short three-segmented antennae are located in pits at the side of the head. The flea has six legs, attached to its thorax. The third pair is much longer than the others and is for leaping when the flea is disturbed or wants to join a host animal. For its size, the flea is among the best jumpers of the animal kingdom. The abdomen consists of 10 chitinous segments, eight of which are distinct. Lateral from them, on both sides of the flea, there are respiratory pores or spiracles. Two pairs of spiracles are present in the thorax as well. Both sexes have dorsally (on the posterior part of the body) a saddle-shaped sensory organ, the sensilium, covered by small hairs and sheltered with the antesensilial setae located anteriorly to the sensilium (Fig. 8.12). This structure is believed to function in the detection of changes in air currents, and hence may assist the flea in finding a host.

A complex copulatory organ is seen posterioventrally in the rear of the male. The corresponding female organ is a spermatheca, sperm storage (Fig. 8.12). The spermatheca is taxonomically the most important genital structure of the female flea, as the morphology of the spermatheca is sometimes used as aid for distinguishing flea species.

The eggs have a glossy surface and their size is about 0.3–0.5 mm. The larva is light and vermiform, and its size varies depending on the developmental stage between 4 and 10 mm. The size of the cocoon is about 3 × 1 mm (Fig. 8.14).

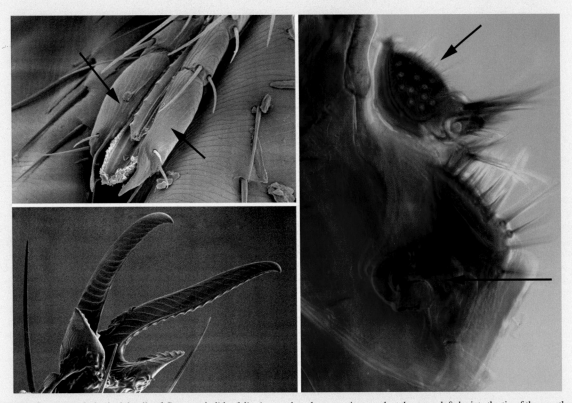

FIG. 8.12 Some morphological details of *Ctenocephalides felis*. A scanning electron micrograph at the upper left depicts the tip of the mouth parts. In the center is the feeding tube consisting of two sawlike stylets or laciniae which cut the skin and is accompanied with the needle-like epipharynx. Together they form the puncturing stylet. On both sides there are two labial palps sheathing the stylet. A scanning electron micrograph at the lower let corner depicts the tip of a flea's leg, which ends in strong claws designed to grasp the host and avoiding dislodgment. A micrograph on the right shows the rear end of the female flea (a micrograph on the left). Dorsally located, saddle-shaped sensory organ or sensilium (*upper arrow*), covered with small hair-like structures, and the spermatheca (*lower arrow*), the sperm storage organ, are clearly seen.

Continued

Morphology of the Flea—cont'd

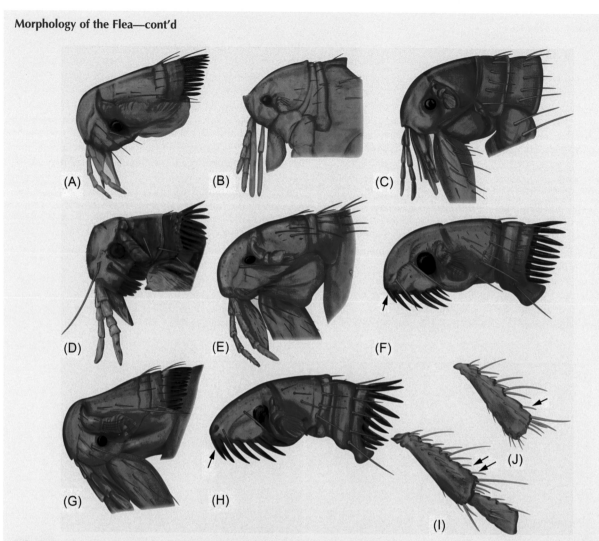

FIG. 8.13 Identification of some flea species found on canine skin. (A) *Monopsyllus sciurorum*, the squirrel flea. Morphology: No genal comb, about 18 spines in the pronotal comb. (B) *Echidnophaga gallinacea*, the hen flea or stickfast flea or sticktight flea. Morphology: Lacking genal and protonal combs. Flattened and angular forehead. Embeds its mouthparts in the skin and feeds at one site for up to 19 days. (C) *Pulex irritans*, the human flea. Morphology: Lacking genal and protonal combs. (D) *Psilopsylla cuniculi*, the rabbit flea. Morphology: Genal and pronotal combs present, angular head. (E) *Archaeopsylla erinacei*, the hedgehog flea. Morphology: A few spines in the genal comb, 2–3 spines in the pronotal comb. (F) *Ctenocephalides canis*, dog flea. Morphology: Distinct genal and pronotal comb, the head is broadly rounded and its length is not twice the height vs. *Ctenocephalides felis*. The first spine of the pronotal comb (*arrow*) is shorter than the second spine. vs *C. felis*, there are two short stout bristles in the interval between the postmedian and apical long bristles on the dorsal margin of the hind tibia (*arrows* in the detail illustration "I"). (G) *Ceratophyllus* spp., the bird flea. Morphology: No genal comb, tightly spaced pronotal comb, about 24 spines. (H) *C. felis*, the cat flea. Morphology: Distinct genal and pronotal comb, streamlined, elongated head length more than twice the height). vs *C. canis*: First two spines of the pronotal comb are approximately equal in length (*arrow*). One stout bristle in the interval between postmedian and apical long bristles on the dorsal margin of the hind tibia (*arrow* in detail illustration "J"). (I) *C. canis*, detail of hind tibia. (J) *C. felis*, detail of hind tibia.

Life Cycle

Only adult fleas (males as well as females) are parasites. Other stages of the life cycle, comprising about 95% of the flea population, reside in the dog's living environment, for instance, in the bed. About one-third of a typical adult population consists of males and the other two-thirds are females. Having found a suitable host animal, the fleas usually stay on the same host for the rest of their lives. Adult fleas start sucking blood within a few minutes after finding a suitable host, and egg productions starts about 24–36h after the first blood meal. Females lay daily dozens of light-colored and glossy eggs among the dog's hairs (Fig. 8.14). At first, the surface of the egg

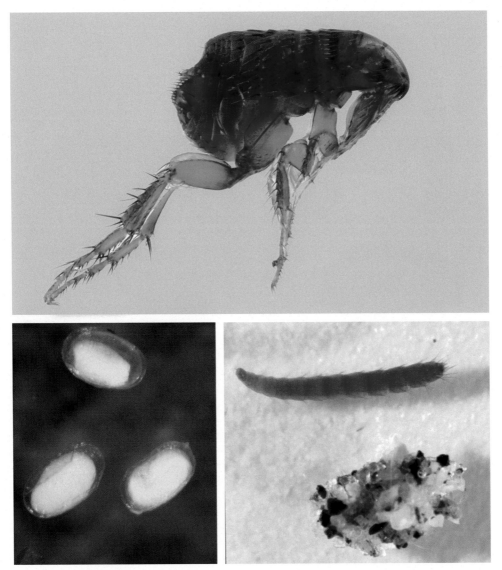

FIG. 8.14 Stages of flea's life cycle. Figure above: adult flea (male); left lower figure: flea eggs; right-side figure: a larva and a cocoon phase. Figures depict *Ctenocephalides felis*, the cat flea.

is sticky. Once the surface dries, the eggs fall into the environment. The egg hatches to produce a larva (Fig. 8.14). Hatching takes, depending on the temperature, from less than 2 days to 2 weeks. In dry conditions and in temperatures below 3°C, the development of eggs stops. All life cycle stages are dependent on temperature and humidity. The larva favors conditions where the temperature is 21–32°C and the relative humidity about 70%. It tends to follow gravity and to keep away from light, moving into an optimally sheltered place. The larvae use all sorts of organic material for nutrition, especially the feces of adult fleas, with contains partially digested nutrient rich blood. The larva molts twice before the pupal phase (Fig. 8.14), which may last from a few weeks up to a year. The actual metamorphosis usually lasts 5–

12days, but before hatching from the pupa, the adult flea awaits signs of the presence of a host animal, for instance trembling, temperature change, or the increase of ambient carbon dioxide concentration. This guarantees a fast blood meal right after hatching. The life cycle of flea is illustrated in Fig. 8.15.

Fleas are not very strict about their host animal. Any suitable species that happens to be available can be a target for a blood meal. Apart from dog and cat fleas, fleas of several wild animal species can cause long-term problems for dogs, when they settle in the dog's living environment. While bird and hedgehog fleas are common in nature, for instance, they do not usually need to be controlled in dogs, since they stop only briefly for a snack (Fig. 8.13).

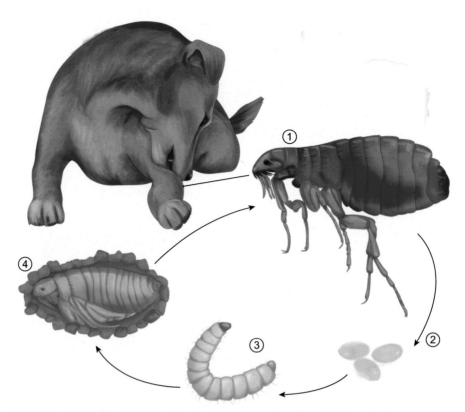

FIG. 8.15   Life cycle of the flea: (1) adult fleas live in the fur coat of the dog, suck blood and copulate; (2) the female lays smooth-surfaced eggs among the dog's hairs. They fall into the environment, for instance, the dog's bed or sites where the dog passes time; (3) the larva hatches from the egg. It feeds on organic material found in the environment, particularly the feces of adult fleas, containing blood. The larva molts twice; and (4) the larva forms a pupa around itself. The pupa phase lasts from a week to up to a year. The adult is released from the pupa, having received a signal of the presence of a host animal, for instance trembling. This improves the chances of reaching a host without delay.

Distribution

Fleas are prevalent everywhere in the world. Their local variety of species varies geographically primarily on the basis of the availability of host species. The cat flea is the most common species in dogs as well as in cats. According to the results of studies conducted in different part of the world, fleas are not very host-specific rather host-preferential. Hence, dogs are affected, apart from the cat flea, e.g., by the rabbit flea (*Spilopsyllus cuniculi*), human flea (*Pulex irritans*), bird flea (*Echidnophaga gallinacea*, *Ceratophyllus* spp.), and dog flea (*Ctenocephalides canis*), which is becoming increasingly rare due to the global emergence of the cat flea. Central heating in houses does not favor the life cycle of fleas, and consequently canine fleas are not a significant problem in cold climate countries with high standards of living.

Importance to Canine Health

The misleading term puliculosis is used for flea infestations in English-language literature. The name comes from *P. irritans*, the human flea. The saliva of fleas contains a histamine-type substance and the bite causes local irritation. In a serious flea infection, the dog self-traumatizes the skin through scratching and expose it to secondary bacterial infection. Small dogs may become anemic, if there are many bloodsucking fleas and the problem continues for a long time. The anemia may even be fatal for small puppies. It has been estimated that an adult female flea consumes blood up to 15 times its own weight daily. In recurrent flea exposures, the dog may become sensitized to flea saliva and develop flea allergy dermatitis (FAD). Signs of FAD can be seen in dogs as young as 6 months, but more commonly the first signs break out when the dog is 3–6 years old. Thereafter, a small scale flea infestation may lead to a severe skin reaction and excruciating pruritus. Dermal signs may include alopecia, erythema, popular dermatitis, lichenization, and pigmentation (Figs. 8.16 and 8.17). Fleas may carry several infectious canine diseases, a range of viruses and bacteria. In addition, they are a host for flea-tapeworm, *D. caninum*, and *Acanthoceilonema reconditum* nematode. Fleas feed also on human blood. Bite marks manifest on human skin as itchy insect bite papulae. They are most

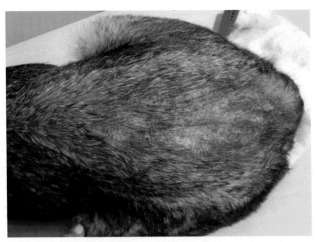

FIG. 8.16   Tail-head pruritus extending to the lumbo-sacral area with erythema, hyperpigmentation, and lichenification are typical findings for flea allergy dermatitis. *(Photo by Svetlana Belova, reproduced with permission.)*

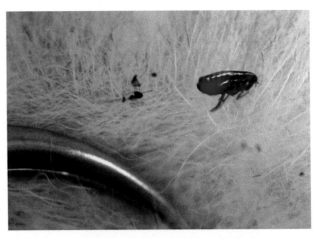

FIG. 8.18   Flea infestation in a dog. A cat flea is depicted together with black flea feces containing blood.

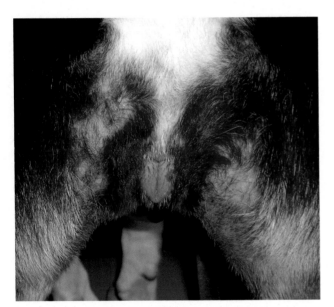

FIG. 8.17   Lesions of FAD in the dog's skin at the rear and medial thighs. *(Photo by Svetlana Belova, reproduced with permission.)*

commonly seen in ankles and wrists. Fleas have been confirmed to be the vector of a number of human pathogens. Historically fleas are notorious as the carriers of plague (*Yersinia pestis*).

Diagnosis

Adult fleas can be seen with the naked eye, when their movements in the dog's fur catch the attention of the dog owner. Sometimes the owner has been bitten too. If the signs are typical of flea infestation, but fleas are not found, black flea feces falling from the fur coat may suggest a diagnosis (Fig. 8.18). The droppings dye wet paper tissue red. Fleas and their dry droppings can be harvested from thick fur with a flea comb. Thanks to its narrow profile, the flea lies down on its side on a microscope slide. When the flea is placed on a microscope slide, its morphology, especially its pronotal and genal comb, is made visible. If lactophenol is dropped on top of the sample, the chitin cuticle of the flea will become transparent within a day (Fig. 8.19). If the slide is warmed, the process is faster. Thereafter the diagnosis is done by searching for species-specific features by microscopy. Since about 2500 flea species are recognized, identification is not always easy. However, the most common canine fleas can usually be distinguished without problems (Fig. 8.13). There are analyses based on ELISA and intradermal testing for diagnosing FAD. Treatment success and alleviation of allergic signs after long-term, effective medicinal flea control is strongly suggestive of FAD diagnosis.

Treatment and Prevention

Some fleas of wild animals visit a dog for a quick bite, and leave its fur coat without a need to resort to treatment. This is usually the case, for instance, for bird or hedgehog fleas. However, if the flea found in the dog is of a type known to cause long-term harm for the dog and is capable of reproduction in the dog's environment, control is needed. Medication has to be continued without interruption, until the problem is solved. Breaking the fleas' life cycle in a home or kennel environment usually requires at least 12 weeks of continuing treatment with a drug efficient against fleas. The most common cause of treatment failure is insufficient duration of treatment or interruptions of the treatment, allowing the flea population to bounce back. All dogs and cats of the household should be treated at the same time.

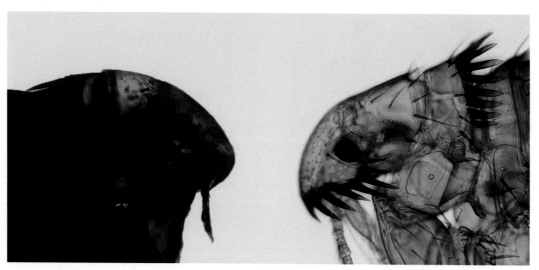

FIG. 8.19   Fleas are not naturally transparent in microscopy. With lactophenol clearing (see instructions in Chapter 11, Diagnostics), the flea is made transparent, allowing the visualizing of morphological details.

There are many antiflea products available. They have important difference in the mode or duration of action and in the speed of killing. Some products are effective against adult fleas, while others kill also larvae and eggs. In addition, there are several products with long-acting adulticidal effect combined with insect growth regulators. The pupa is the most challenging life cycle phase in terms of control. Only about 5% of fleas are adults parasitizing the dog. The rest are eggs (about 50%), larvae (about 35%), and pupa-phase fleas (about 10%). Therefore, the fleas found in the dog constitute only a tip of the iceberg, and the problem is hiding elsewhere in the home. Since most of the flea life forms stay in the dog's surroundings, flea control must be extended to curb this population seriously. Especially places where the dog sleeps and spends its time should be thoroughly cleaned. The bed, and possibly also the car, deserves special attention. Mechanic cleaning is important. Washable materials are machine washed. It may be practical to replace old bedding with new. It may be beneficial to spray insecticide into places of difficult access, such as the cracks between the floor and wall close to the dog's bed. All phases of the cat flea life cycle die in subzero temperatures ($-1°C$) within few days. The larvae cannot survive in relative humidity under 50%. Fleas may be transmitted between dogs or from the natural surroundings, for instance, while hunting. Kennels and other places where the dog density is high are a transmission risk, even without direct contact. If a dog is taken to a country where the flea prevalence differs from home, it is advisable to commence preventive treatment before traveling and continue it during the whole trip. In many countries where flea season continues through the year, dogs should be kept under constant preventive treatment. If an infection of *D. caninum* canine tapeworm is diagnosed in a dog, it has to be treated also against fleas, its intermediate hosts, to prevent reinfection.

Tunga penetrans, Chigoe Flea or Jigger

The chigoe flea (Fig. 8.20) is an oddity among fleas, a species living in the tropical areas of America and Africa. It causes a parasitic infection caused tungiasis. After copulation, the female flea, about 1 mm long, jumps onto a suitable host animal and penetrates its skin so that the rear parts of the body remain outside the skin. The perforation enables the flea to get air and secrete feces and provides the eggs with access to the environment. The circumference of the flea's rear end grows and it forms a balloon of about 6 mm circumference. The swelling is made possible by the elastic membrane between the chitin segments. The end-result is an abscess-like skin lesion, which may be secondarily infected. The eggs fall on the ground and larvae hatch from them in a few days. The lesion caused by the chigoe flea is recognized as tungiasis, when flea eggs are found at the skin perforation in microscopy. The treatment aims for the removal of the flea and control of the secondary infection if present. The flea can be excised by stretching the perforation and cautiously removing the flea. The bloated flea is difficult to remove, and it is often necessary to cut it out surgically, together with surrounding tissue.

TABANIDAE, Horseflies

- Horseflies are dipteran flies.
- They are often large and agile, only females bite animals to obtain blood.
- They are active in sunlight.
- A nuisance especially for grazing animals, but they may suck blood from dogs as well and cause irritation.

Adult horseflies feed on nectar and plant exudates; the males have weak mouthparts and only the females bite

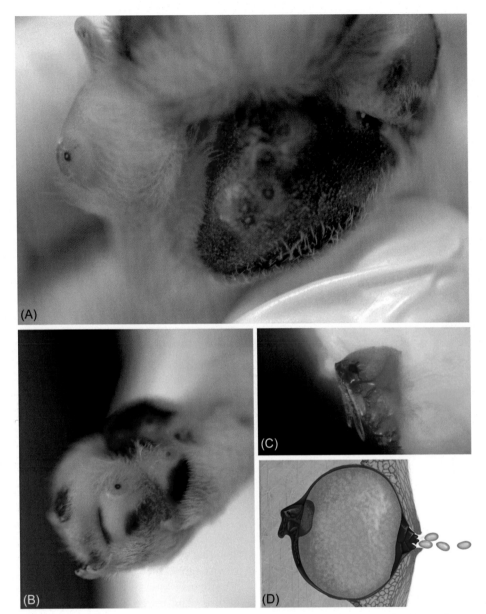

FIG. 8.20 (A–B) Skin lesions associated with *Tunga penetrans* infestation in paw pad of the dog. The penetration sites can be seen as pale nodules with centrally locating genital opening seen as a black dot. The surrounding skin is erythematous. These lesions are usually painful. (C) *T. penetrans* excised from a paw lesion. (D) Female *T. penetrans* buried in the skin. An illustration is based on illustration depicting jigger flea, British Museum of Natural History, 1909. *((A–C) Reproduced with permission from Klaus Earl Loft.)*

animals to obtain enough protein from blood to produce eggs. The mouthparts of females are formed into a stout stabbing organ with two pairs of sharp cutting blades, and a sponge-like part used to lap up the blood that flows from the wound. The larvae are predaceous and grow in semiaquatic habitats.

Female horseflies can transfer blood-borne diseases from one animal to another through their feeding habit. In areas where diseases occur, they have been known to carry equine infectious anemia virus, some trypanosomes, the filarial worm Loa loa, anthrax among cattle and sheep, and tularemia. As well as making life outdoors uncomfortable for humans, they can reduce growth rates in cattle and lower the milk output of cows if suitable shelters are not provided.

Identification

Horseflies (family Tabanidae) are large (6–30 mm) and robust dipteran (two-winged) insects. The horsefly family has over 4000 species. Horseflies are generally dark and their posterior body is often striped or spotted. The head is much broader than it is long. Their compound eyes are often spotted and colorful (Figs. 8.21 and 8.22).

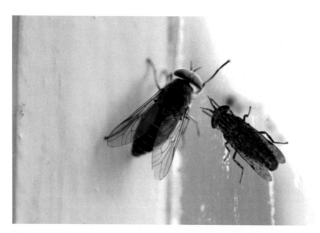

FIG. 8.21 Examples of tabaniid flies: *Tabanus* sp. (larger horsefly on the left) and *Haematopota* sp. (a cleg, on the right).

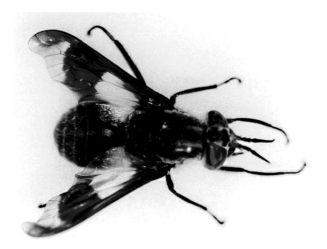

FIG. 8.22 A deer fly, *Chrysops* sp. is recognizable by the triangular shape, mottled wings, and the metallic sheen of its eyes.

Life Cycle

Only female horseflies suck blood from a wide range of hosts, males feed on nectar only. The female pierces the skin with its sharp mouthparts and sucks the blood seeping into the lesion. Especially the beginning of the sucking action is painful to the host animal, and the horsefly must often change the point of attack on the host, having been interrupted by the host's actions. The interruption of the attack is, indeed, the reason why horseflies are important factor in spreading contagious diseases. Once the female has got the taste for blood, it will try to find a less recalcitrant target as soon as possible. When the female reaches a new victim, it secretes an anticoagulant substance from the salivary glands and continues sucking despite interference. The female horsefly lays its eggs on plant leaves and on rocks in a moist, earthy, or watery environment. Horsefly larvae are primarily carnivores that feed on small invertebrates. The larvae of *Tabanus* genus participate in the control of horsefly population themselves, since they

do not hesitate to eat their own species. The horseflies pass the winter while at the larval stage, and form pupae in the spring. For some horsefly species, the pupal stage may last for years, but usually the adult hatches in couple of weeks.

Importance to Canine Health

Horseflies are a nuisance especially for grazing animals, such as horses and ruminants. When the opportunity arises, they may suck blood from dogs as well and cause irritation.

MUSCIDAE, Stable Flies, and FANNIIDAE, Lesser Houseflies

Muscidae or stable flies and Fanniidae, lesser houseflies, are genera belonging to the suborder Brachycera flies, which further belong to two-winged insects (Diptera). Many species belonging to these families are blood-sucking infection vectors or nuisance species for humans and domestic animals. The taxonomy of flies is often based on their favorite food source. Alternatively, flies can be also classified as either stinging or nonstinging flies on the basis of their mouthparts. Stinging flies have mouthparts adapted for piercing the skin and for acquiring blood and tissue fluids for nutrition. The species-level identification is based on size, mouthparts, coloring, the presence of stripes and spots, and the patterns of wing veins. Flies annoy grazing animals in particular—and dogs, when the opportunity arises. The biting house fly (*Stomoxys calcitrans*) is classified as a parasite and it can suck blood also from dogs. The length varies between 5 and 7 mm. Since biting house flies are blood suckers, they have a distinctly forward-pointing proboscis. In the posterior part of the body, otherwise gray, there are seven round-edged black spots. The female biting fly lays eggs especially in sites with rotting plant fibers. The larvae are found, for instance, in wet straw bedding, rotting hay, and composted lawn grass. Dung heaps and plant material are also favored by biting flies. The fly sucks blood once daily, and each blood meal takes a few minutes. The bite results as a painful lesion, and animals bothered by the flies are typically very restless. A large and distinct swelling grows into the bite spot.

OESTRIDAE, Bot Flies, Warble Flies, Heel Flies, Gadflies

- Dipteran flies.
- The larvae are internal parasites of mammals.
- *Dermatobia hominis* and *Cuterebra* spp. are the species of botfly known to parasitize dogs.
- Causative agents of migratory and furuncular myiasis.

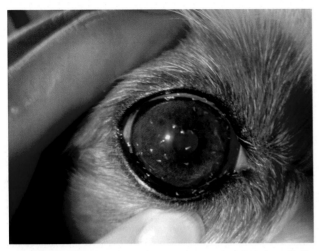

FIG. 8.23 Reindeer throat bot (*Cephenemyia trompe*) is a botfly belonging to the Oestridae and parasitizing reindeer. Here a female *Cephenemyia* has mistaken the host and laid eggs in a dog's eye. *(Photo by Annette Brockmann, reproduced with permission.)*

Bot flies are about 150 species family of parasitic flies belonging to the order Diptera and the suborder Bracycera. The larval forms are parasites and many bot fly species have been named after the animal, which the larvae parasitize. With some exceptions, bot flies are not very host-specific but may demonstrate host preferences (Fig. 8.23). They are usually large and hairy flies. An adult lays the eggs on the skin or the fur of the host, and after hatching, the larvae penetrate the subcutis. Bot flies species, parasitic for the dog, live in the subcutaneous tissue, but the family includes many species, which larvae live in the alimentary tract or in the nasal cavities and the pharynx. The larva feeds on the tissues or tissue fluids of the host and exits the host, once it is ready to form a pupa. *Cuterebra* spp. is endemic especially in the Americas. The larvae usually parasitize lagomorphs, but they can also be found in dogs. The female flies often lay eggs on surfaces and vegetation along the paths used by lagomorph animals and at the opening of their burrows. The larvae grasp the hairs of the host fur and use the natural orifices of the body for entry. They do not usually penetrate the skin. Most commonly, the larvae enter through the nostrils, migrate via nasal sinuses and pharynx into the thorax and further via the thoracic and abdominal cavity in the typical site, the subcutis. In the subcutaneous tissue, they form a cavity-like lesion and pierce an opening to the covering skin. The subcutaneous stage lasts a few weeks, during which the larva grows substantially bigger. Once ready to form a pupa, the larva exits the host though the hole in the skin.

The signs caused by *Cuterebra* depend on the number of larva and the migration route in the dog's body, and on the way the canine immune defense reacts to the larvae. The most common sign is a cutaneous and subcutaneous cyst with a 2–4 mm orifice on the surface. Larvae migrating in the respiratory tract may cause respiratory signs, such as dyspnea. Analogically, larvae straying to the nervous tissue cause nervous signs. *Cuterebra* larvae are usually removed surgically. The species diagnosis is primarily based on the morphology of the air vents (spiracles) in the larva's posterior.

CALLIPHORIDAE, Blowflies

- Blowflies are dipteran flies often metallic in appearance.
- Attracted to decaying meat and are typically the first organisms to come into contact with dead animals.
- Their larvae may infest living tissues of the dog, especially sores, wounds and decomposing flesh, causing wound myiasis.

The family Calliphoridae, blowflies, consists of moderately large flies that lay eggs into fresh or cooked meat or into dung. They are also able to lay eggs into living animals.

As examples genera *Lucilia*, "green bottle flies," and *Calliphora* are introduced. Green bottle flies are have a metallic green sheen, and *Calliphora* are larger (length 10–14 mm) and blue and black. *Calliphora* flies make a clear buzzing noise while flying. *Calliphora* cause fly strike, or myiasis. They interfere in parasitological fecal examination by laying eggs very quickly in fresh canine feces. The eggs are big enough (about 1.5 mm) to be seen with a naked eye of the dog owner in feces. The larvae hatch in less than 12 h and can cause a suspicion of an endoparasite infestation. It is assumed that *Calliphora* eggs can pass undamaged through the canine intestine, for instance, if a dog has eaten meat or a carcass with blowfly eggs, and the larvae hatch in the canine feces soon after defecation. The dog is not harmed by this passage. The problem arises, when the dog is poorly managed and the blowfly lays eggs, for instance, in a festering wound or feces-stained fur. Part of the larvae may enter the fecal mass in the rectum or the end of the large intestine. From large traumatic skin lesions, the blowfly larvae may migrate into the subcutis and perforate the intact skin from the inside. Many blowfly females only ingest dead tissue. They can be used in medicine for cleaning out the granulation tissue that grows in wounds.

Cochliomyia hominivorax (Figs. 8.24–8.26) is a screwworm fly that lives in the southern USA and Central and South America. It usually lays eggs in the desiccated surfaces of wounds that are a few days old. The larvae hatch from the eggs in about a day. They penetrate the skin and use healthy tissue for food. When bothered, they penetrate deeper in the tissues. The larval stage lasts only a few days, after which the larvae exit the host animal and pupate in the ground. A severe *Cochliomyia*-myiasis may be fatal for a dog. The diagnosis is based on the morphology of the

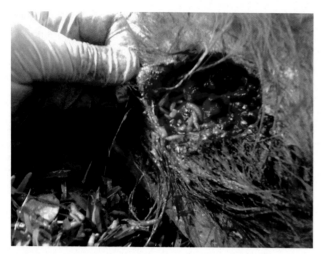

FIG. 8.24   Larvae of *Cochliomyia hominivorax* blowfly in a wound. *(Photo by Arlett Perez, reproduced with permission.)*

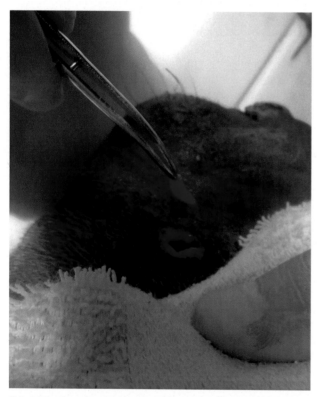

FIG. 8.25   Removing larvae of *Cochliomyia hominivorax* blowflies from the wound. *(Photo by Arlett Perez, reproduced with permission.)*

larvae. Their surface is clearly segmented with ring-shaped thicker parts, which give the larvae the name screw-worm. The shape and dimensions of the larva's mouthparts and spiracles can be used to diagnose the cause of myiasis. For treatment, the affected skin areas must usually be shaven. The lesions are washed with antiseptic shampoo. The wounds are flushed and the blowfly larvae removed as thoroughly as possible. Many substances of the avermectin group and nitenpyram are effective against fly larvae.

Myiasis

A condition where flies lay eggs in a living vertebrate host animal's skin or cavities and the hatching larvae eat the surrounding flesh is called myiasis. This can be detected in eyes, ears, nasal and oral cavities, skin, alimentary tract, and urogenitals. The larvae can be two types: maggots or bots. Maggots are long and slender (*Calliphora*, *Cochliomyia*, *Lucilia* (Figs. 8.27 and 8.28), *Musca*, *Phaenicia*, *Phormia*, and *Sarcophaga* spp.) and typical associated with wound myiasis and typically wounded, unhealthy, or dirty and moist body parts are affected. Bots are large and rotund (e.g., *Cuterebra* and *Dermatobia* spp.) and manifested as so-called furuncular and migratory myiasis. In addition, myiasis can be classified as obligatory, facultative, or accidental. In the obligatory myiasis, the larvae of the parasitic fly species (e.g., bots) require the host for nutrition and development for larval development. The facultative form is a consequence of an opportunistic behavior of nonparasitic flies that use organic material for laying eggs and an open wound or soiled hair just happens to be available for them. Accidental myiasis is actually a pseudoparasitosis when ingested larvae are present in feces or vomit without any clinical signs—the larvae are not able to develop further in the intestines if they are eaten.

The diagnosis of myiasis is made by the finding of fly larvae in tissue. Identification to the genus or species level is based on travel history of the dog and certain morphological structures, especially on posteriorly locating spiracles of the mature (third-stage) larva (Fig. 8.29). In addition, the differences in mouthparts, tracheal trunks, and cuticular spines may aid in differentiation from other myiasis maggots. It may take a while for the owner to realize the situation if the area affected is covered with hair coat, even though there might be stinking odor and pus secretion involved. Animals that are not individually handled on a daily basis may suffer from a hidden myiasis.

The treatment of myiasis is based on the manual removal of the larvae (especially in wound myiasis), blocking the respiration (occlusion) of the larva (especially in furuncular myiasis), and/or using larvicidal antiparasitics. The larvae must be mechanically removed without breaking them. This needs anesthetizing the dog and clipping the hair around the area for better visibility and healing. The damaged area is then cleansed thoroughly. Removing necrotic tissue aids the healing process. Because secondary bacterial infections are common, a proper wound management is advised to the owner and antibiotics administered if necessary. Larvicidal antiparasitics may be used for killing the possible existing larvae and to discourage further myiasis. To ensure prevention, environmental conditions of the dogs should be clean and dry. No fecal or urine contamination of the hair coat is allowed. Any damaged skin should be treated carefully and weak animals kept indoors. Regular grooming and daily handling the dogs reveal the myiasis quickly, and the treatment can be started without delay.

In some circumstances, living fly larvae can be used in wound therapy by inducing myiasis artificially and under control. This procedure is known as maggot therapy and usually the larvae of *Lucilia sericata* are utilized for this indication as they are known for their strong dietary preference on necrotic tissue while clean and healthy tissues seem to be unsuitable for them.

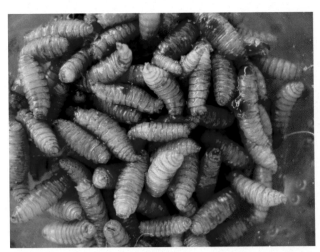

FIG. 8.26 Mature *Cochliomyia hominivorax* blowfly larvae. All the larvae have been removed with forceps from the dog patient. *(Photo by Arlett Perez, reproduced with permission.)*

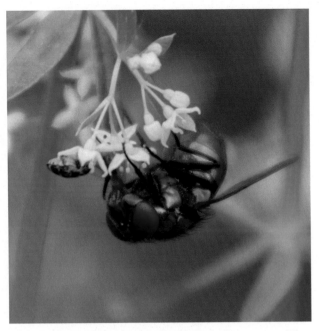

FIG. 8.28 An adult greenbottle fly (*Lucilia* sp.) feeding on nectar. *(Photo by Olli Immonen, reproduced with permission.)*

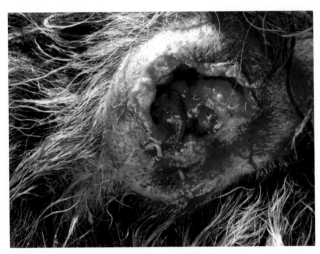

FIG. 8.27 Wound myiasis caused by a blowfly (probably by *Lucilia* sp.) in a dog. *(Photo by Kirsti Schildt, reproduced with permission.)*

CULICIDAE, Mosquitos

- Culicidae consists of 1000 of species.
- Mosquitos need water in their life cycle as the larvae of all species are aquatic.
- In addition to local irritation and hypersensitivity reaction in the bite site, mosquitos can act as vectors for infectious diseases.
- Vectors of the canine heartworm.

Identification

Mosquitos are dipteran flies containing 1000 of species. The most important mosquito genera are the *Aedes, Culex,* and *Anopheles*. Mosquitoes are rather small and slender flies. They have a narrow body and two wings, and their length varies between 2 and 10mm (Fig. 8.30). They have long, thin legs and compound eyes that are large in proportion to the size of the head. The complex chitin structures of the body, such as the chitin plates and the hair-like protrusions of varying size, create a coloring and pattern characteristic for each mosquito species. While at rest, the mosquito holds its narrow wings tightly pressed onto the posterior of the body. Adult mosquitos have scales on their wings (Fig. 8.31) and body. Long and striated antennae are attached between the compound eyes. The male antennae are typically covered with dense and voluptuous "fur." Downy antennae of the male (Fig. 8.32) facilitate locating the female, which makes a whining sound with its wings. The long proboscis, the sucking rostrum, is structurally complex and pointing forward. The proportional lengths of flagellomeres, attaching to the proboscis, and the vein patterns of the wings are used for identification of mosquitos up to the family and species level. Only females suck blood.

The sand fly, *Phelobotomus* sp., a vector for canine leishmaniosis, is not a mosquito. It is a small, sand-colored blood sucker belonging to the family Psychodidae (Fig. 2.26).

Life Cycle

The females of the majority of mosquito species lay 150–300 eggs into ditches, bonds, rainwater containers, or any stagnant water, either as single eggs or in groups.

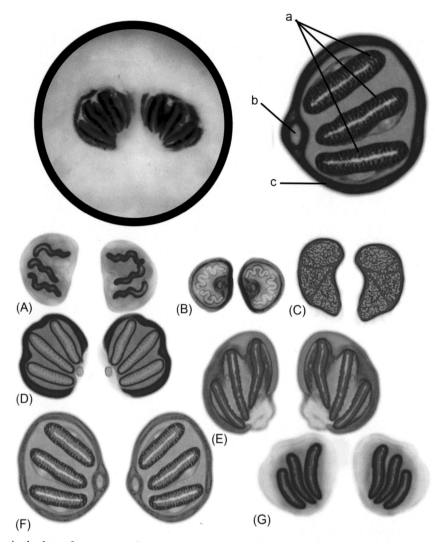

FIG. 8.29 Posterior spiracle plates of some mature dipteran larvae that may cause myiasis or the dog. In the round figure, a micrograph depicts the posterior spiracles of *Cochliomyia hominivorax*. The illustration at the upper right corner shows the key morphological elements of the spiracular plate: (a) slits; (b) button; (c) peritreme. (A) *Cordylobia* sp. with three curved spiracular slits without peritreme. (B) *Musca* sp. showing three sinuous spiracular slits and heavily sclerotized distinct D-shaped peritreme and distinct marginal and medially pointing button. (C) *Cuterebra* sp. showing kidney shaped spiracular plates divided into subplates with a lot of curved tightly packet slits. (D) *Cochliomyia* sp. with distinct but incomplete peritreme; button adjacent to the open peritreme. (E) *Sarcophaga* sp.: Posterior spiracles in cavity with distinct but incomplete peritreme; three vertical rather straight slits pointing towards the peritreme opening. (F) *Lucilia* sp. with well-developed peritreme surrounding also the button; three straight or slightly curved slits. (G) *Dermatobia* sp. with poorly defined and thin peritreme and three slightly curved slits. *(Round figure: Photo by Arlett Perez, reproduced with permission.)*

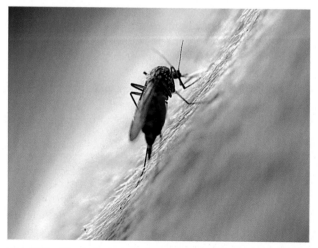

FIG. 8.30 Female forest mosquito sucking blood.

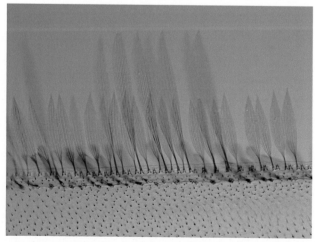

FIG. 8.31 A micrograph depicting a detail of feather-like scales on the mosquito's wing.

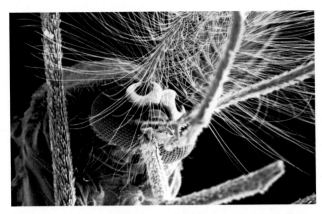

FIG. 8.32 A male mosquito in scanning electron microscopy. Downy antennae of the male facilitate locating the whining sound of the female. The signal of the vibrating flagellomeres is relayed to the Johnston's organ, a doughnut-shaped structure located at the basis of the antenna.

The hatching of larvae depends on the temperature: at the quickest it can happen within a few days after eggs are laid. Eggs of some mosquito species can survive over winter without hatching. The development of larvae requires that at least a thin layer of water remains as their environment. Although the larvae live in water, they need ambient oxygen. Many mosquitoes acquire oxygen though the spiracles, the air vents in the posterior part of the body. The larvae of *Culex* mosquitoes have a tube structure in their rear, through which they breathe. The larvae have a distinct head. Compound eyes, antennae, and brush-like ridge structures, which the larva uses for obtaining nutrients, can be seen in the head. The larval stage consists of four stadia, which can be completed in 3–20 days. On the other hand, the larvae of some species survive over winter and do not continue development until next summer. The larval stage is followed by the pupal stage, during which the head and the middle part of the body are conjoined. The comma-shaped pupa is capable of movement with posterior protrusions that resemble paddles. It has a transparent outer surface. Access to oxygen in the pupal stage is provided by two horn-shaped tubes, which start from the junction of the head and body and are directed towards water surface. The pupal stage lasts from a few days to weeks, again depending on the temperature and the mosquito species. During this stage, the mosquito transforms from the aquatic larva into the flying adult. To finish the pupal stage, the adult mosquito, when ready to hatch, swallows air. This causes the mosquito to swell and the exoskeleton to be torn open. Young adult mosquitoes (males as well as females) store energy by feeding on flower nectar. Copulation soon follows. The hormonal changes that make the ovarian and thereafter egg development possible in the female mosquito, however, cannot start before a blood meal. Blood protein is also necessary for the energy storage of the eggs.

Distribution

Mosquitoes are endemic in all continents. About 3500 mosquito species are known.

Importance to Canine Health

Mosquitoes act as vectors for many important parasites as well as viral pathogens. They may transmit pathogens mechanically but also through biological transmission. The most important one for dogs is the *Dirofilaria immitis* nematode. Mosquitoes do not only spread diseases. They also annoy dogs and may cause cutaneous hypersensitivity reactions. Sucking blood causes the proteins of mosquito saliva to get into contact with skin. After repeated exposure, an immunological reaction starts to develop against the saliva proteins. In a type I hypersensitivity reaction an IgE-mediated skin reaction, caused by histamine secreted from mast cells, develops in a few minutes. A cell-mediated type IV immune reaction, with a more delayed onset, is even more pronounced. Both reaction types cause pruritic maculae to develop. The type IV reaction takes about a day to start, and the maculae are usually larger than those in type I reaction. They may remain on the skin for up to 1 week. Individual dogs react to mosquitoes in a different way.

Treatment and Prevention

If a dog reacts strongly to mosquito stings, they can be prevented with repellent spot-on products or a collar containing insecticides. Pyrethrin and ectoparasite drugs containing pyrethroids, such as permethrin and deltamethrin, have repellent action against mosquitoes.

SIMULIIDAE, Black Flies, Gnats

- Black flies are a large group of small dipterans.
- Water is needed for the life cycle.
- In addition to local irritation in the bite site, black flies can act as vectors for infectious diseases.

Identification

Black flies are small dipteran flies. Their length varies between 1.5 and 5 mm. The family consists of large number of species; at least 1700 have been described to date. Black flies have a small and stubby body, with the mid-body arched so that looking from the side, the insect seems hump-backed. The wings are colorless, and the vein pattern is typically denser in the front edge of the wing. A resting black fly holds its wings tightly squeezed together.

The male and female resemble each other. The most distinct morphological difference is seen in eyes. The male eyes are large and almost cover the whole head area, touching at the center of the head. The female has smaller eyes that are clearly separated from each other. The antennae are small and stumpy, usually consisting of seven to nine segments.

Life Cycle

Black flies need running water in their environment. Only the females are blood suckers—they must have blood for the development of eggs. The black fly pierces the skin with its saw-like mouthparts and sucks the blood seeping into the wound. Once the female has got the taste of blood, it is resistant to outside interference, usually continuing the blood meal for some minutes despite disturbances. It lays eggs as a sticky mass that attaches to vegetation and rocks in running water. In a warm environment, the eggs hatch in a few days and produce larvae. The development is slower in cool conditions, and the eggs of some black fly species do not continue development until after winter. The larva undergoes several molts, until it moves into slowly streaming water and pupates. The adult fly crawls out of the pupa and ingests flower nectar as its first feed. Having eaten, the males swarm in groups, often around prominent landmarks. These swarms are joined by females, which are immediately harassed by males.

Distribution

Black flies are endemic all over the world.

Importance to Canine Health

Black flies are mostly an annoyance for grazing animals, but they can also suck blood from dogs. They are most active in the morning of warm and cloudy days. They especially disturb animals that are kept outside and do not enter houses. Typical skin regions favored by black flies include hairless sites, especially on the abdomen, legs, and head. Around the head, they prefer the inside of pinnae and the ear canal. The visit of a black fly causes a painful dermal trauma, which may bleed even after the insect's blood meal. The pinnae may develop a severe dermatitis, associated with exudation, encrustation and thickening of epidermis. Some dogs react to the bite with a ring-shaped lesion, with typically a small, reddish spot at the sting site and a slightly swollen, light ring around it. Since black flies move in swarms, the dog can be a subject of a massive fly attack. Fatal cases of black fly attacks against dogs have been reported in the literature. Black flies can also act as vectors for infectious diseases. The best known is river blindness in humans, caused by the *Onchocerca volvulus* nematode.

Treatment and Prevention

Dogs can be protected from black flies with repellents containing pyrethrin or pyrethroids.

CULICOIDES, Biting Midges

- Culicoides are small blood-sucking insects that can be identified by their wing spots.
- They cause itchy and painful stings.
- There are fewer midges in a windy spots than in shelter

Identification

Midges are flying insects with a length of 1–2 mm. They have long antennae with 15 segments in their heads. The vein patterns of the wings are used to identify the species. Although midges are small, the colors of the wings, characteristic for this genus, can be seen with the naked eye (Fig. 8.33).

Life Cycle

A female midge, depending on the species, lays a few dozens to hundreds of eggs to moist ground. The midge larvae often develop in the vicinity of watering holes of grazing animals, where the soil is continually wet due to splashing water and mixed with organic fecal material. The larvae feed on small invertebrates, bacteria, fungi, algae, and other living material in its environment. The energy source for adult midges is flower nectar. However, in order to produce eggs, the female must have blood. Female midges are active in windless and warm periods at dusk and night. On the other hand, some are clearly more active during the day. The most resilient species remain active long into the autumn, and they survive in temperatures down to about 4°C.

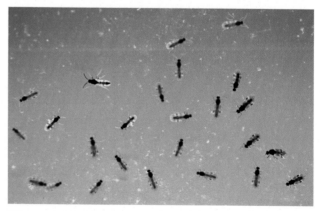

FIG. 8.33 The midge is a small blood sucker that can be identified based on its wing spots.

Importance to Canine Health

Midges are mostly a nuisance species for grazing animals, but they can also annoy dogs. Some species are blood suckers, and some damage skin with their mouthparts and feed on blood and tissue fluids seeping into the wound. After they leave, an itchy and painful sting remains. As a result of pruritic signs and scratching, skin trauma and restlessness are common observations among dogs bothered by midges. Usually, however, great swarms of midges rapidly disperse and the dog has a chance to recover.

Treatment and Prevention

Due to their small size and proportionally big wings, midges find it difficult to fly in the wind. Thus, there are typically fewer midges in a windy spot than in a sheltered landscape. Pyrethrins and pyrethroides are the most commonly used repellents.

HIPPOBOSCA LONGIPENNIS, Dog Fly and *LIPOPTENA CERVI*, Deer Ked

- Blood sucking flying dipteran insects.
- Adults spend most of their time in the host's fur, whereas other life stages live in the environment.
- *Hippobosca longipennis'* habitat is warm and humid, *Lipoptena cervi* is a louse fly of temperate zones, e.g., Europe and northern Asia.
- Both cause itchy bite marks; *H. longipennis* may act as vector to Filaria-nematodes.

Identification

Louse flies or keds (Hippoboscidae) are dorso-ventrally flat, about 1 cm long insects of the family Diptera. The somewhat flexible chitin cover of the posterior body enables the posterior to expand when the ked sucks blood or when the larva grows inside the female. Strong legs are attached to the mid-body, and the pit of each extremity has two claw-like structures. Both *Hippobosca longipennis* and *Lipoptena cervi* (Fig. 8.34) have large compound eyes and short antennae located in a recess in the head. Although some keds living on host animals have no wings, both dog fly and deer ked have very long and well-developed wings. When resting, the ked keeps the wings tightly pressed along the posterior body. *H. longipennis* can be distinguished from other keds based on its wing vein-pattern. The vein network is loose except in the front edge of the wing, where it is very dense.

Life Cycle

Both male and female keds are blood suckers. The blood meal causes the flying muscles to disintegrate while the leg muscles simultaneously grow stronger. For instance, when the deer ked finds a suitable host animal, its wings break of from the base and only small stubs are left. Keds are larviparous, meaning that they give birth to larvae, not eggs. The egg embryonates and hatches in the uterus. The development of the larva also takes place in utero, and the larva is fed by the uterine glands. The birth takes place, when the larva has become mature enough to pupate. *H. longipennis* typically gives birth to a larva in a sheltered place, for instance a burrow, crevice or hidden by vegetation. Having given birth, the female returns to the skin of the host. The female may live for up to 4–5 months and produce 10–15 larvae during that period. The larva pupates soon after being born, and the pupal stage lasts from less than 3 weeks to up to 5 months. Environmental conditions influence the duration of the pupal phase, which is longer in unfavorable conditions. The deer ked is an ectoparasite of deer and elks, but it is also a blood-sucking nuisance for dogs and humans. It has a reputation for being a lazy flier. Deer keds pass their time on the branches of fir trees, waiting for a host animal of suitable size to pass by. If the ked is lucky, the chosen target is a deer or elk, because a blood meal from Cervids is necessary for its reproduction.

Distribution

H. longipennis lives in moist and warm climate and favors carnivores, especially canids and felines, as hosts. It is found infrequently in Europe. *Lipoptena cervi* is a louse fly of temperate zones. It is endemic in Europe, Siberia, northern Asia, and North America. As keds are sluggish flyers, they are mostly concentrated in areas with a dense Cervid population.

Importance to Canine Health

In a dog, *H. longipennis* favors the ventral side of neck and the region of the armpits. The bite of a dog fly can be painful. The fly can act as a vector for several diseases. From the group of nematodes producing *Microfilaria*, the dog fly can spread *Microfilaria auguieri* and *Acanthoceilonema dracunculoides*. Deer keds may cause itch and bite trauma, which can be secondarily infected with bacteria.

Treatment and Prevention

Louse flies are often difficult to manage. Pyrethrin and pyrethroids (e.g., permethrin and deltamethrin) probably have some repellent activity against louse flies.

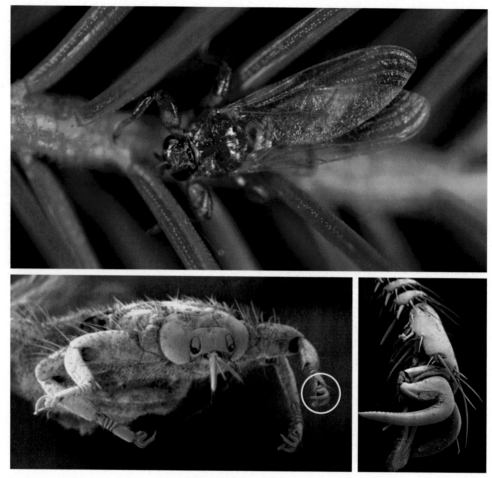

FIG. 8.34 The deer ked has a characteristic louse fly morphology. The upper photo shows the deer ked stalking by-passers on a spruce branch. The micrographs below show the same insect seen in the SEM and the morphological detail of deer ked tarsus.

FURTHER READING

Blagburn B, Dryden M: Biology, treatment, and control of flea and tick infestations, *Vet Clin North Am Small Anim Pract* 39:1173–1200, 2009.

Companion Animal Parasite Counsil, CAPC, Recommendations: Fleas. http://www.petsandparasites.org/dog-owners/fleas/. (Accessed May 2018).

Day MJ, editor: *Arthropod-borne infectious diseases of the dog and cat,* ed. 2, Boca Raton, FL, 2016, CRC Press.

Deplazes P, Eckert J, Mathis A, von Samson-Himmelstjerna G, Zahner H: *Parasitology in veterinary medicine,* ed 1, Wageningen, 2016, Wageningen Academic Publishers.

Dryden MW, Rust MK: The cat flea: biology, ecology, and control, *Vet Parasitol* 52:1–19, 1994.

European Scientific Counsel Companion Animal Parasites (ESCCAP): *Control of ectoparasites in dogs and cats,* Guideline 3, ed 6, March 2018. https://www.esccap.org/uploads/docs/gm7zb43y_0720_ESCCAP_Guideline_GL3_update_v6.pdf. (Accessed May 2018).

Gunn A, Pitt SJ: Arthropod parasites. In *Parasitology, an integrated approach,* Chichester, 2012, Wiley-Blackwell, pp 137–179.

Hellenthal RA, Price RD: Phthiraptera: chewing and sucking lice. *In Encyclopedia of insects,* ed 2, San Diego, 2009, Academic Press.

Hwang S, Svoboda T, DeJong I, Kabasele K, Gogosis E: Bed bug infestation in an urban environment, *Emerg Infect Dis* 11:533–538, 2005.

Khan H, Rahman M: Morphology and biology of the bedbug, *Cimex hemipterus* (Hemiptera: Cimicidae) in the laboratory, *Dhaka Univ J Biol Sci* 21:125–130, 2012.

Krinsky W: True bugs. In Mullen G, Durden L, editors: *Medical and veterinary entomology,* Orlando, FL, 2002, Academic Press, pp 67–86.

Mathison BA, Pritt BS: Laboratory identification of arthropod ectoparasites, *Clin Microbiol Rev* 27:48–67, 2014. https://doi.org/10.1128/CMR.00008-13.

Miller W Jr, Griffin C, Campbell K: *Muller and Kirk's small animal dermatology,* ed 7, St. Louis, 2012, Saunders-Elsevier.

Pampliglione S, Fioravanti ML, Gustinelli A, et al: Sand flea (*Tunga* spp.) infections in humans and domestic animals: state of the art, *Med Vet Entomol* 23:172–186, 2009. https://doi.org/10.1111/j.1365-2915.2009.00807.x.

Russel R, Otranto O, Wall R: *The encyclopedia of medical and veterinary entomology,* Wallingford & Boston, 2013, CABI.

Rust M, Dryden M: The biology, ecology, and management of the cat flea, *Annu Rev Entomol* 42:451–473, 1997.

Saaed S: *Ctenocephalides felis*, University of Michigan, Museum of Zoology. https://animaldiversity.org/accounts/Ctenocephalides_felis/. (Accessed May 2018).

Saari S, Nikander S: Kirput yleistyvät—katsaus Suomessa koirista tavattaviin kirppulajeihin ja niiden morfologisiin eroavaisuuksiin, *Suom Elainlaakaril* 97:362–366, 1991 (in Finnish).

Saari S, Nikander S: Lähikuvassa koiran täi (*Linognathus setosus*) ja väive (*Trichodectes canis*), *Suom Elainlaakaril* 100:372–378, 1994 (in Finnish).

Seago JM: *CDC: Fly larvae: pictorial key to some common species*, p 124. https://www.cdc.gov/nceh/ehs/docs/pictorial_keys/flies.pdf. (Accessed June 2018).

Taylor M, Coop R, Wall R: *Veterinary parasitology*, ed 4, Oxford, 2016, Blackwell Publishing Ltd.

Thomas J, Reichard M: *Managing maggots & bots in dogs & cats,* 2018, Vet Team Brief. https://www.veterinaryteambrief.com/article/managing-maggots-bots-dogs-cats. (Accessed September 2018).

Zajac AM, Conboy GA: Diagnosis of arthropod parasites. In *Veterinary clinical parasitology*, ed 8, Chichester, 2012, Wiley-Blackwell.

Chapter 9

Arachnida

Arachnida is a class of Arthropoda together with Insecta (insects). It includes subclass Acari, ticks, and mites, which are important in veterinary medicine. The arachnid species strongly resemble insects in appearance and in morphology. Arachnida have two body parts: cephalo-thorax and abdomen. Sometimes the body parts are called gnathosoma (mouthparts) and idiosoma (the main body). The adults have eight legs. There are no antennae. The metamorphosis is hemimetabolic, incomplete, with eggs, six-legged larvae, and immature nymph stages before adulthood.

Arachnida have digestive tract similar to insects: a tube from mouth to anus. The nervous system consists of supraesophageal ganglion (brain) connected to a ventral nerve cord. The eyes are missing or there might be several of them—not always attached to the head. The gas exchange happens through openings called stigmata, which lead to lamellar book lungs. The circulatory systems consists of a tubular vessel or heart pumping the hemolymph. Females and males have differing sexual organs.

Parasitic acari are true parasites that spend the whole life on the host animal, or facultative parasites that only take their meal from the host and spend the rest of the life cycle in the environment. Some acari suck blood and the others use epidermal material or tissue fluid as food. The clinical signs associated with acari parasites are reactions by the host to their bites and secretions. Ticks act as vectors for infectious diseases, such as anaplasmosis, babesiosis, and erlichiosis.

The medical treatment or prevention of acari have multitude of choices nowadays. Many dog owners want to protect their pet from ticks for the whole season, especially if the ticks are common in the area. Mite infestations are typically acquired from another dog/animal and they are treated when diagnosed.

IXODES RICINUS, Castor Bean Tick

- Large, obligate blood-feeding ectoparasites.
- Distributed in Europe.
- Common in humid habitats.
- Three blood meals from the hosts are needed to the transformation from larva to adult.
- Vector for bacterial and viral diseases.
- Acarisidic medication is recommended in the areas of dense tick population.

Identification

The morphology of *Ixodes ricinus* is characteristic for ixodid ticks. In Europe, it is essential to be able to distinguish the castor bean tick from the ticks of *Rhipicephalus* and *Dermacentor* genera, which are the other most important hard tick genera in canine medicine (Fig. 9.1). The *Ixodes* tick (Figs. 9.2–9.7) has characteristically long mouthparts. Anchoring to the host skin is facilitated by a sword-like structure, or hypostome, that has backward-pointing chitin barbs (Fig. 9.3). On the dorsal surface of the basis capituli (base of the head), round, and somewhat triangular porous areas can be seen in a female (Fig. 9.4). The dorsal shield, or scutum, lacks the marble pattern, and the shield's edges lack festoons that give some other tick species a pie-crust look. *I. ricinus* has no eyes. The best morphological feature for distinguishing *Ixodes* from *Rhipicephalus* and *Dermacentor* is found on the ventral surface: the anus is surrounded by a U-shaped groove, which arches anterior from the anus (Fig. 9.3). Another morphological feature characteristic for *Ixodes*-genus ticks and found on the ventral side is the set of sharp spur-like protrusions seen proximally (coxae) in the first pair of legs (Fig. 9.4). The female tick is 3–3.6 mm long until it sucks blood. After a blood meal, it is much bigger, up to more than 1 cm. The male tick is smaller (2.4–2.8 mm) and evenly coffee-brown in color (Fig. 9.2).

Life Cycle

Like most of its close relatives, the castor bean tick has a three-host life cycle, meaning that it needs three blood meals from three different hosts during its life cycle to be able to continue its development to the next phase (larva to nymph, nymph to adult, and for females, prerequisite for egg production). The castor bean tick spends most of its life separated from its host animals.

In order to find a host, *I. ricinus* climbs up vegetation up to the height of 1.5 m, where it scans the environment with the front pair of legs raised high and with Haller's organ (Fig. 9.7) exposed, looking for a suitable passer-by. In

Canine Parasites and Parasitic Diseases. https://doi.org/10.1016/B978-0-12-814112-0.00009-X

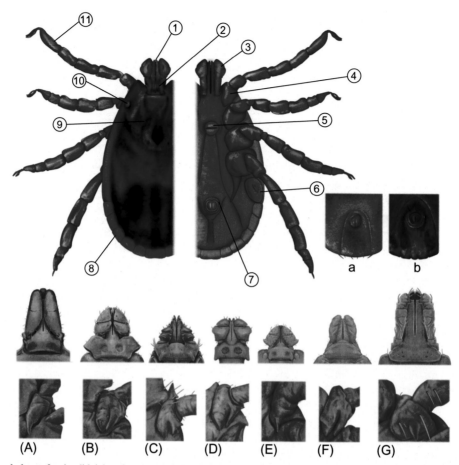

FIG. 9.1 Basic morphology of an ixodid tick and some morphological differences in the most important ticks genera. Ixodid female tick; dorsal view on the left and ventral view on the right. (1) Hypostomum, (2) basis capituli, (3) palps consisting of three segments, (4) coxa I, (5) genital opening, (6) stigmatal plate (spiracles), (7) anus and anal groove, (8) festoons, (9) scutum, ornamented, (10) eye, and (11) tarsus with Haller's organ. (a) Anus and anal groove of *Ixodes* type: U-shaped anal groove arching anus anteriorly and (b) anal groove arching the anus posteriorly. (A) *Ixodes*: Mouthparts are significantly longer than basis capituli. Well-developed internal spur in coxa I. (B) *Rhipicephalus*: Short mouthparts are shorter than the width of basis capituli but longer than hypostomum; basis capituli is hexagonal with distinct lateral projections. Well-developed paired spurs present in coxa I. (C) *Boophilus*: Short palps that do not reach the tip of hypostomum and with sharp ridges between the segments. Small paired spurs present in coxa I. (D) *Dermacentor*: Rectangular basis capituli, short palps. Large paired spurs present in coxa I. (E) *Haemaphysalis*: Rectangular basis capituli, short palps; base of palpal segment II with distinct lateral projection. Single large internal spur present in coxa I. (F) *Hyalomma*: Long mouthparts, II and III palpal segments about equal in length. Large equal spurs present in coxa I. (G) *Amblyomma*: Long mouthparts, palpal segment II about twice as long as segment III. Coxa I with small unequal paired spurs.

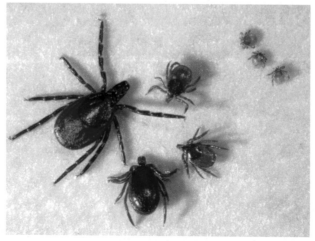

FIG. 9.2 Developmental stages of a castor bean tick (*Ixodes ricinus*): a female at the extreme left, a male below, two nymphs in the center, three larval stages at the upper right corner.

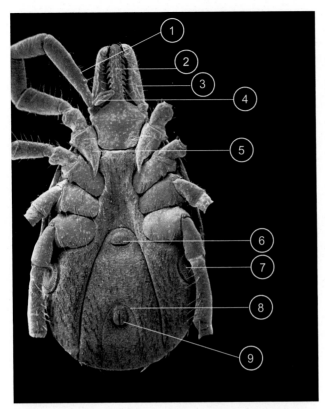

FIG. 9.3 Female *Ixodes ricinus*, ventral view: (1) tarsus with Haller's organ; (2) hypostomum lined with backward-pointing chitin barbs that help anchoring into skin; (3) palp consisting of three segments; (4) pulvillus with claws; (5) well-developed internal spur in coxa I; (6) genital opening; (7) stigmatal plate (spiracles); (8) U-shaped anal groove arching the anus (9).

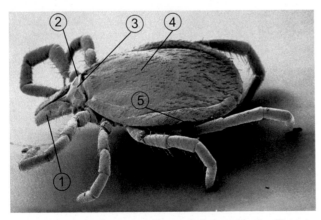

FIG. 9.4 Female *Ixodes ricinus* dorso-lateral view: (1) palp; (2) porous area of basis capituli (3); (4) scutum; and (5) stigmatal plate (spiracles).

the grass-tops, the tick may suffer from dryness and it often has to climb down closer to the moisture of the ground to revive its fluid homeostasis.

After it has clutched onto a host animal, the castor bean tick seeks a suitable skin area, pierces the surface with its mouthparts and anchors tightly into the skin with the barbed

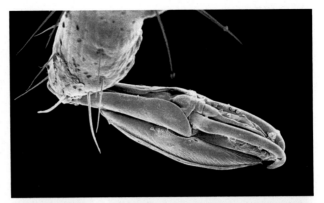

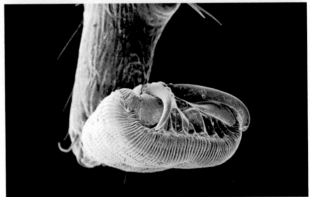

FIG. 9.5 The distal end of the tick tarsus with its hooks and pulvillus. The leg has hook structures and the pulvillus, which the tick can fan out.

hypostome and the adhesive substance it secretes. During the first few days after attaching, the female prepares for blood sucking. Little blood is ingested during this time. An adult female stays attached in the skin for about 1 week. The pheromones it secretes attract male ticks. There are conflicting data regarding the blood sucking activity of the male castor bean tick. Some sources claim that the male is a blood sucker that sucks blood only briefly each time. Other sources state that the male gets its blood meal while being attached to the female. Yet none of the authors has observed a male castor bean tick attached to the skin.

When the male tick finds a female, it crawls into the ventral side of the female and pushes its mouthparts into the genital pore. The male mouthparts spread 90° sideways. The male tick is often found under the female stuck in this position (Fig. 9.8). A result of the union, the male transfers its spermatozoa-containing capsule (spermatophore) into the female genital pore.

At the end of the blood sucking activity, an abscess-type cavity forms in the sucking site of the host's skin. It loses the skin tissue, enabling the fully engorged female to disengage (Fig. 9.9). The female falls onto the ground and lays about 2000 eggs into the detritus layer. The last weeks or months of the female's life are spent tending the eggs (Fig. 9.10). In the following spring, eggs hatch into small, six-legged tick larvae. By then, the female is dead.

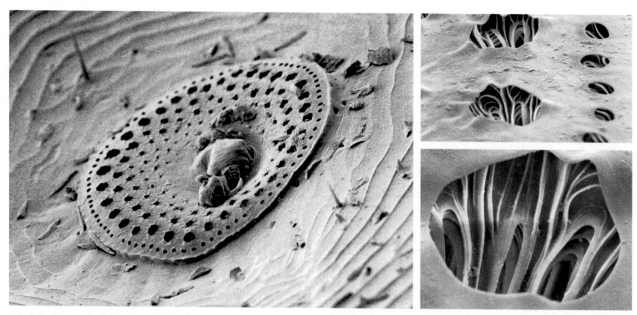

FIG. 9.6 Oxygen intake happens through a sieve-like stigmatal or spiracular plate located on both sides of the abdomen. The holes, stigmata (spiracles), are of varying size and connected to the book lungs with thin folds of membrane.

After hatching from the egg, the larva stays together with its siblings for a while, until the chitin structures of scutum have sclerotized (Fig. 9.11). In order to be able to molt to the next developmental stage, the larva must have a blood meal. The mouthparts of a larva are substantially shorter and more delicate than those of an adult castor bean tick. That is why larvae usually suck blood from thin-skinned small mammals or birds. After the blood meal, the larva is released and creeps into the detritus layer for molting. This phase lasts a few weeks, longer in cool conditions. The eight-legged nymph must also feed on blood. It

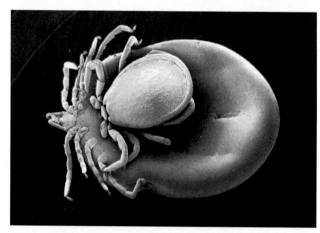

FIG. 9.8 Having found a blood-sucking female, the male tick crawls to its ventral side and pushes its mouthparts into the female genital pore. The male mouthparts bend 90 degrees laterally. Males stuck in this position are often found under a female tick.

climbs up the vegetation and catches a host animal passing by, sucks blood for 5–7 days, disengages, molts and passes the winter as an adult tick. If a suitable host does not pass the nymph's hunting site, it spends the winter as a nymph and continues the ambush the following spring. An illustrated lifecycle of *I. ricinus* is presented in Fig. 9.12.

Distribution

The castor bean tick is drought-intolerant. Its essential requirement is rather high ambient humidity, preferably over 80%, sufficient rainfall and enough vegetation to maintain a moist microclimate. In temperate zones, ticks'

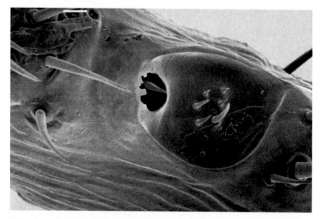

FIG. 9.7 A tick, typically for Arachnids, does not have antennae. The duties of antennae are handled by the complex sensory organ, Haller's organ, located on the dorsal surface of the first pair of legs at the terminal segment. The organ enables host detection and mate seeking by sensing temperature, odors, humidity, chemical substances, and carbon dioxide. Haller's organ is formed by a tiny chamber with a pit and a capsule and several sensory setae.

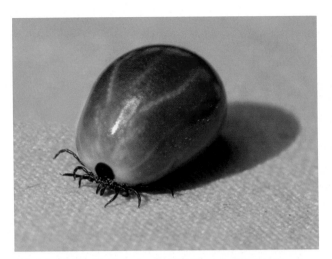

FIG. 9.9   After a blood meal, a female tick can be the size of a pea.

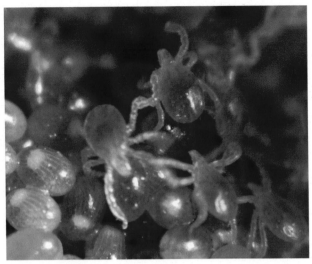

FIG. 9.11   After hatching from the egg, the tick larva spends time with its siblings, until the chitin structures of its surface have hardened.

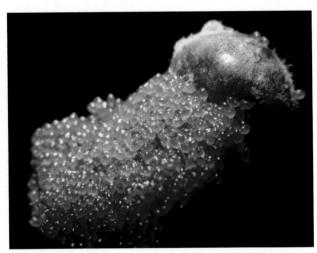

FIG. 9.10   After sucking blood, the female falls onto the ground and lays about 2000 eggs in the detritus. The female spends the last weeks of its life taking care of the eggs. The amber-colored eggs have a shiny and smooth surface. The female, in the background the figure, is already partially covered by mold.

preferred environments are moist shore pastures, broad-leaf woodland and shady forests. During the dry and hot periods of high summer, host animals are relatively safe from ticks' attachment attempts, because the castor bean ticks hide in the moisture of earth surface waiting to get active, after the rain has ensured the proper moisture. Thanks to the limitations caused by climate, it takes years for the castor bean tick to complete the stages of its life cycle. Temperatures of few degrees over the freezing point are sufficient to activate the castor bean tick and trigger its thirst for blood.

Importance to Canine Health

The clinical importance of the castor bean tick is not limited to blood sucking, while in regions of high tick population density, dozens of ticks may be found attached to a dog. The more important role in pathogenesis is the ticks' ability to act as vectors for many feared contagious diseases. For dogs, the most important are borreliosis (*Borrelia burgdorferi* infection) and anaplasmosis (*Anaplasma phagocytophilum* infection). Tick-borne encephalitis (TBE) caused by Flavi-virus can also affect dogs, although a clinical disease is very rare. Tick attachment typically produces a zone of erythema of a few millimeters' diameter on the skin. This often becomes a lesion that is somewhat elevated from the surrounding skin. Repeated exposure to castor bean ticks may lead to a hypersensitivity reaction, where the skin reaction is much more severe and may involve pruritus and secondary trauma due to scratching. Removal of a recently attached tick almost always leads to a situation where pieces of mouthparts are torn off and remain in the skin. This is not dangerous, as the host removes the mouthpart remnants with an inflammatory reaction similar to that against a foreign object.

Salivary glands of some tick species produce toxic proteins that may cause paralysis in host animals. The best known of these species is *Ixodes holocyclus*, the cousin of *I. ricinus* and endemic in the eastern coast of Australia. It can cause several types of signs, such as disorders of coordination and sight, abnormally copious salivation, vomiting, and respiratory problems. Notably, while tick paralysis may be fatal in dogs, it is not seen in Australian native fauna.

Diagnosis

The diagnosis is based on recognizing the typical morphology of ticks found in dogs.

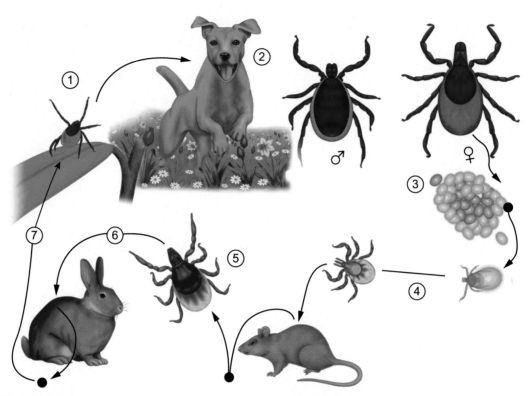

FIG. 9.12 Life cycle of *Ixodes ricinus*: (1) *I. ricinus* waits for a suitable host animal to pass by, clinging onto vegetation and holding the front pair of the legs high; (2) having grasped the host animal, the castor bean tick finds a suitable skin site and anchors itself tightly into the skin with its barbed hypostome and adhesive substance it secretes onto the skin. An adult female stays attached for about 1 week. The pheromones it secretes attract male ticks. The male pushes its spermatophore into the female genital pore; (3) the fully engorged female drops onto the ground after copulation and lays about 2000 eggs into the detritus; (4) the eggs hatch next spring to produce small, six-legged tick larvae. Since the mouthparts of the larvae are short and delicate, they usually suck blood from thin-skinned small mammals and birds. After the blood meal, the larva detaches and crawls into the detritus layer for molting; (5) molting results in an eight-legged nymph, which in temperate climates often does not continue the life cycle until the next summer. The nymph needs a blood meal too. After feeding, it molts and spends the winter as an adult; and (6) in the following summer, the adult castor bean tick (7) continues its life cycle. The tick has a three-host life cycle, the length of which is dependent on the climate.

Treatment and Prevention

Ticks attached in the skin should be immediately removed from as close to the skin as possible. Several special instruments are available for the removal to avoid the manipulation of the swollen abdomen of the tick. If castor bean ticks are abundant in the dog's environment, the dog should be protected during the entire tick season with continuous medication without treatment gaps. To reduce the risk of vector-borne pathogen transmission the tick product should have a rapid onset of activity following administration, it should protect all areas of the treated dog, and the product should maintain its efficacy throughout the retreatment interval.

Most Important Canine Infectious Diseases Transmitted by *Ixodes ricinus*

Borreliosis is a tick-borne infectious disease. Many mammalian, avian, and reptilian species can be infected, but few get sick with clinical borreliosis. *Borrelia* are elongated, thin, and helical rod-shaped spirochete. They are difficult to detect even in light microscopy. *B. burgdorferi sensu lato* forms a group of genetically diverse subgenera, of which only some are pathogenic.

The transfer of *Borrelia* spirochete between ticks and mammals has been investigated mainly with rodents. Attachment to the host causes an increase in the number of *Borrelia* in the tick's alimentary tract. Soon after they migrate to the tick's salivary gland and further, when blood sucking takes place, to the host. *Borrelia* transfer usually happens 1–2 days after the tick has attached, at the earliest. *Borrelia* do not survive free in the environment. Their survival requires them to be passed from one host to another by blood-sucking ticks. Ixodid ticks have a three-host life cycle, and a blood meal is obligatory for the larval, nymphal, and adult development stages. The tick obtains *Borrelia* in its body while having a blood meal during the larval or nymphal stages.

Canine *Borrelia* infection is usually subclinical. The incubation period of borreliosis is poorly known. In experimental infections, clinical signs do not manifest until 2–6 months after infection. The clinical signs of borreliosis include fever, inappetence, somnolence, lameness that varies between legs, joint swelling, and enlarged lymph nodes. Renal insufficiency (immunomediated glomerulonephritis) and hypoproteinemia due to proteinuria have also

Most Important Canine Infectious Diseases Transmitted by *Ixodes ricinus*—cont'd

been described. Bernese mountain dogs seem to be prone to infection by *Borrelia* bacteria. There is no totally reliable test for diagnosing borreliosis. Increased antibody titers indicate that the dog has got the infection at some point, but do not ascertain that the dog's clinical signs are caused by borreliosis. Many dogs without signs are seropositive in endemic areas.

Clinical signs, a rise in antibody titers seen in paired serum samples, and therapeutic response to treatment may help to define whether canine borreliosis is in an active state. The progressively widening ring-shaped erythema migrans around the attachment site, common in human borreliosis, is a very rare finding in dogs.

Anaplasmosis, also known as granylocytic anaplasmosis, is a rickettsial infectious disease caused by *A. phagocytophilum* in dogs, humans and many other species. The bacteria, earlier known as *Ehrlichia phagocytophila/equi*, is Gram-negative, immobile, and coccoid or ellipsoid. *Anaplasma* lacks a cell wall and it lives inside cells, favoring mature neutrophilic granulocytes, and more rarely eosinophilic granulocytes, as its environment.

Ixodic ticks are the most important vectors for *A. phagocytophilum*. *Anaplasma* is infectious to many species, apart from the dog, for instance, to horses, cats, cattle, small ruminants, and humans. Wild ruminants and rodents are significant reservoirs of *Anaplasma* in nature.

The transfer of *Anaplasma* from the castor bean tick to a mammal happens, according to studies conducted on mice, 24–48 h after the tick has attached. *Anaplasma* remains infectious in the tick's salivary gland. If the bacteria are in an infectious stage in sufficient numbers in the gland, the transfer to the mammal may happen even faster.

Round, basophilically stained morula stages of the bacteria can be found in neutrophilic granulocytes in a stained blood smear. PCR is more sensitive in analysis of anaplasmosis than blood smear. Antibodies against *Anaplasma* can be detected from a blood sample, but it is important to note that many dogs without clinical signs of anaplasmosis are seropositive in endemic areas.

TBE is a tick-borne infectious disease with central nervous signs caused by Flavi-virus. *I. ricinus* and *Ixodes persulcatus* ticks are considered the most important vectors for the viral disease. Clinical TBE affects humans especially, but the clinical disease has also been described in dogs and other mammals. The disease is usually geographically limited.

Results from studies on serological prevalence, conducted in endemic areas, indicate that the TBE virus infects dogs quite commonly. To date, it is not known why the clinical disease is very rare in dogs. Whenever TBE manifests in dogs, it is, however, severe and often fatal.

TBE virus can infect the host within a few minutes after the tick has attached. When the blood meal continues, the risk of transmission increases, because the virus multiplies after the tick has attached.

Pulling the tick off or killing it soon after attachment is not an effective method of preventing TBE infection.

The seropositivity of infected animals can be analyzed with a test. Since many dogs without disease signs may be seropositive in endemic areas, not even the combination of seropositivity and manifest central nervous signs constitute proof of TBE. Increased antibody concentrations in paired serum samples suggest a recent infection. Proof of the virus can also be found with the PCR methods. Clinical TBE is usually a rapidly progressive disease and the diagnosis can often only be confirmed at autopsy and by subsequent histopathological and immunohistochemical examination.

Tick Paralysis

About 70 tick species are known to be able to cause tick paralysis with their salivary neurotoxins. Australian *I. holocyclus* causes the most serious paralysis with up to 10% mortality. The toxicity is not necessarily related to the amount of ticks or the duration of the attachment, but the secretion of toxin and the immunity and sensitivity of the host. Even one tick may cause the death of a large dog. The signs usually appear about 4–7 days after the attachment and worsen rapidly over the following 24–48 h. At the beginning lethargy, dilated pupils and incoordination might be seen. Later there is respiratory distress and the dog is not able to stand or swallow; in these cases, the prognosis is guarded. For diagnosis the history of attached ticks or traveling in the endemic area are essential, because there are no specific tests. The ticks are removed as a treatment and the dog is kept in nonstressful conditions. It might be beneficial to sedate the dog, to keep it calm. In the endemic areas tick antiserum for the toxin is available. Tick prevention is recommended.

Classification of Tick Paralysis Signs in Dogs by Atwell

Neuromuscular Score

Stage 1: Dysphonia (noticed retrospectively), weakness and incoordination, but can still stand and walk. Best assessed walking up stairs.

Stage 2: Can stand, but unable to walk (obvious ataxia/paresis).

Stage 3: Cannot stand, but can right itself.

Stage 4: Cannot right itself.

Respiratory Score

(A) Normal—no clinical respiratory compromise.

(B) Mild compromise—increased heart rate and respiratory rate.

(C) Moderate compromise—restrictive breathing, gagging, retching. Cannot stand but can right itself.

(D) Severe compromise—expiratory grunt, dyspnea, cyanosis. Cannot right itself.

Ticks Manipulate the Host's Immune Defense and the Pathogens Manipulate the Tick

Salivary secretions of *I. ricinus* contain immunomodulating substances that have a direct effect on the host's immune defense (Fig. 9.13). The known effects include

- weakening of the complement cascade
- tying down of histamine
- disruption or inhibition of the action of NK cells, dendritic cells and neutrophilic granulocytes
- diminishing antibody concentrations
- inhibiting cytokine production
- inhibiting lymphocyte production

Thanks to these effects, the ticks can suck blood from the same host repeatedly. Meanwhile, the tick-borne pathogens also benefit: the local immunosuppression effected by the tick increases the infection risk.

The pathogens are known to affect ticks as well. According to studies, castor bean ticks attaching to a host animal carry tick-borne pathogens with a higher likelihood than other endemic ticks in general. For instance, a tick carrying *Borrelia* withstands dry conditions better than infection-free ticks. A more drought-resilient tick can concentrate better on stalking by-passing host candidates, since they do not have to keep returning to the moist detritus to amend their fluid homeostasis, unlike those more sensitive to drought. This currently poorly known mechanism benefits the *Borrelia* bacteria as well as the castor bean tick.

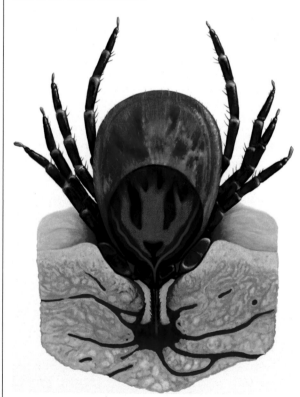

FIG. 9.13 Ticks manipulate hosts' immune defense. *(Illustration by Tom Björklund, reproduced with permission.)*

DERMACENTOR RETICULATUS, Marsh Tick

- Common in central Europe.
- Moisture is needed in the habitat, adapted also in parks and other cultivated environments.
- Festoons, ornamentation of the scutum and the shape of basis capituli can be used for identification.
- Important vector of *Babesia canis*.

Identification

The basic morphology of *Dermacentor* (Fig. 9.14) is characteristic of ixodid ticks. *Dermacentor* has relatively short mouthparts. The base of the head (basis capituli) is rectangular, and wide, oval, and porous sites can be seen on the dorsal surface of a female (Fig. 9.15). The dorsal shield (scutum) of *Dermacentor* has a distinct, ornamental and light-colored marble pattern (Figs. 9.14 and 9.15). The eyes are at the back, laterally, at about the level of the second pair of legs (Fig. 9.15). The posterior edge is characterized by festoons, which create a pie-crust appearance (Fig. 9.16). Usually there are 11 festoons. *Dermacentor* is one of the largest ticks. The female is 3.8–4.2 mm long and significantly larger after a blood meal, up to 15 mm. The male is also big: 4.2–4.8 mm long.

Life Cycle

Larvae hatching from the eggs typically suck blood from thin-skinned rodents, rabbits, and birds. Adults may parasitize many animal species. They suck blood, for example, from wild ruminants, horses, humans, and dogs. As a species with a three-host life cycle, *D. reticulatus*

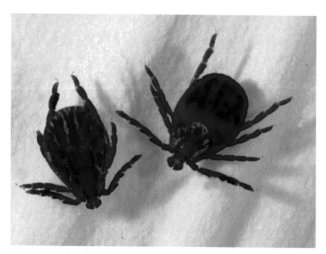

FIG. 9.14 *Dermacentor reticulatus*, male (left) and female (right). The dorsal shield has a distinct and ornamental, light marble pattern. The posterior edge is skirted by a pie-crust pattern created by festoons.

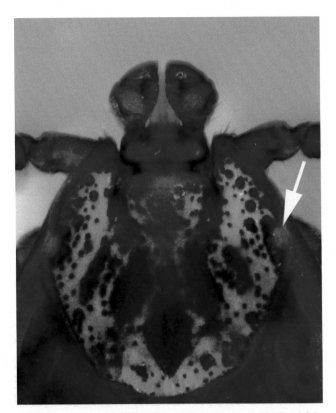

FIG. 9.15 *Dermacentor* has relatively short mouthparts. The base of the head is shaped like a rectangle. In a female tick, wide, oval, and porous areas can be seen on its dorsal surface. The eyes (*arrow*) can be seen at the back of *Dermacentor* laterally, approximately at the level of the second pair of legs.

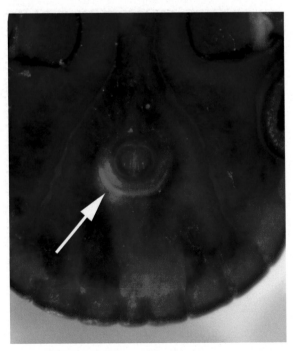

FIG. 9.16 The posterior edge of *Dermacentor* is skirted by a distinct pie-crust pattern created by festoons, of which there are usually 11. The *arrow* points to an anal groove, which does not extend to the front of the anus.

needs a blood meal three times during its life cycle. After the final blood meal and copulation, the adult female lays up to 4500 eggs. Hexapod larval stages hatch from eggs in 1–2 weeks. In optimal circumstances, two generations of D. reticulatus can complete their life cycle during 1 year. *Dermacentor* finds its host animals in the similar manner as *Ixodes*: by spending most of its life stalking in grass and waiting for an opportunity to get hold of an animal passing by. Copulation takes place on the dog's skin. The female starts the blood meal and secretes pheromones to attract males. The sucking of blood continues during copulation and beyond it. The engorged female disengages and descends into a sheltered place to lay eggs. It dies soon after. The male can copulate with several females.

Distribution

Dermacentor reticulatus lives in the central Europe mostly on relatively moist and open pastures that grow deciduous trees and bushes. It especially favors riverside woods and pastures close to forests. *Dermacentor* is well adjusted to manmade environments and it is common in parks, which have been converted to recreational areas by conserving original vegetation and waterways. Generally, *D. reticulatus* thrives and is expanding its endemic areas in Europe.

Importance to Canine Health

A severe *Dermacentor* infestation may cause anemia in a small dog. In sites where blood has been sucked, swelling, pruritus, and other signs of inflammation can be seen. In the same manner as with other ticks, the clinical importance of *Dermacentor* is primarily based on its ability to act as a vector for many infectious diseases. In European conditions, it is a significant source of canine babesiosis (piroplasmosis), caused by *Babesia canis*. It can likely also infect dogs with borreliosis and tularemia.

Diagnosis

The diagnosis is based on identifying morphologically characteristic ticks in dogs.

Treatment and Prevention

Attached ticks should be removed as soon as they are detected. In areas of abundant tick populations, dogs can be given continuous antitick treatment for the entire tick season.

RHIPICEPHALUS SANGUINEUS, Brown Dog Tick

- Widely distributed due to its ability to survive in dry conditions, including human dwellings.
- Festoons and the shape of basis capituli can be used for morphological identification.
- Transmits several vector-borne diseases.
- May require pest control visits in the kennel/household.

Identification

The basic morphology of *Rhipicephalus* is characteristic of Ixodidae hard ticks (Figs. 9.17–9.20).

It is essential to be able to distinguish it from the ticks of *Ixodes* and *Dermacentor* genera. The mouthparts of the brown dog tick are relatively short. The base of the head (basis capituli) is hexagonal. It has lateral protrusions, and on the dorsal surface of the female head, round and porous spots are seen (Figs. 9.18–9.20). The coloring of the brown dog tick is reddish brown. It has light-colored rings at the leg joints. There is no marble ornamentation in the dorsal shield (scutum). The shield is laterally grooved at approximately the first and second pair of legs. The eyes of *Rhipicephalus* are visible laterally on the back, at about the level of the second pair of legs. The posterior edge of the brown dog tick is skirted by festoons, forming a pie-crust pattern. The female is 3–4.5 mm long and substantially larger after having had a blood meal.

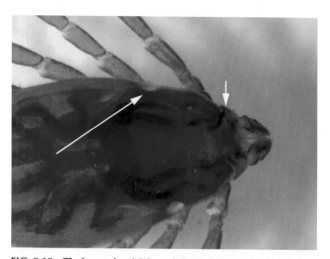

FIG. 9.18 The brown dog tick has relatively short mouthparts. The base of the head (*short arrow*) is hexagonal. It has lateral protrusions, and on the dorsal surface of a female tick, round and porous sites can be seen on its dorsal surface. The eyes (*long arrow*) are located laterally, approximately at the level of the second pair of legs.

Life Cycle

Since the brown dog tick has a three-host life cycle, it needs three blood meals to be able to finalize its development (from larva to nymph, from nymph to adulthood and for females, as a prerequisite for egg production). The tick spends most of its life separated from the host animal. Its preferred host is a canid, but it can suck blood from other animals as well. The brown dog tick is a hunter, which moves actively searching for a suitable blood source. This characteristic sets it apart from *Ixodes* and *Dermacentor*, which spend

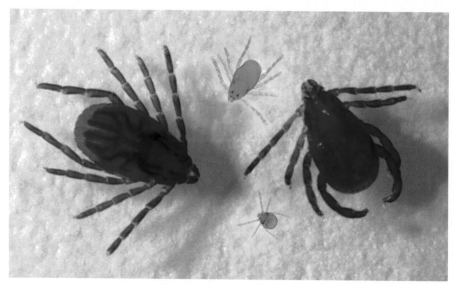

FIG. 9.17 Developmental stages of the brown dog tick (*Rhipicephalus sanguineous*): female (left), male (right), nymph (center above), and larva (center below).

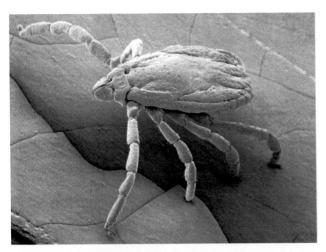

FIG. 9.19 A female brown dog tick in scanning electron microscopy. The dorsal shield has grooves at the level of first and second pair of legs. The posterior edge is skirted by distinct pie-crust pattern formed by festoons. The female is 3–4.5 mm long, and much bigger after a blood meal.

most of their lives waiting for a host in grass. Skin penetration is achieved with the hypostomum and chelicerae organs. *Rhipicephalus* pierces the epidermis with its short mouthparts, covering the skin, but can only reach the distal layer of dermis. The tick augments attachment by secreting a hardening substance on the area. The mouthparts damage the dermal veins, and the brown dog tick ingests blood that seeps into the pool forming at the vascular trauma area. The blood meal lasts from a few days for larvae, up to weeks for females. The male is also a blood sucker, and can have repeated blood meals. Copulation takes place on the dog's skin. The absence of male ticks prolongs the blood meal

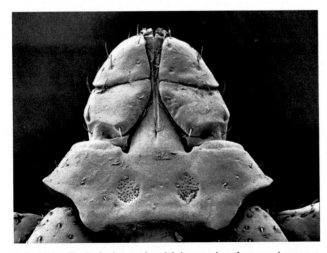

FIG. 9.20 Head of a brown dog tick in scanning electron microscopy. The mouthparts are shorter than those of *Ixodes*. The hexagonal basis capituli with its lateral spur-like projections and round porous areas can be seen.

of the female. In contrast, the presence of males speeds up the blood meal, including that of the larval and nymphal stages.

The engorged female disengages, searches for a sheltered place and lays up to 4000 eggs during the following weeks. Delicate, hexapod larvae hatch from the eggs in about a week to a few weeks. The larvae have to harden the chitin that covers their exterior for a few days, before they are ready to suck blood. After a blood meal, the larva moves to a sheltered place to molt. The nymph developing from the molting must again acquire a blood meal, so that the life cycle can continue. The life cycle of *Rhipicephalus sanguineus* is illustrated in Fig. 9.21.

Distribution

The brown dog tick is probably the most geographically widely spread tick in the world. In Europe, it is especially abundant in Mediterranean countries. Thanks to its original environment, it is well adjusted to hot and dry conditions. This has enabled the brown dog tick to migrate to cooler climates, where it thrives in dwellings. Today it is endemic also in temperate zones, where it may become a nuisance and difficult to get rid of. The tick can be active the year around thanks to the stable environment in households, even during very cold weather. While *I. ricinus* needs 3–4 years to complete its life cycle due to winter-related constraints, the brown dog tick enjoys life indoors safe from climatic alterations and completes up to four generations per year in ideal conditions.

Importance to Canine Health

Interdigital skin, the insides of the ear pinnae (Fig. 9.22), and the outer ear are skin areas that the brown dog tick especially favors. Early developmental stages are found particularly at the neck. Several attached ticks are usually found on one inspection. Some dogs appear to be more attractive for brown dog ticks than others, and it is common to find dogs with many ticks, while others in the same household play host to hardly any. Generally tick infestations are more abundant in young dogs than in adults. Some breeds are known to be more susceptible to severe infestations; for instance, the cocker spaniel is more favored than the beagle as a blood source for brown dog ticks.

A severe tick infestation may cause anemia for the dog. Swelling, itching, and other inflammatory signs may manifest in the suction site. In the same manner as with other ticks, the clinical importance of the brown dog tick is primarily based on its ability to act as a vector for many infectious diseases. The bacterium *Ehrlichia canis* causes a disease called canine monocytic ehrlichiosis. Other *Ehrlichia* species spread by the brown dog tick are *E. ewingii*

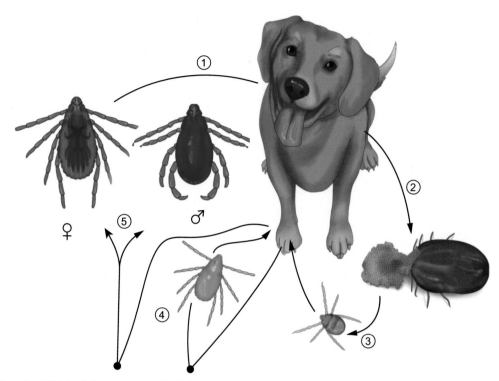

FIG. 9.21 Life cycle of *Rhipicephalus sanguineus*: (1) adult brown dog ticks feed and copulate on the dog's skin; (2) the engorged female tick disengages, moves into a sheltered place and lays thousands of eggs; (3) in a few weeks, the eggs hatch to produce hexapod larvae. The larva sucks blood from a thin-skinned host or from a thin spot on canine skin. After the blood meal, the larva moves into a sheltered site to molt; (4) the nymph, uncovered from the molting, must have a blood meal in order to complete the life cycle and reach adulthood; and (5) brown dog ticks spend most of their life separate from a host animal, moving actively and searching for a blood source. They withstand drought well and are suited for surviving and reproducing in human dwellings.

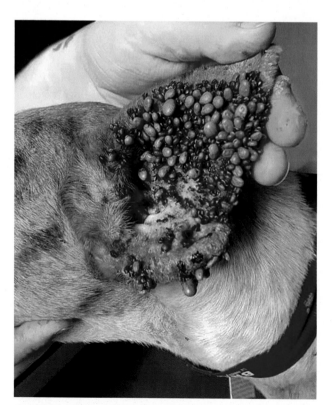

FIG. 9.22 A dog ear-flap with a heavy tick infestation. (*Photo by Jennifer Gerner/CLAW/South Africa, reproduced with permission.*)

and *E. chaffeensis*. The brown dog tick also acts as a vector for Rickettsia ricksettsii that causes Rocky Mountain spotted fever, and for Rickettsia conorii, which is the causative organism of Mediterranean spotted fever in humans. Of parasitic diseases, the brown dog tick spreads *Hepatozoon canis* protozoa and allegedly certain strains of *Babesia canis* and *B. gibsoni*.

Diagnosis

The diagnosis is based on identifying morphologically characteristic ticks in dogs. It is important to identify the species, because a population of brown dog ticks that has settled indoors is very difficult to eradicate. Eradication should be started immediately.

Treatment and Prevention

Ticks attached to a dog are immediately removed and the dog is given a long-term tick control treatment, lasting up to 6 months. The treatment should not be interrupted before the *Rhipicephalus* life cycle has been broken and ticks have been destroyed from the dog's environment. Commercial pest control is often needed indoors.

AMBLYOMMA AMERICANUM, Lone Star Tick

- *Amblyomma* has long hypostome, festoons are present in the rear, anal groove is posterior to anus.
- Dorsal scutum of the female has a light-colored spot (lone star).
- Endemic in North America.
- Vector for diseases, causes local skin lesions.
- Preventive treatment is recommended in areas with high prevalence.

Identification

Amblyomma ticks have long hypostome and palps (Fig. 9.23). The basis capituli is almost rectangular. Festoons and eyes are present. The dorsal scutum of the female A. americanum has a single light-colored spot-like mark, from which the tick has got its common name: lone star tick. The males have two pale spots close to the hind margin and other pale marks at the lateral margins. The anal groove is located posterior to the anus. The engorged female is about 1 cm long and bean-shaped, while the male is smaller. Nymphs are less than 2 mm and larvae less than 1 mm in size.

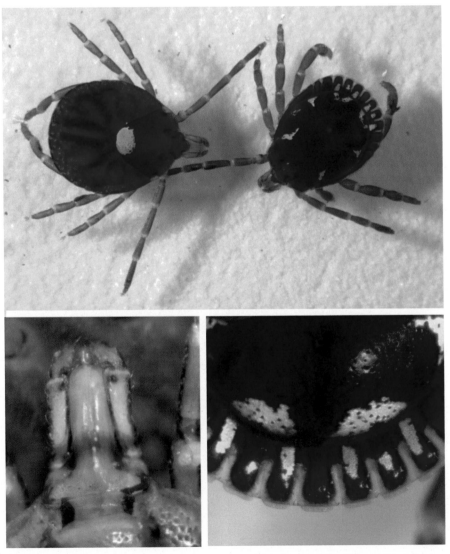

FIG. 9.23 *Amblyomma americanum* ticks, upper picture female (left) and male (right). Characteristics of the species are long mouthparts, the legs with pale rings, distinct festoons and a white spot with red and green tinge on the back of the female, the inspiration for the name "lone star tick." The figure at the lower left shows the long mouthparts with palpal segment II about twice as long as segment III. The figure at the lower right depicts the festoons.

Life Cycle

Amblyomma is a three-host tick, three blood meals and 3 years are needed for the full life cycle. Female lays eggs to the ground and the next year the larvae are hatched. After the blood meal, they drop to the ground, over-winter, and molt to nymphs, before adulthood in the following year.

Distribution

There are about 140 *Amblyomma* species mainly in tropical and subtropical regions, but not in Europe. The best-known *Amblyomma* species in canine parasitology, *Amblyomma americanum*, lone star tick, is found in North America. It is found in woodlands with dense underbrush, and the populations especially dense in the transition zones between the forest and meadow.

Importance to Canine Health

The bite site of the tick might be inflamed and painful; bite site necrosis might even be seen. *Amblyomma* is a vector for many vector-borne diseases such as ehrlichiosis and rickettsiosis.

Diagnosis

Diagnosis can be made after finding ticks with typical morphology attached to the dog's skin. Vector-borne diseases are diagnosed with the clinical appearance and the specific antibody results from serological tests.

Treatment and Prevention

Tick attachment should be prevented medically in the areas with high prevalence. All ticks found on the dog should be removed without delay (Fig. 9.24).

ORNITHODORUS MOUBATA

- Soft tick endemic in Africa, but spread with humans elsewhere too.
- Vector for diseases, may cause skin reaction in the bite site.
- Many acarisidic substances may be used for control.

Identification

Ornithodorus (synonym *Ornithodoros*) *moubata*, the African hut tampan or the Eyeless tampan, belongs to the family Argasidae or soft ticks. The significant morphological features of the nymph or adult stage, distinguishing Argasidae ticks from the Ixodicae, are the ventrally located head, invisible from the dorsal side, and the lack of chitin dorsal shield (scutum). Unlike hard ticks, pulvilli are not present at the tip of tarsi in adult and nymphal stages. The surface of *Ornithodorus* is leather-like, wrinkled, and covered by small nodules. Unlike many ticks of the same family, *O. moubata* has no eyes. Other morphological features that distinguish Ornithodoros from other soft ticks include the lack of a "suture line" at the border of dorsal and ventral surfaces, typical to the soft ticks of Argas genus,

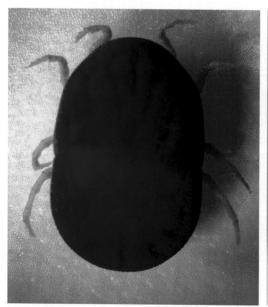 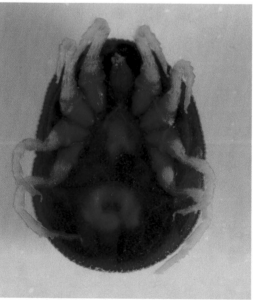

FIG. 9.24 *Ornithodorus moubata.* The significant morphological features of the nymph or adult stage, distinguishing Argasidae ticks from the Ixodicae, are the ventrally located head, invisible from the dorsal side, and the lack of chitin dorsal shield.

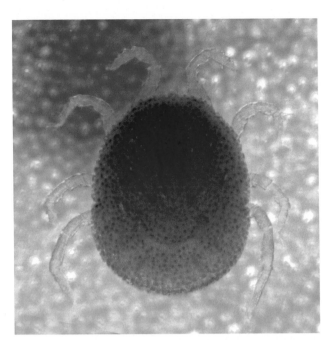

FIG. 9.25 The surface of *Ornithodorus* is leathery, wrinkled, and covered with small nodules. The photo depicts a nymph.

and long mouthparts (hypostomum), equipped with long and backward-pointing chitin barbs, which *Ornithodorus* uses to pierce the skin of the host animal. The female is about 10 mm and the male 8 mm long (Fig. 9.25).

Life Cycle

A hexapod larval state hatches from the egg of *O. moubata* after about 1 week. It molts a few days later and develops into a nymph stage without a blood meal. Nymphs are blood suckers, and the blood meal takes less than half an hour. There are several nymph stages. Those ticks developing to be males go through four nymph stages, and the females go through five. Copulation takes place when the female has received a blood meal. Copulation stimulates ovarian development, and the female typically lays eggs about 2 weeks after copulation. The female can copulate and lay eggs several times during its lifetime, producing a total of about 500 eggs.

Ornithodorus is a nocturnal tick that hides during days in the cracks and crevices of human and animal habitation, and hunts for blood at night.

Distribution

O. moubata is endemic especially in East and South Africa. It often leads an evasive life in mud huts and other primitive human dwellings. It is able to parasitize many vertebrate species, including dogs and humans. The preferred host species of many *Ornithodorus* are artiodactyls. The species has spread along with humans outside Africa.

Importance to Canine Health

O. moubata is an important infestation vector for humans and many domestic animals. A severe *Ornithodorus* infection may cause anemia, bite-site swelling, itching, and inflammation in dogs.

Diagnosis

Diagnosis is based on identifying morphologically characteristic ticks found in dogs.

Treatment and Prevention

Many products intended for tick control, including novel isoxazoline compounds, are effective against *Ornithodorus*.

OTOBIUS MEGNINI, Spinose Ear Mite

- Soft tick endemic in North America, Africa, and southern Asia.
- Adults are nonparasitic and they do not feed; larvae and nymphal stages are parasites.
- Low host-specificity, infests dogs too.
- Causes irritation, damage, and inflammation in the ear canal.

Identification

Otobius megnini (Fig. 9.26) is also known as the spinose ear mite. The unfed larva is 0.6 mm and the capitulum is visible in both dorsal and ventral views and over one-third of the length of larva consists of mouthparts. As a result of feeding on blood, the larval stage grows to be about 4 mm long and molts, developing into a nymph. There are two nymphal stages. The nymph has a general morphology typical to soft ticks. Their body has a constriction in the middle giving them a shape of a violin and they are four-legged. The second nymphal stage is the stage that is usually found in the ear of the host. The nymphs are widest at the middle. Their skin is covered with nodular lumps and has numerous spine-like processes. The body is bluish gray, while the legs, mouthparts, and spines are yellowish. There are four pair of legs. Adults are nonparasitic.

Life Cycle

Eggs of *O. megnini* are laid on the ground. After hatching, the larvae crawl up vegetation or rocks, waiting for a suitable host to come along. Finding one is easier in animal shelters.

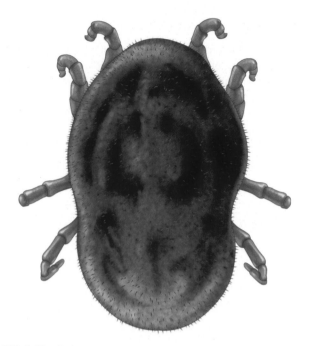

FIG. 9.26 *Otobius megnini*, the spinose ear mite.

When on the host, the larva moves to the outer ear canal. Feeding on blood enables the larval stage to engorge and to molt into a nymph. There are two nymphal stages. The immature stages of Otobius can spend long times parasitizing the ear canal. At its shortest, this period may last 5 weeks, but some mites spend months in the ear. When it leaves the host, the Otobius is 8 mm long. It moves into a sheltered place to molt and mature to adult stage.

Distribution

The spinose ear mite is a soft argasiid tick endemic especially in arid areas of American mainland, but it is endemic in Africa and southern Asia as well. It favors horses, cattle, and llamas as host animals, but can suck blood from dogs as well. It is only parasitic in the larval and nymphal stages.

Importance to Canine Health

The spinose ear mite can cause severe irritation in the dog's external ear canal and the infestation may be complicated by tympanic damage or a secondary bacterial infection.

Diagnosis

O. megnini is rather large tick and hence, readily visualized, e.g., with the aid of an otoscope. A cotton swab may be used to sample the exudate from the ear canal.

Treatment and Prevention

Tick control products can be used in the treatment and prevention of *O. megnini* infestation.

PNEUMONYSSOIDES CANINUM, Nasal Mite

- Endemic especially in Scandinavia, elsewhere constant long-acting ectoparasite treatments probably limit the survival.
- Transmits through direct contact, but may survive in the environment for days.
- Causes loss of scent, reverse sneezing, irritation of nose and sinuses and nasal discharge.
- Rarely seen; diagnosis is usually based on treatment trial and vanishing of the clinical signs.
- Macrocyclic lactones can be used for treatment.

Identification

Pneumonyssoides (synonym *Pneumonyssus*) *caninum* belongs to order Mesosigmata and has an oval shape and yellowish white color (Figs. 9.27 and 9.28). The length of the mite varies between 1.0 and 1.5 mm, while the width is about 0.5–0.9 mm. The adult stage has four distinct pairs of legs, of which the anterior one is more developed than

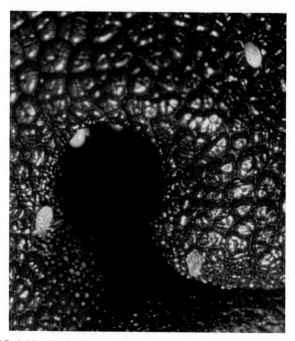

FIG. 9.27 Nasal mites on a dog's nose. *(Photo by Bengt Ekberg/SVA, reproduced with permission.)*

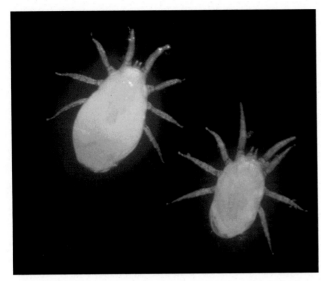

FIG. 9.28 Female nasal mite (left) and male (right). *(Photo by Bengt Ekberg/SVA, reproduced with permission.)*

the rest. The tips of front legs have paired, strong, and curved claw-like structures (Fig. 9.29). The tips of the second, third, and fourth pair of legs have a long-stemmed pad-like pulvillus, to which two claw structures are attached. They are much weaker than those in the first pair of legs (Fig. 9.29). The larval stage is somewhat smaller (length usually about 0.7 mm and width 0.5 mm) than the adult and has three leg pairs, with the morphological features described before.

Life Cycle

The nasal mite lives in the nasal cavity and nasal sinuses of the dog, especially in the area of sinus frontalis. Developmental stages of nasal mite this far discovered are the adult—especially females, as males are very rare—and larval stage. Several investigators have found highly advanced larval stages already inside the eggs that are inside the female. The eggs are large and fill a major part of the female's abdominal cavity. The larva hatches already in the female. The nymphal stage, common for most arachnids, has not been described. It is possible that either the stage does not exist at all, or the nymphal stage lasts only a very short time. Since the larvae move actively and the mites seen on the dog's nose or environment are usually larvae, infestation is assumed to take place via direct contact, as larval stages move from one dog to another. In laboratory conditions, nasal mite has been observed to be attracted by expired air rather than move away from light, for instance. The nasal mites survive for almost 3 weeks separated from the host animal in cool and moist conditions. The life cycle of *P. caninum* is illustrated in Fig. 9.30.

Distribution

Nasal mites are endemic in the Nordic countries in particular. Several prevalence studies have been conducted in Sweden, using autopsy findings. Nasal mites have been found in 20%–23% of the autopsied dogs. The parasite is

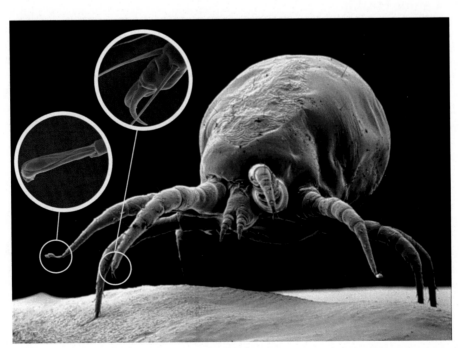

FIG. 9.29 Female nasal mite in scanning electron microscopy. The tip of the anterior pair of legs has hook-shaped structures (upper close-up). Other pairs of legs have small hooks as well (lower close-up). *(Photo of a nasal mite in the background by Tapio Nikkilä SVA/SLU, reproduced with permission.)*

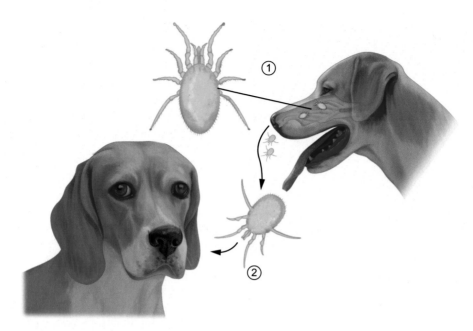

FIG. 9.30 Life cycle of *Pneumonyssoides caninum*. (1) *P. caninum* mites live in the nasal cavity and sinuses. Developmental stages discovered this far are only the adult and the larval stage. (2) Larvae are actively mobile. Infestation is assumed to take place via direct contact, as larval stages move from one dog to another, or indirectly by larvae that have strayed to the environment.

found also in Norway (reported prevalence 7%) and in Finland. In the rest of the world, the nasal mite is either rare or underdiagnosed. Apart from dogs, the mite parasitizes foxes. It seems to prefer large dog breeds.

Importance to Canine Health

The nasal mite is generally considered be a relatively harmless canine parasite. The infestation is subclinical in many dogs. The most common signs are a sniffle and reverse sneezing, a cramp-like condition of the upper airways. The symptoms may be due to the hypersensitivity reaction associated with the infestation. Pruritus of the muzzle is common and the dog shows this by scratching the rostrum with its paws or against, for instance, a rug. The nasal discharge associated with the invasion is usually clear, but epistaxis can also be seen. Many dog owners and practitioners have claimed that the clinical signs are quite often getting worse a couple of days after effective treatment followed by rapid clinical cure. The infestation may weaken the dog's sense of smell. Many working dogs whose skills are dependent on smelling are known to lose their ability to work almost completely. Submandibular lymph nodes and tonsils may react as a result of nasal mite infestation.

Diagnosis

It is rare to be able to confirm the diagnosis of nasal mite infestation. Mites that hide in the sinuses can seldom be seen, and to date there is no confirmatory laboratory test. The infestation is associated with antibody response, but even though there are some promising study results, no commercial diagnostic test has emerged. With some luck, nasal mites can be found in endoscopy of upper airways.

Lavage of the canine nasal cavity with saline has been proposed as a diagnostic method in literature. The lavage solution is harvested and analyzed for the presence of mites. The procedure is tedious and requires sedation. The sensitivity is poor. Because nasal mites seem to avoid inhalation anesthetics, the best chance for most veterinarians to see nasal mites is when the mites exit the dog's nostrils during anesthesia. Nasal mite infestations are occasionally associated with eosinophilia. The eosinophilic reaction on the nasal mucosa, sometimes observed, can be discovered in the cytological analysis of nasal discharge.

Alleviation of signs after antiparasitic treatment suggests a correct diagnosis of nasal mite infestation. Many dog owners and practitioners consider that the transient worsening of signs on the days immediately after treatment indicate a correct diagnosis, because dying mites are believed to release reactive allergenic substances.

Treatment and Prevention

Macrocyclic lactones, such as selamectin, milbemycin oxime, and moxidectin, are commonly used to treat nasal mite infestation. The treatment should last for a long time, preferably weeks. Since the infestation takes place via direct contact, symptomatic dogs should not be in contact with healthy ones. It is difficult to prevent infestation by mites living free in the environment. The efficacy of isoxazolines remains unclear.

DERMANYSSUS and *ORNITHONYSSUS* GENERA, Poultry and Rodent Mites

- Mites of birds and rodents.
- May cause skin problems to dogs and also humans, if prevalent in the environment.
- The clinical signs disappear, when the mites are eradicated from the environment.

Identification

Birds and rodents are parasitized by many species of the Mesostigmata order. Some of them, despite their certain host preference, are weakly host-specific and may bother dogs as well. Identifying the species requires expertise and is difficult, because there are many morphologically similar, harmless mites in the canine environment. Typical examples include numerous storage mites and mites, which use plant extracts or decomposing organic detritus for nutrition. Identification often relies on the structures and dimensions of skin-piercing mouthparts, the size and shape of the chitin plates on the outer surface, and the number and localization of sensory hairs. Mites of this group are about 1 mm long, long-legged, actively moving, and light colored, but after a blood meal the color is tinted red. There is a pulvillus and double claw present at the tip of each leg. Stigmata (spiracles) are located ventrolaterally in the mid-abdomen (hence the order name Mesostigmata). The larval stage has six legs, whereas the nymph and the adult have eight. It should be noted that the canine nasal mite, *P. caninum*, belongs to the same Mesostigmata order and morphologically resembles avian and rodent mites.

Life Cycle

Most of the life cycle takes place in the environment, for instance, in a chicken house or pet rodent cage, but in order to have a blood meal, mites must visit the skin of the host animal. The life cycle is hemi-metabolic, lacking the pupa stage. Eggs hatch to reveal hexapod larvae, which molt twice to become octapod nymphs before reaching adulthood. All stages after the egg stage suck blood. Poultry and rodent mites are nocturnal. Since the complete

life cycle can be completed in 1 week in ideal conditions, the mite population is able to multiply rapidly.

Distribution

Poultry and rodent mites are endemic everywhere in the world. The chicken mite, *Dermanyssus gallinae*, is a significant hindrance to egg production everywhere. It is also well known to use mammals for the source of blood meals. In addition, wild animals' mites, such as the northern fowl mite, *Ornithonyssus sylviarum*, very common among the native birds of Nordic countries, and the tropical rat mite, *Ornithonyssus bacoti*, a parasite of laboratory and pet rodents, can cause skin problems in dogs.

Importance to Canine Health

Poultry and rodent mites are not canine parasites per se, but their visits and blood sucking in dogs can cause annoyingly itchy dermatitis. Very severe infestations have been reported in dogs. The most common sign is pruritus, with associated scratching and, consequently, alopecia, skin damage, and risk of secondary bacterial infection.

Diagnosis

When examining the cause of canine itch, very small red mite bites may be discovered on the skin. Similar pruritic erythematous spots or macules can be seen on the owner as well. If birds or rodents are kept in the dog's vicinity, the search for mites can be concentrated in their dwellings. For instance, corrugated cardboard kept overnight in a rodent or birdcage may act as a mite trap. In the morning, mites hide away from daylight in the crimps of the cardboard, from where they can be shaken off for microscopic analysis. Lactophenol treatment makes the mites transparent and facilitates observation of morphological details (see Chapter 11, Diagnostics).

Treatment and Prevention

The dog's clinical signs disappear when exposure to the parasite ends. Thus, it is important to find out the source. Mite problems are common in henhouses and pet shops. They are difficult to get rid of, since the mites hide in bedding and structures. Many acaricidal treatments are effective against mites, if treatment is needed to support the management of the skin condition, while mites are being eradicated from the surroundings (Fig. 9.31).

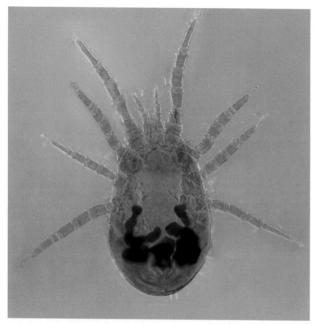

FIG. 9.31 Red chicken mite (*Dermanyssus gallinarum*) is one of the many morphologically similar Mesostigmata mites. They are long-legged and have tarsi with pulvillus and double claw at the tip. The group consists of a large number of avian and rodent parasites. Most species exhibit a host preference but are not very host-specific, and they can be a nuisance for dogs. Distinguishing mites of this group is based on structural differences of the skin-piercing mouthparts (slender chelicerae with scissor-like chelae) and the cuticular plate structures of the thin chitin surface.

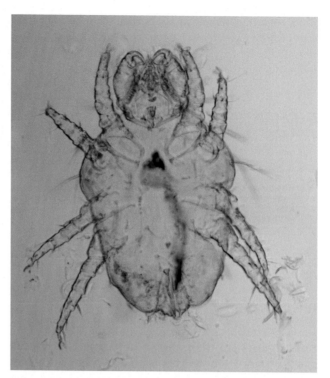

FIG. 9.32 The length of the *Cheyletiella yasguri* female is 0.5mm. The narrow "waist" of the mid-body is characteristic. The well-developed pedipalps, with prominent hooks at the end, are features that distinguish *Cheyletiella* from other mites.

CHEYLETIELLA YASGURI, "Walking Dandruff"

- Mite with prominent clawed pedipalps and comb-like tips of the extremities.
- Clinical signs usually seen in puppies, especially in caudal back.
- "Walking dandruff" (excessive dandruff with mites and their excretions) and pruritus are the most common signs.
- Diagnosis with microscopy, treatment possible with several ectoparasiticides.
- May cause itching spots to humans in contact.

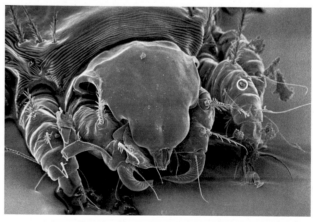

FIG. 9.33 Scanning electron microscopy image of *Cheyletiella*. The photo clearly shows the pedipalps equipped with claw-like hooks. The sensory organ, solendo, in the right front leg is marked with a *white circle*.

Identification

Cheyletiella yasguri is a relatively large, light yellowish, oval, rather angular mite (Figs. 9.32 and 9.33). The female is usually about 0.5mm long and 0.3mm wide. The male is smaller (0.35mm × 0.22mm). When observed the outline of the mite, the waist-like narrowing at the midriff is characteristic (Fig. 9.32). In contrast to other mite species, *Cheyletiella* has very prominent (pedi)palps, which have strong, hook-formed structures in the end (Fig. 9.34).

Another distinguishing feature in contrast to other mites is seen in the tip of the legs: *Cheyletiella* has comb-like structures at their ends. In other parasitic mites, the legs end in a sucker or a claw-like structure.

A good-quality microscope is necessary for a species-specific diagnosis. *C. yasguri* can be distinguished from other members of *Cheyletiella* genus by the Y-shaped sensory organ (solendo), which can be seen at the dorsal

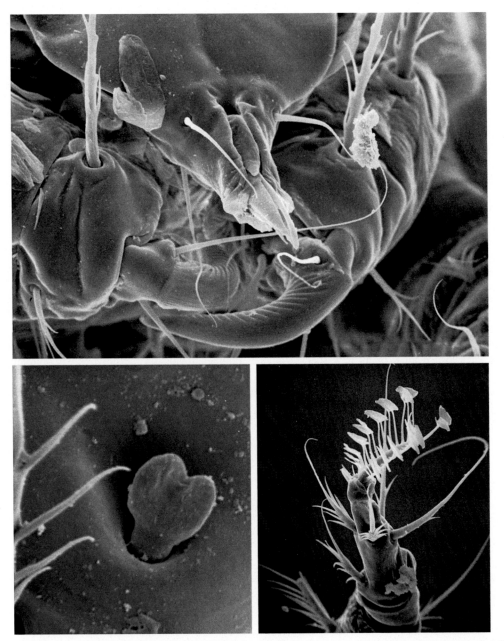

FIG. 9.34 Some morphological details of *Cheyletiella* in scanning electron microscopy. Upper photo shows the mouthparts of *Cheyletiella*. The hooks of the pedipalps are at seen both sides of the piercing mouthparts. The photo at the bottom left shows a close-up of the sensory organ (solendo). The species-level morphological diagnosis of *Cheyletiella* is based on the shape of the solendo located at the level of the first pair of legs. In *Cheyletiella yasguri* it is Y-shaped. The photo at the bottom right depicts branched, comb-like structures in the end of Cheyletiella's tarsi. Other parasitic mites have funnel-shaped or pad-like pulvilli or claw-like structures.

side of the first pair of legs (Fig. 9.34). The sensory organ of the cat's *C. blakei* is shaped like a peg, and that of the rabbit's *Cheyletiella* (*C. parasitovorax*) like a sphere.

Life Cycle

Cheyletiella attaches to the skin with its well-developed jaw extremities. By flexing its muscles it pushes the stylet-like mouthparts into the skin, to the depth of about 10–20 μm.

When pressed together, these stylets form a hollow, needle-like organ, used by the mite to inject salivary secretion into the skin (Fig. 9.34). The mite then sucks the saliva with the digested tissue into its intestine.

The complete life cycle of *Cheyletiella* takes place on the skin of the host. Its larval and nymphal states have been found to die within 2 days when separated from the host species. Females are more robust, and they have been experimentally noted to survive 10 days in refrigeration temperature. Eradication of *Cheyletiella* has been shown to be difficult, especially in kennel conditions. It can be assumed that in conditions favorable for the mite, in a sufficiently humid environment and in the presence of dog hair and dandruff, the mites could survive even longer.

The female fastens the egg to the dog hair one by one. In light microscopy, the *Cheyletiella* egg resembles that of a louse, but it is substantially smaller and attached to the hair loosely with fibrous material at the full length of the egg (Fig. 9.35). In contrast, the louse egg is not only larger but also characteristically fastened only by its posterior tip.

The life cycle of *Cheyletiella* comprises five stages: egg, hexapod larval stage, two nymphal stages, and the adult stage. The cycle from egg to adulthood lasts about 3 weeks.

Distribution

Cheyletiellosis was first described in animals in the late 1800s. Until the 1950s, it was assumed that the *Cheyletiella* genus has only one poorly host-specific species, *C. parasitovorax*, which causes dermatological signs in several mammalian species. Since then, many new species have

been added to the genus, of which *C. yasguri* is adapted to parasitizing dogs. Opinions about the degree of host-specificity still differ: *Cheyletiella* species do transfer easily from one host species to another and cause symptoms in humans as well. The prevalence of *Cheyletiella* is global, and the parasite is especially common in kennels and pet shops. *Cheyletiella* seem to be particularly common in countries, where regular flea control with long-acting antiparasitic products is not routine.

Importance to Canine Health

Cheyletiella is a highly contagious ectoparasite, and it is common that the whole litter and all dogs in a household are infested. Direct contact is the most important route of infestation. The infestation can spread between dogs also via grooming equipment, such as combs and brushes. Since *Cheyletiella* have been observed riding larger parasites, such as lice and fleas, it is assumed that they may help spread cheyletiellosis.

Clinical cheyletiellosis is especially a skin disease of puppies. Typically the diagnosis is done at the veterinary

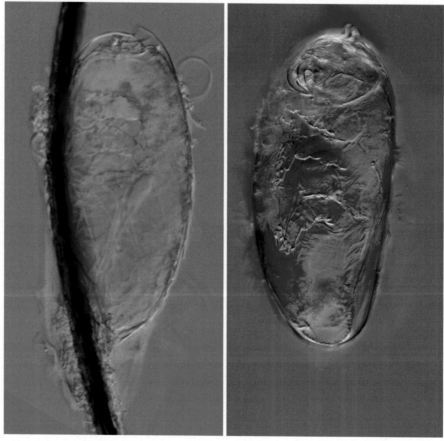

FIG. 9.35 The *Cheyletiella* female attaches its eggs one by one onto the dog's hairs. In light microscopy, the egg resembles a louse egg, but it is much smaller and loosely fastened with delicate fibers along the full length of the egg. The shape of the larva can often be seen inside the egg, and it can be identified as *Cheyletiella*.

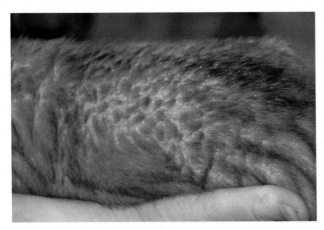

FIG. 9.36 Typical clinical manifestation of *Cheyletiella* infestation in a puppy. Dandruff is plentiful, especially on the back. *(Photo by Erja Juvakka, reproduced with permission.)*

inspection either at the first check-up of puppies or when they are about to be vaccinated. Copious dandruff on the puppy's back is a warning sign for the veterinarian. Dandruff (seborrhea), varying from dry to oily, can be considered the most important manifestation of clinical cheyletiellosis. The changes typically start from the caudal dorsum and advance towards the neck and head (Fig. 9.36). Generalized cheyletiellosis, with lesions all over the body, is rare. In exceptional cases, macules are seen. Pruritus is common. The severity of itch varies and a serious disease without any signs or pruritus is possible. In dogs over 6 months of age, cheyletiellosis is often subclinical or manifested by mild dandruff and pruritus.

Diagnosis

Dandruff and pruritus at the caudal side of a puppy's back is a strong reason to suspect cheyletiellosis. A carefully obtained scrape sample is needed for confirming the diagnosis. A scalpel dipped in mineral oil is first used to scrape the keratin layer of the skin. The yield is analyzed by microscopy for *Cheyletiella* mites and eggs. The alternative technique is to press a transparent tape against the affected skin, thus collecting mites and eggs for microscopy. When the skin and dandruff obtained from an infected dog is placed on paper and observed closer, it is possible to see keratin particles that move while the *Cheyletiella* move under them. This is the origin of the term "walking dandruff."

When there are few mites on the dog, it may be necessary to investigate a greater amount of material from the skin keratin layer, collected with a louse comb, for instance. The obtained mass is put into a centrifuge tube with earlier added 1 mL of 10% potassium or sodium hydroxide solution. The tube is kept in a warm water bath, until the keratin and the hair have broken down (in practice about 30 min). After this, the tube is filled with saturated

sugar solution and centrifuged at $270 \times g$ for 10 min. The sample is carefully taken for microscopy from the surface of the liquid.

Diagnosis can also be reached by collecting mites with negative pressure. A tested method is to use an ordinary vacuum cleaner. Several layers of gauze are placed between the nozzle and the tube. When the dog's fur is vacuumed, the mites get stuck in the gauze and they are easily collected for analysis with a stereomicroscope, for instance.

It should be noted that a very itchy dog with cheyletiellosis will chew its fur and in the process swallow mites and their eggs. Thus, they can be accidentally found in fecal analysis with the flotation methods. However, it is not rare that no mites are found on the skin in cheyletiellosis. In such cases, diagnosis is made by judging the typical clinical signs and the results of a treatment trial.

Treatment and Prevention

Many ectoparasiticides have good effect against *Cheyletiella*, but there are few products registered for the purpose. Macrocyclic lactones, such as selamectin, moxidectin, and milbemycin oxime, are most commonly used. Fipronil and pyrethroids have a reported efficacy as well. Controlling *Cheyletiella* is difficult especially in kennels, where the mites seem to survive for long times when separated from their hosts. It is important to pay attention to the cleaning of the premises and see that all dogs in the kennel are treated with effective ectoparasite treatment for at least 6–8 weeks. Asymptomatic carriers have an important role in maintaining *Cheyletiella* infestations.

Cheyletiellosis Is a Zoonosis

When dealing with cheyletiellosis, the ability of the parasite to cause human infestations and severe dermatitis should always be kept in mind. It has been estimated in literature that the probability of *Cheyletiella* causing dermatitis symptoms in humans who deal with pets' cheyletiellosis is 25%–80%. When the diagnosis of canine cheyletiellosis is made, the dog owner should be informed about the zoonotic character of the parasite. It is often difficult for the dog owner and the human dermatologist to discover the causality between a recently introduced puppy and simultaneously appearing dermatitis of the owner. The symptoms of cheyletiellosis in humans are most often seen on arms, feet, and the abdominal skin. The early stage is manifested by the appearance of macules (reddish spots), which quickly grow into papules (slightly elevated pimples) (Fig. 9.37). Later the lesions may develop into blisters, pustules, or vesicles. Necrosis starting from the middle is typical of an old cheyletiellosis lesion. Regardless of the manifestation, the skin lesions caused by *Cheyletiella* are almost always severely pruritic. Since *Cheyletiella* is unable to complete its life cycle on the human skin,

Continued

Cheyletiellosis Is a Zoonosis—cont'd

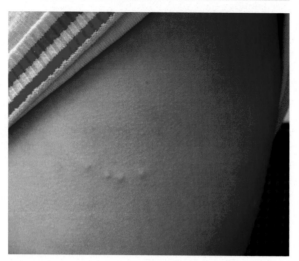

FIG. 9.37 *Cheyletiella* is a zoonotic mite. The symptoms of cheyletiellosis in humans are most often seen on arms, feet and the abdominal skin. The early stage is manifested by the appearance of macules, reddish spots, which quickly grow into papules, slightly elevated pimples. *(Photo by Leena Saijonmaa-Koulumies, reproduced with permission.)*

the infestation is self-limiting. If *Cheyletiella* are successfully eliminated from household dogs, the human skin lesions will disappear within a few weeks.

DEMODEX CANIS, DEMODEX INJAI, and DEMODEX CORNEI

- In most dogs, harmless commensal mite of the skin, clinical disease is dependent on the immunological status of the dog and is seen in young dogs.
- Clinical signs in local demodicosis: a few hairless skin patches—spontaneous recovery without medical intervention.
- Generalized demodicosis: severe and sometimes fatal skin disease with large areas of skin affected—medical treatment is necessary.
- The most practical treatment options nowadays are macrocyclic lactones and products from the isoxazoline group.

Identification

Demodex canis (Fig. 9.38) is the most important and best known of the three canine *Demodex* species. The two others are *D. injai* (Fig. 9.39) and *D. cornei* (Fig. 9.40). The former is much longer than *D. canis* and the latter much shorter. The three mites are easily identified to the genus level thanks to their distinctive morphology.

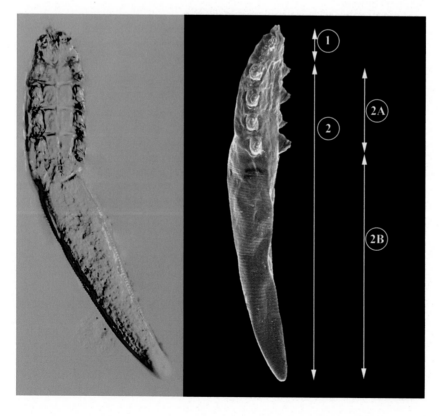

FIG. 9.38 *Demodex canis* in light and scanning electron microscopy. The length of mites varies between 150 and 285 μm. Similarly to other mites, the general structure of *Demodex* consists of the head, or gnathosoma, with its mouthparts (1), the trunk or idiosoma (2), and the extremities. The idiosoma includes the podosoma (2A), into which the legs are attached, and opistosoma (2B), distal to the legs. The elongated, cigar-like idiosoma, ring-like segmentation of opisthosoma, and very short legs are characteristic *Demodex* features.

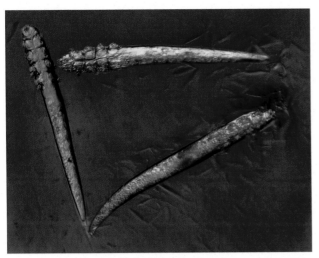

FIG. 9.39 *Demodex injai* is clearly the longest of canine *Demodex* mites (330–370 μm). This species has an exceptionally long opisthosoma.

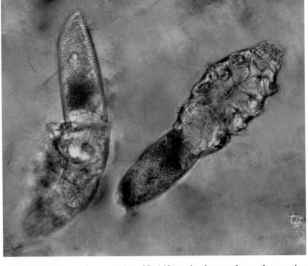

FIG. 9.40 *Demodex cornei* at 90–140 μm is shorter than other canine *Demodex* mites. *D. cornei* is possibly a morphological variation of *D. canis* species. *(Micrograph by Kirsti Schildt, reproduced with permission.)*

Morphology of *Demodex* spp. found in Dogs

Similarly to other mites, the general structure of *Demodex* (Fig. 9.38) consists of the head, or gnathosoma, with its mouthparts, the trunk (idiosoma) and the extremities. The idiosoma includes the podosoma, into which the legs are attached, and opistosoma, distal to the legs. The elongated, cigar-like idiosoma, the ring-like segmentation of opisthosoma and very short legs with claw-like hooks at the tips are characteristic *Demodex* features (Fig. 9.41). The gnathosoma is trapezoid and wider than its length. The slit-like genital pore of the female is located ventrally at the level of the fourth pair of legs, extending slightly caudal past it. The male genital, or aedeagus, is located dorsally in the genital pore that is at the level of the second pair of legs. The width of female *D. canis* is about 40 μm and the length varies between 165 μm and 285 μm. Males are shorter (150–210 μm) with a shorter and sharper opisthosoma that that of females. *D. injai* is longer than *D. canis* (330–370 μm) and *D. cornei* is shorter (90–140 μm). Molecular biological studies have indicated that *D. cornei* may not be an independent species, but rather a morphological variant of *D. canis*. The egg is spindle-shaped and sized 80–105 μm × 32–54 μm (Fig. 9.42)

Life Cycle

The life cycle of *Demodex* includes, apart from the adult mite, egg, larva, protonymph, and tritonymph stages. The most common estimate of the length of life cycle in literature is 3–4 weeks. The puppy is infected by the dam during the first days of life. The infestation is preceded by the multiplication of the mites on the dam's skin (Fig. 9.43). The mechanism, which accelerates the multiplication just before whelping, is not known. It is possible that prepartum hormonal or immunological changes somehow signal the mites about the impending arrival of puppies. *Demodex* have been found from the hair follicles of rostral area of as young as 16-h-old puppies. All life cycle stages of *D. canis* live in the follicles (Fig. 9.41), more rarely in sebaceous glands. In cases of generalized demodicosis, mites can also be detected in lymph nodes and even visceral organs, but they are dead individuals transferred elsewhere in the body by blood or lymph circulation. Unsuccessful attempts have been made over the years to infect dogs via oral, intraperitoneal, and intra-tracheal routes. Keeping dogs with clinical demodicosis signs in contact with healthy dogs

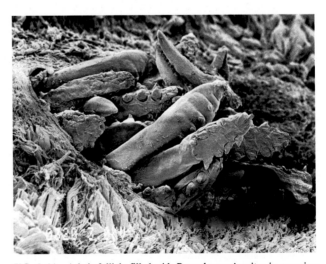

FIG. 9.41 A hair follicle filled with *Demodex canis* mites in scanning electron microscopy. A sample from a young Australian terrier suffering from generalized demodicosis.

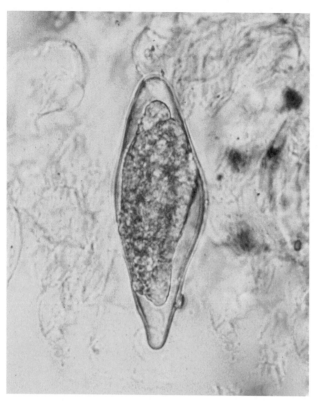

FIG. 9.42 The egg of *Demodex* is spindle-shaped and of size 80–105 × 32–54 μm.

has not led to transmission of the infestation—or at least the disease. The close contact between the dam and the puppy appears essential for *Demodex*. The mites are very common species-specific commensal organisms for mammals, using the follicle contents, such as the host's cells, keratin, and sebum for nutrition. Most dogs harbor single, latent *Demodex* mites in their hair follicles, living in quiet seclusion. In some individuals and in some circumstances the mites can start to multiply uncontrollably, leading into the symptomatic of demodicosis. The life cycle of *D. canis* is illustrated in Fig. 9.44.

Distribution

D. canis mites and the disease they cause are ubiquitous everywhere where dogs are kept. *Demodex* are species specific. Almost all mammals, including marsupials, have their own *Demodex* species. In most animals, *Demodex* mites have managed to develop their relationship with the host to perfect commensalism. The coexistence of *Demodex* mites and host animals has lasted tens of millions of years. Of the canine *Demodex* species, *D. canis* is the most common and most important.

Importance to Canine Health

The dog is one of the few species in which *Demodex* mites can cause clinical demodicosis. The dermatitis can be found in all dog breeds, but some are known to be more susceptible than others. In particular, Shar Pei, several terrier breeds, bulldogs, great Danes, Tibetan mastiffs and Weimaraners are considered sensitive for *Demodex*. It is still poorly known in which situations and through which mechanisms lead to disease. *D. canis*, a normally harmless commensal mite commonly found in healthy dogs, causes hairless skin patches in some dogs (Fig. 9.44) and, to some, a severe (Fig. 9.45) and sometimes fatal skin disease. It is acknowledged that the canine immune defense system is, despite the absence of clinical signs, aware of the presence of *Demodex* mites. Toll-like receptors in dermal cells recognize the mites' chitin, but the subsequent immune reaction is usually that of tolerance. In some circumstances in young dogs, but also in adults with some generalized disease, *Demodex* mites start to multiply uncontrollably. When the number of mites in the hair follicles has grown, hairs detach simultaneously, creating bald skin areas. The immune defense responds, often limiting the multiplication of mites and facilitating new hair growth on the alopecic patches. This is the typical picture of localized demodicosis (Fig. 9.44).

Some dogs, due to the genetic deficiency of immune system, generalized disease, or immunosuppressive medication, fail to respond to the multiplication of mites. The situation leads to the exhaustion of T lymphocytes. As a result, the production of cytokines that maintain immune defense diminishes, while the production of immunosuppressive mediators increases. The host's ability to regulate the mite population is severely limited. In addition, the mites invade new hair follicles and cause epithelial damage. As a result, the contents of the follicle are absorbed into skin. This causes a chronic and purulent foreign body-type reaction with associated secondary bacterial infection. The situation may escalate into a severe dermatitis, generalized demodicosis (Fig. 9.45). Bacteria, usually of the genus Bacillus living in the gut of the *Demodex* mites, may also contribute to the pathology of *Demodex* infestation.

In order to optimize treatment, it is important to be able to distinguish local and generalized demodicosis. According to the most common classification, localized demodicosis manifests as six or fewer alopecic skin patches of smaller than 2.5 cm in diameter. Focal alopecia seldom harms the dog: the lesions are neither itchy nor erythematous. Demodicosis is classified as generalized when the hairless patches number 12 or more, or in cases where the lesions cover a body part, for instance, the dog's muzzle or head. Severe *Demodex* infestation of paws, or podo-demodicosis, is classified as generalized (Fig. 9.46).

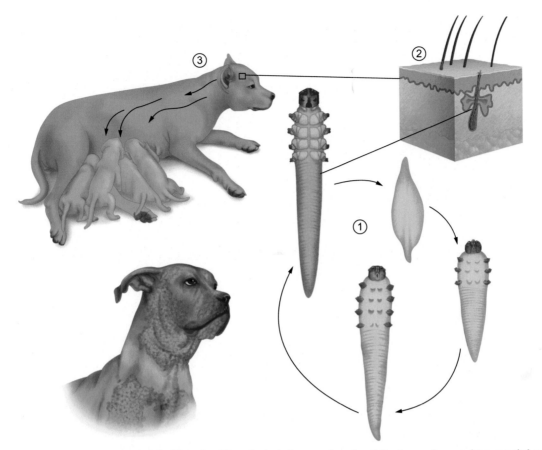

FIG. 9.43 Life cycle of *Demodex canis*: (1) the life cycle of *Demodex* includes, apart from the adult mite, egg, larva, and two nymphal stages; (2) the lifecycle happens in hair follicles. The puppy is infected by the dam during the first days of its life. The infestation is preceded by the multiplication of the mites on the dam's skin (3). The mechanism, which accelerates the multiplication just before whelping, is not known. Most dogs harbor single, latent *Demodex* mites in their hairfollicles, living in quiet seclusion. In some individuals and in some circumstances the mites can start to multiply uncontrollably, leading into the symptomatic demodicosis.

The middle ground between six and twelve skin lesions represents the group of unclassified cases. It is up to the veterinarian to decide in which category they belong. Apart from the character of lesions, the age of the dog at the time of disease onset is another source for classification. The term "juvenile onset demodicosis" describes cases that manifest in small dogs before the age of 12 months, in larger dogs before the age of 18 months, and in giant breeds before the age of 24 months. Dogs that develop signs at the age of 2–4 years have usually had dermatitis problems earlier as well. The term "adult onset demodicosis" is used when the skin signs manifest only when the dog is over 4 years old. The diagnostic emphasis in these cases is to find out what is impairing the dog's immune defense. The reasons include leishmaniosis, hyperadrenocorticism, glucocorticoid therapy, hypothyroidism, and malignant tumors and their treatment. Occasionally demodicosis localizes at the external ear, causing

abnormal cerumen production and possibly signs of otitis externa. This sort of ear infestation often requires treatment.

Skin lesions associated with demodicosis can be very varied. The localized form, especially in short-haired dogs, manifests most often as "moth-eaten" fur. The skin is otherwise unaffected. The lesions are occasionally misdiagnosed as fungal infections. In some dogs the common manifestation is papulo-pustular dermatitis, which can closely resemble bacterial folliculitis. The skin of some dogs flakes out as dandruff or becomes pigmented, and the lesions may include the comedo formation (blackheads). In generalized demodicosis, lesions typical for deep pyoderma are often dominant, such as furunculosis and crust-covered dermal lesions.

Demodex injai usually causes a scaling dermatitis of dorsal skin. Terriers, especially the Scottish and West-Highland terrier, are overrepresented in reports on

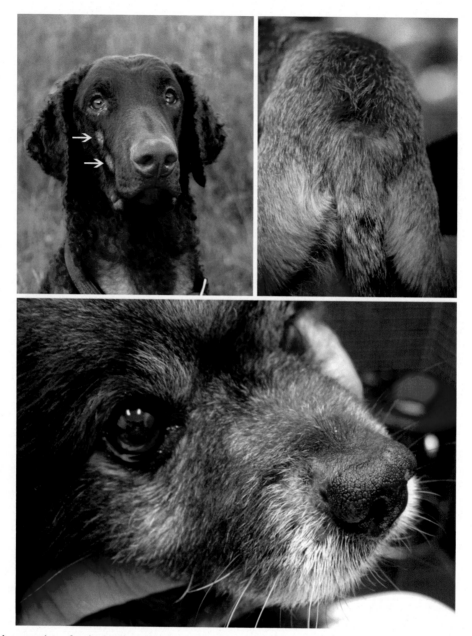

FIG. 9.44 Typical presentations of canine localized demodicosis. The photo at the upper left shows local demodicosis (*arrows* point at skin lesions) of a curly-coated Retriever. The photo at the upper right depicts local demodicosis dorsally at the base of the tail in a Border terrier. The photo at the bottom shows a mild case presented with nonpruritic skin lesion with partial hair loss adjacent to the nose. *(Upper left: photo by Marja Lehtiö. Bottom: photo by Leena Saijonmaa-Koulumies, reproduced with permission.)*

D. injai, but this mite is also found in other breeds. The dog often has a history of thyroid insufficiency or long-term treatment of atopy or other allergic dermatitis, preceding a sudden aggravation of clinical signs.

Diagnosis

Diagnosis of demodicosis is usually based on finding mites in skin scrapings of the affected skin area. When taking a sample, the skin is squeezed between the thumb and the index finger and the contents of the follicles milked towards the surface. Material is scraped from the surface with a scalpel, until the skin capillaries start to bleed. Care is taken not to slash the skin. The yield is spread on a slide and viewed with microscope for mites and parasite eggs. If the yield is small or it is dry, it can be mixed with paraffin oil. An alternative to the scrape sample is using sticky transparent tape. After squeezing the skin to bring forth the mites, the tape is pressed on the site and then placed on a slide for microscopy. The third option is a hair plucking

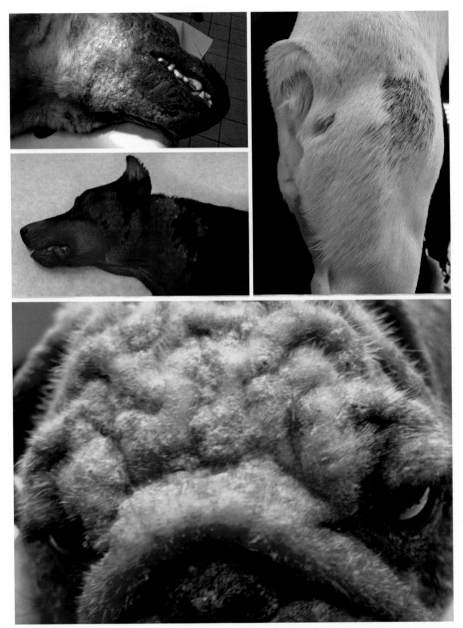

FIG. 9.45 Five dogs presented with canine generalized demodicosis and associated secondary pyoderma. *(Upper left: photo by Sofie Alakoski. Middle on the left: photo by Marika Tenhunen. Right: photo by Kirsti Schildt. Bottom: photo by Leena Saijonmaa-Koulumies, reproduced with permission.)*

technique: trichography (Fig. 9.47). Whatever hairs remain at the lesion site are plucked and viewed along with their roots and examined with microscope. Again, mites and their eggs are searched for. Isolated *Demodex* mites are considered to belong to normal skin fauna, since demodicosis diagnosis required finding several mites. Diagnosis is usually obtained without a skin biopsy (Fig. 9.48). On the other hand, finding *Demodex* mites in biopsies seldom poses problems. Especially in cases of pododemodicosis, in which taking scrape, sticky tape, or trichography samples is often difficult or futile, analyzing a skin biopsy may be

indicated. Molecular biological methods have also been developed recently for *Demodex* diagnostics. They are specifically used to study the relationships between *Demodex* species of different mammal species.

Treatment and Prevention

How demodicosis is treated depends on whether the disease is localized or generalized, and whether it is of the juvenile or adult onset type. About 90% of dogs are cured without treatment thanks to their own immune defense. Localized

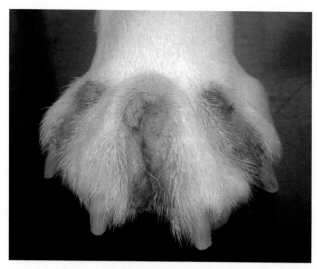

FIG. 9.46 Severe *Demodex* infestation of paws is classified as generalized and is often referred as pododemodicosis. *(Photo by Kirsti Schildt, reproduced with permission.)*

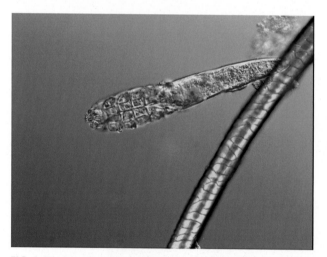

FIG. 9.47 *Demodex canis* seen in a trichography sample.

demodicosis should not be treated, but the dog should be monitored for flare ups, for instance with veterinary visits taking place at 4-week intervals. It should be noted that a dog that has visited the veterinarian for single hairless patch and has not been treated may later develop more alopecic skin patches. The regeneration of fur on bald skin sites may take up to several months. Therapy is only initiated if the diagnosed skin condition emerges to generalized demodicosis.

Only a few years ago, it was very difficult to treat generalized demodicosis. Many cases eventually led to euthanasia. With modern medication, generalized demodicosis can almost certainly be cured. Although some type of genetic deficiency or immune defense problem probably contributes to the pathogenesis, the disease rarely recurs in dogs that have been appropriately treated. Nor are dogs that have undergone demodicosis more susceptible to other contagious diseases than the rest. Treatment aims to eradicate the mites, giving the tired T cells an opportunity to recover and reassume their immune defense duties. Antimicrobial therapy must often be given for the secondary purulent skin infection.

A long-term treatment, often lasting for months, is always required for generalized demodicosis. In the past, amitraz was the most frequently used drug. Amitraz bathing is, however, very tedious, and the treatment has been mostly replaced with systemically acting substances. Most treatment regimens are based on the use of macrocyclic lactones, for example, milbemycin oxime, ivermectin, moxidectin, or doramectin. Drugs of isoxazoline group have also shown themselves to be very effective against demodicosis. The duration of treatment depends on the case. Scrape samples are taken in about 4-week intervals during treatment and the follow-up. Treatment can be terminated when the skin is clearly recovered and the samples are free of *Demodex* mites in two successive

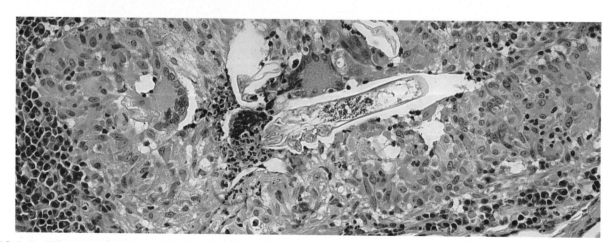

FIG. 9.48 Histopathological tissue section of the skin of a dog suffering from demodicosis. The hair follicle has been torn releasing the mite and keratin from the follicle to the surrounding skin. This has resulted in foreign body granulomatous reaction with multinucleated giant cells, with haphazardly arranged nuclei. These giant cells are fused macrophages. The smaller cells in the periphery are plasma cells.

monthly analyses. A bitch with demodicosis should be neutered as part of the treatment, because cycling is apparently associated with relapse risk, especially in association of pseudopregnancy. A case of adult-onset demodicosis is treated in the same manner as a juvenile disease, but it is important to find the factors making the dog susceptible to demodicosis and control them as well as possible.

TROMBICULIDAE and LEEUWENHOEKIIDAE MITES (Chigger Mites, Harvest Mites)

- Only the hexapod larvae are parasites.
- Prevalent all over the world, clinical signs typically during late summer or autumn.
- Mites cause erythematous and pruritic spots in the skin areas that are in contact with the ground and vegetation; orange mites may be seen with the naked eye.
- Treatment: many antiparasitic agents are effective.

Identification

Trombiculidae and *Leeuwenhoekiidae* mite families are parasitological curiosities in the sense that only their hexapod larval stages are parasites. Octapod nymphs and adults live in the environment and are not parasitic. *Trombiculidae* larvae are reddish in color and 150–300 μm in size. The size of *Straelensia* larvae, which parasitize dogs and belong to the family *Leeuwenhoekiidae*, is 700 × 425 μm.

Life Cycle

Adults and nymphs of *Trombiculidae* and *Leeuwenhoekiidae* genera are predatory living free in the environment (Fig. 9.49). Only the larvae are parasitic. Adult mites typically lay eggs in spring or early summer. The larvae (Fig. 9.50) hatch about 10 days later, but as parasites they are at their most active later, in summer and autumn. Despite being small, they move quickly as they seek a suitable host animal. The activity of the species living in Mediterranean countries depends on the temperature. They are most lively during the afternoon hours, when the temperature of the ground is 25–30°C. The larvae search for a skin area, which is sheltered and thin, and, having pierced the skin with their mouthparts, they attach. The larvae secrete salivary proteolytic enzymes that digest host tissue for nutrition. Meanwhile, the skin hardens around the mouthparts. The mite sucks the tissue fluid for feed and leaves the host 3–4 days later.

The larvae of *Straelensia* mites live within the skin, attached to the inner surface of hair follicles, and form solid

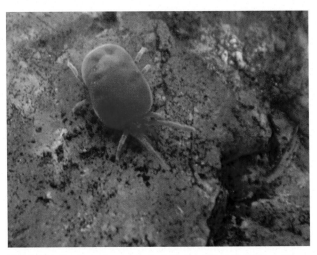

FIG. 9.49   A velvet mite, a typical adult mite of *Trombiculidae* and *Leeuwenhoekiidae*-type. The adult mite is predatory, but the larval stages are parasites.

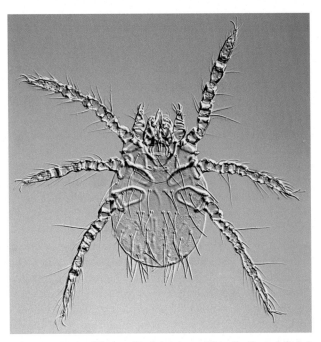

FIG. 9.50   Larva of *Neotrombicula inopinata. (Photo by Alexandr Stekolnikov. Stekolnikov A, Santibáñez P, Palomar AM, Oteo JA: Neotrombicula inopinata (Acari: Trombiculidae)—a possible causative agent of trombiculiasis in Europe, Parasit Vectors 7:90, 2014, http://www.parasitesandvectors.com/content/7/1/90, reproduced with permission.)*

nodules in the host skin. Larvae molt in the environment via the nymphal stages (protonymph, deutonymph, and tritonymph). The tritonymph finally develops into an adult chigger mite. The adults copulate and the female lays eggs to the environment. The hatched larvae need a meal from a host animal, which can be, for many chigger mite species, apart from vertebrates, one of the many arthropods.

Distribution

Dozens of *Trombiculidae* and *Leeuwenhoekiidae* species have been identified, and many probably still await identification. These mites are ubiquitous in all parts of the world. Species found in dogs include *Eutrombicula alfreddugesi*, *Neotrombicula autumnalis*, and *Straelensia cynotis*. *Straelensia* invasions have been reported especially in Spain, Portugal, and France. In practice, a species-specific identification is seldom attempted. Larval stages (Fig. 9.50) found on the skin are often grouped as belonging to chigger mites or roughly into the *Neotrombicula* subgenus. *Straelensia* mites, living in the hair follicles, form another group. Larvae are not especially host-specific, but certain mites are often found in some preferred hosts. This is probably more a result of shared environments of mites and the hosts than choice. The larvae usually acquire the meal from wild animals. However, domestic animals or humans are not safe from them, although invasions are infrequent.

Importance to Canine Health

Clinical signs usually appear during the late summer or in the autumn. The chigger mite and harvest mite are synonymic. *Trombiculidae* and *Leeuwenhoekiidae* mites typically affect those skin areas that are in contact with the earth and vegetation. Macules appear in the skin likely as a result of trauma caused by mouthparts and the reaction against the salivary substances of the mite. The spots are red and itch severely. Scratching the skin breaks the surface and exposes it to secondary bacterial infection. *Neotrombicula* can often been seen with the naked eye in clusters that resemble tiny orange grits. In prolonged and repeated exposure, the animal may be sensitized to mite saliva and develop an allergic reaction even to a small number of mites. Pruritic signs often continue when the mites have left the host. *Straelensia* infestations are known to be less pruritic than those caused by *Trombiculidae*, but the macules can be sensitive to touch. In a skin biopsy, the follicular epithelium is thickened often associated with perifollicular edema and mucinosis. A chronic perifolliculitis and perivasculitis are additional nonspecific findings.

Chigger mites have no role as pathogen vectors, because their life cycle includes only one parasitic meal. As a result, any pathogens that the mite potentially ingests never get a chance to be transmitted to other dogs.

Diagnosis

The timing of skin signs in late summer and autumn, and staying in a chigger-infested environment, are suggestive of mite invasion. The dog may easily scratch the mites off its skin, and they stay with the dog briefly anyway, up to a few days. That is why the mites are rarely found in skin scrapings. *Straelensia* mites are especially difficult to find, thanks to their location inside the hair follicle. The preferred way to diagnose *Straelensia* is by analyzing a skin biopsy.

Treatment and Prevention

When a diagnosis has been made, it is important to ensure that the environment and the sleeping place of the dog are not a source of mite invasion. Several parasiticides and antimicrobials have been used treat mite dermatitis with variable results. It has been reported that a systemic treatment of avermectins has reduced the number of nodules in many dogs. Despite repeated exposure, the dog recovers spontaneously within 2–12 months (median 3 months), when the activity of host-seeking and blood-sucking larvae ends, but there have been severe cases that have had poor response to treatment and have led to the death of the dog. The infestation is not passed between dogs, because the larvae feed only once during their lifetime and the rest of the life cycle takes place in the environment.

OTODECTES CYNOTIS, Ear Mite

- Infests dogs but is more common in cats.
- Clinically seen plenty of dark brown cerumen and pruritus in the ear canal.
- Diagnosis is easy with the microcopy of the cerumen and identifying the mites.
- Treatment with macrocyclic lactones or isoxazolines and cleansing the ear canal.

Identification

Ear mites (Figs. 9.51–9.54) are relatively large, white mites, which move freely along the ear canal. They have four leg pairs, which extend beyond the profile of the abdomen, except the atrophied fourth leg pair of the female (Fig. 9.54). The anus is located at the rear. The male mite has suction cup type structures (pulvillae), shaped like a wine glass, at the tip of all legs, on the end of short and unsegmented stalks (Fig. 9.55). The female has corresponding structures on the two most anterior leg pairs (Figs. 9.53 and 9.54). The third pair of the legs ends in two very long hair-like setae (Figs. 9.52–9.55). In addition, the male's and tritonymph's posterior body part has peg-shaped protrusions that enable copulation (Fig. 9.55). The size of adult females is 350–450 μm and that of males is 275–360 μm. The eggs are large in relation to the body: about 200 μm long.

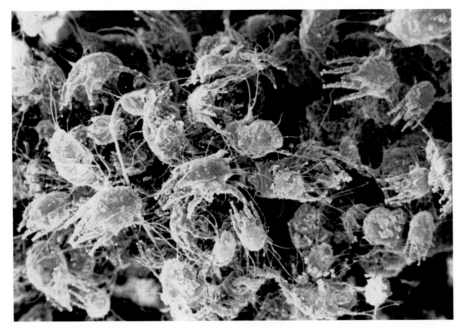

FIG. 9.51 A sample from the ear canal exudate from an ear with a severe mite infestation, via scanning electron microscopy. The secretion consists almost entirely of ear mites of different developmental stages.

Life Cycle

Ear mites live their entire life in the ear canal of the host, but do occasionally wander out to the dog's skin. Apart from the adult mite, the life cycle includes the egg, larva, and protonymph as well as the tritonymph (a.k.a. deutonymph) stages.

Ear mites use skin secretions, tissue fluids, and flaked dead tissue for nutrition. The male mites grasp onto the tritonymph-stage mites (Fig. 9.55). It is not possible to distinguish male and female tritonymphs morphologically from each other. It appears that the male ear mite cannot tell the

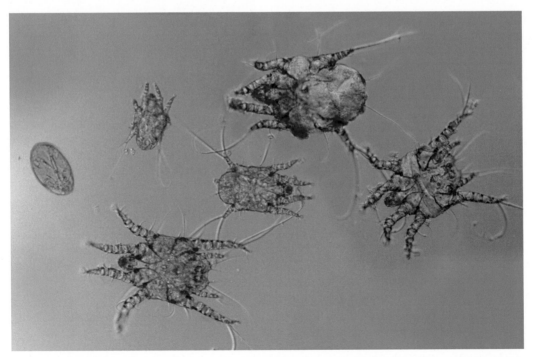

FIG. 9.52 Developmental stages of an ear mite (*Otodectes cynotis*): an egg, a larva (the smallest mite), a nymph (protonymphal stage, in the middle), and two males and a female (on the top).

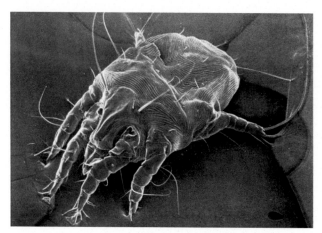

FIG. 9.53 A female ear mite in scanning electron microscopy.

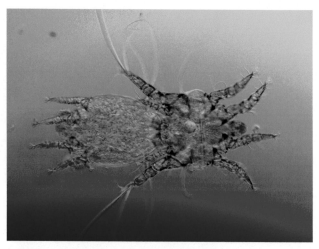

FIG. 9.55 A male (on the right) grasped onto the tritonymph-stage mite (on the left). Copulation takes place, when the tritonymph has developed into an adult female through molting. The attachment has to happen between the adult male and the tritonymph as only the male and the tritonymph possess the copulatory appendages enabling the attachment.

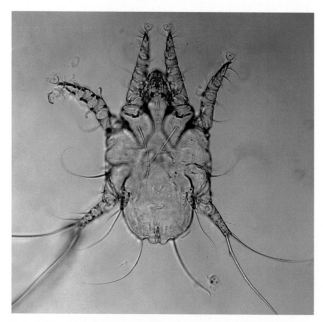

FIG. 9.54 A female ear mite in light microscopy. Female have four leg pairs, which extend beyond the profile of the abdomen, except the atrophied fourth leg pair. The anus is located at the rear. The pulvillae, shaped like a wine glass, can be seen at the tip of all legs, on the end of short, unsegmented stalks, on the two most anterior leg pairs. The third pair of the legs ends in long, paired, hair-like setae. The size of adult females is 350–450 μm.

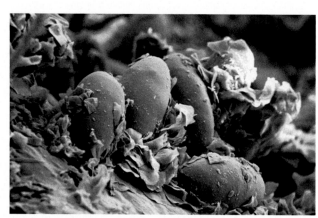

FIG. 9.56 Ear mite eggs in the keratin layer of the external ear canal in scanning electron microscopy.

difference between genders either. Copulation takes place, when the tritonymph has developed into an adult female through molting. If the female reaches this stage before the male has attached to it, the female remains infertile. If, on the other hand, the tritonymph molts to become an adult male, the other male has wasted its time waiting for the molting to happen. The female lays 15–20 eggs during its lifetime of a few weeks. It fastens the eggs to the keratin of the ear canal (Fig. 9.56). Eggs hatch to become hexapod larval stages, which through molting first become eight-legged protonymphs and thentritonymphsand finally adults. The life cycle usually lasts about 3 weeks. The transmission often happens between the dam and puppies or otherwise in direct contact between dogs or other pets.

Distribution

Many carnivore mammals worldwide harbor ear mites. In veterinary practice, the most common animal with ear mite infestation is the cat, but dogs and ferrets are often infected as well.

Importance to Canine Health

Clinical signs may be innocuous or mild in adult dogs. Younger dogs have more severe infestations and manifest clinical signs. The manifestation of ear mite infestation, typical for cats, is a copious coffee-ground-like discharge with large numbers of mites. However, this is rare in dogs. There are usually few mites in a dog's ear, but they do cause irritation and inflammation. Mites moving around in the ear canal, and their secretions, may cause (besides itching) otitis externa, which can be purulent. The dog may damage the skin by scratching, causing a secondary infection. Scratching and head shaking can also lead to an othematoma, an internal bleeding of the pinna. The dog may become hypersensitive to mite secretions and start to react to even small mite numbers. In exceptional cases, ear mites can cause dermatitis elsewhere on the dog's skin. According to some reports, ear mites have infrequently caused skin and ear problems in humans. Considering that ear mites are very common in dogs and cats, human cases are probably highly exceptional.

Diagnosis

When the ear canal is packed with an earthy, dark brown secretion, and a close inspection reveals ear mite movement with the naked eye, the diagnosis is almost certain. The presence of ear mites is confirmed with microscopy. Dogs usually have much fewer mites in their ears than cats, and dogs can show clinical signs of infestation already at the early stage, when the mites are too scarce to be sampled.

Treatment and Prevention

Macrocyclic lactones have a good effect on ear mites, as long as the treatment lasts long enough. They can be given systemically as spot-on treatments and tablets, or locally as ear drops. Isoxazolines have shown to be effective and also fipronil have been used. The other dogs, cats, and ferrets of the household must be treated concomitantly. Cleaning the dog's bed thoroughly of loose ear mites helps prevent reinfestation. The mites can survive for over 2 weeks in cool and moist conditions.

SARCOPTES SCABIEI VAR. *CANIS* and VAR. *VULPIS*, Sarcoptic Mange

- Scabies mites live in the tunnels dug in the epidermis.
- Common infestation in dogs; may be transmitted from wild carnivores in their habitat.
- Clinical manifestation vary from slight itch to severe life-threatening hyperkeratotic skin condition with systemic signs.
- Skin scraping may reveal the mites, but it is not a very sensitive method.
- Treatment (and treatment trial) with macrocyclic lactones for example, but the length of the course must be long enough (several weeks).

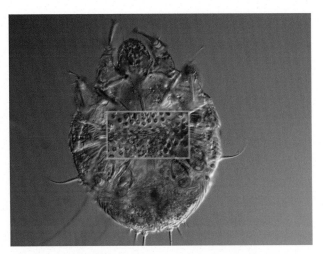

FIG. 9.57 A sarcoptid mite in light microscopy ventral view. The female is 0.3–0.5 mm long. The mite is oval and has four pairs of legs. The third and fourth pairs are located so ventrally that they do not extend beyond the mite's silhouette. The two first pairs have a sucker in the end of a long and straight stalk. The white rectangle borders a photo from the mite's dorsal side, and triangular chitin spikes can be seen with light microscopy. The anus is terminally located.

Identification

The sarcoptid mange mite is a microscopic arachnid belonging to the family Sarcoptidae. Identification of *Sarcoptes* requires light microscopy, where the typical features of the species, such as the size, length of legs, sucker-like pulvillus at the tip of legs, and grooves and the triangular protrusions of the exterior surface can be observed (Figs. 9.57–9.59).

Today parasitologists commonly agree that *Sarcoptes scabiei* is one species, although there is variation in size, host specificity, and even morphological features among the itch mites. Some subspecies exist, adapted for life in

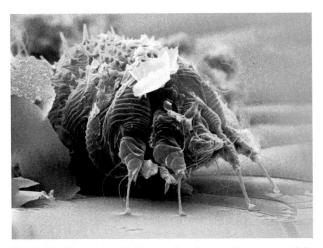

FIG. 9.58 *Sarcoptes scabiei* in scanning electron microscopy partially covered by keratin flakes. The triangular chitin spikes of the dorsal surface and the suckers of the foremost leg pairs are clearly visible.

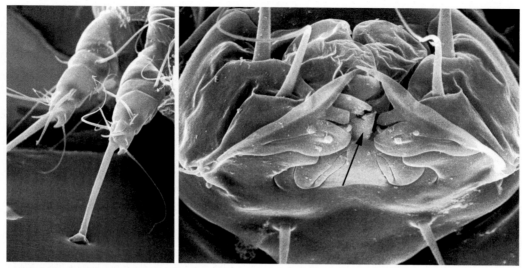

FIG. 9.59   Some morphological details of the sarcoptic mite. On the left: the Sarcoptic mite's two first leg pairs have a pad-like pulvillus in the end of a long and straight stalked empodium. Two spur-like claws are located at the base of the shaft. On the right: the head (gnathosoma) of the Sarcoptic mite is equipped with plier-like mouthparts (*black arrow*).

different host species. The most common subspecies found in dogs are *S. scabiei* var. (varietas) *canis* and the causative organism of fox mange, *S. scabiei* var. *vulpis*.

Life Cycle

The *Sarcoptes* mites live in burrows, which they dig into the keratin layer and the superficial layer of the epidermis. All developmental stages, except the adult females, can also be seen on the skin surface. The mite burrows by secreting saliva dissolving the keratin and by moving its head and mouthparts. It uses the two front leg pairs to expand the tunnel. The mite eats part of the skin material that the digging produces, but a major part is compacted into the tunnel walls. The mite penetrates the stratum granulosum and spinosum of the epidermis and feeds on the tissue fluids seeping into the tunnels. Due to the continuing renewing of epidermis, a major part of the tunnels, eggs, larvae, and mite excrement ends up in the keratin layer. The older parts of the burrows are scaled off from skin surface along with keratin. Male *Sarcoptes* are more mobile than the females, and they are found on the skin and in the burrows dug by females searching for a copulation partner. There are probably pheromones associated with the mate seeking as there are often only few mites present in one canine host, but male and female mites seem to be able to find each other and copulate. The female lives for 4–6 weeks. It digs up to 5 mm of a new tunnel each day and lays two to four eggs daily. The eggs hatch in 50 h, at the earliest, producing six-legged larval stages that are substantially smaller than the adults. The larva seeks to exit its birth tunnel by digging one of its own, often all the way to the skin surface. From the surface, it digs a sheltered place in the keratin layer for

molting. The larval stage lasts 3–4 days. The larva molts to create an actively moving eight-legged protonymph. This life cycle stage lasts 2–3 days. The next molting produces a tritonymph (a.k.a. deutonymph) that molts 2–3 days later into an adult mite. In experimental conditions on a rabbit, the entire life cycle of the itch mite, from egg to adult, lasted at least 10 days. According to literature, a typical life cycle lasts 2–3 weeks. The life cycle of *S. scabiei* is illustrated in Fig. 9.60.

Sarcoptes may become separated from their host animals. Their chances for survival depend on the ambient temperature and humidity. *Sarcoptes* mites are known to survive in human dwellings (21°C, relative humidity 40%–80%) for 24–36 h. In cool and humid conditions, they can survive much longer. In 10°C and in the relative humidity of 97%, Sarcoptid mites can survive up to 18 days. High temperature and dryness kill the mites in a few hours.

Scabies is easily passed between dogs, almost always through direct contact. Since the mites survive only briefly outside the host, the transfer may also happen indirectly via cages, bedding, or grooming equipment. Wild foxes and raccoon dogs may act as a source for infestation as well (Fig. 9.61). The infestation does not require direct contact with the wild animal. Instead, a visit in burrows, culverts, or any places where mangy wild animals have spent time may led to infestation.

Despite a thoroughly investigated history, the infestation source cannot often be determined. Although *Sarcoptes* mites are readily transmitted, all exposed dogs do not manifest clinical scabies. In households with multiple dogs, it is common that only one dog or some dogs become symptomatic.

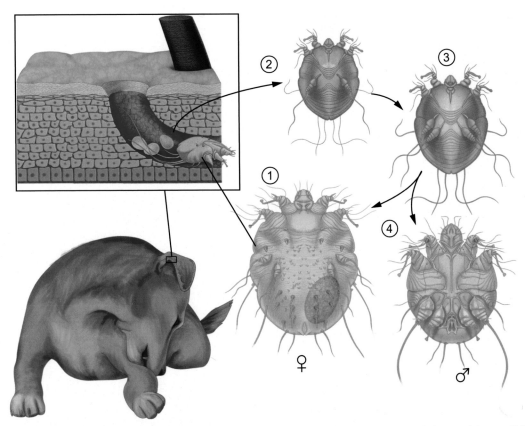

FIG. 9.60   Life cycle of *Sarcoptes scabiei*. (1) The *Sarcoptes* mites live in burrows, which they dig into the keratin layer and the superficial layer of the epidermis. The female lays two to four eggs daily. (2) The eggs hatch and producing six-legged larval stages that are substantially smaller than the adults. The larva seeks to exit its birth tunnel by digging one of its own, the larva molts to create an actively moving eight-legged protonymph. This life cycle stage lasts 2–3 days. (3) The next molting produces a tritonymph that molts 2–3 days later into an adult mites (4). In experimental conditions on a rabbit, the entire life cycle of the itch mite, from egg to adult, lasted at least 10 days. According to literature, a typical life cycle lasts 2–3 weeks.

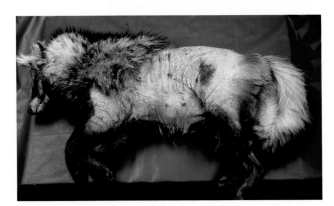

FIG. 9.61   Wild animals, especially foxes and raccoon dogs can act as a source of *Sarcoptes* infestation for dogs. A raccoon dog suffering from a generalized sarcoptic mange.

Distribution

Scabies is common in dogs of all ages and breeds all over the world. Dogs used for cave hunting are particularly often exposed to infestations originating from foxes and raccoon dogs.

Morphology of *Sarcoptes scabiei*

The Sarcoptic mite is oval shaped. Its dorsal surface is convex and the ventral side flat. The general coloring is creamy yellow. Legs and mouthparts contain more chitin and consequently have a brownish color in light microscopy (Fig. 9.57). The female is 0.3–0.5 mm and the male 0.2–0.4 mm long. The chitin shell is thin and grooved. Typical for arachnids, the adult stage has four pairs of legs. The third and fourth pairs are located so ventrally that they are not visible when the mite is observed from above. Two most anterior leg pairs have a long-stalked empodium that terminates in a pad. There are two claw-like protrusions at the base of the shaft (Figs. 9.57–9.59). The pad-like structures are missing from the two last leg pairs of the female and from the third pair of the male. Triangular chitin spikes at the dorsal surface of the mite and often an oval egg, which is quite large (150–200 × 175–250 μm) in contrast to the size of the mite, are visible even with a light microscope. The head (gnathosoma) has plier-like mouthparts. The mite's anus is located terminally.

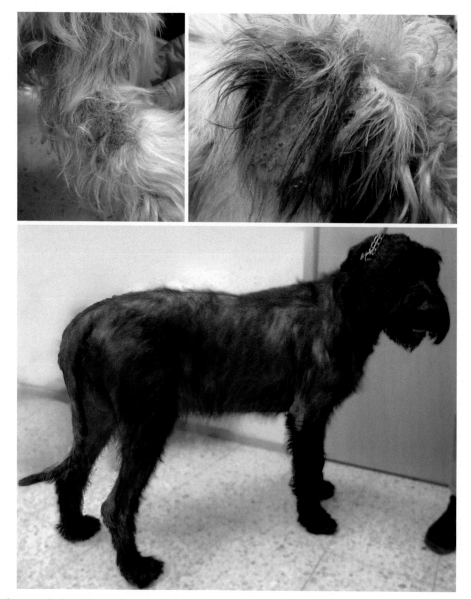

FIG. 9.62 Sarcoptic mange in dogs. Upper left: A pruritic hyperkeratotic skin thickening, in a dog's elbow. Upper right: a classical manifestation of sarcoptic mange in a dog: intensely pruritic, crustous and scaly lesion in the pinnal margin. Below: severe scabies in a dog. *(Upper left: photo by Leena Saijonmaa Koulumies. Upper right: photo by Mirja Kaimio. Below: photo by Lotta Pänkälä, reproduced with permission.)*

Importance to Canine Health

S. scabiei infestation, or scabies or sarcoptic mange, is usually a very pruritic skin disease (Fig. 9.62). The itch is at its worst in warm conditions and at night. For example, a warm bath can exacerbate the signs. The signs typically start 2–4 weeks after infestation, but they also can start earlier or later. If the dog has already been sensitized to Sarcoptic infestation, severe pruritus can commence as early as 1 day after infestation. The mechanical skin damage and irritation of burrowing mites has a minor role in causing the pruritic signs. The hypersensitivity reaction to the mites, and especially to their secretions, explain why only a few

itch mites can cause severe pruritic signs, why only some infected dogs become symptomatic, and why the pruritus can last long after the infestation has been treated. The classical early signs of a Sarcoptic infestation include erythematous and papulomatous dermatitis of urticarial character especially in the edges of the pinnae, elbows and hocks. Lesions are also often seen on the ventral skin and on the sides. When the infestation develops further, lesions may spread to the skin of the entire head and legs. They are seldom seen on the dorsal skin. Scratching causes the skin lesions to become bloody and hairless. The skin at the edges of pinnae and the on the elbows can be covered with dry and scaly crusts. Thickening, hyperkeratosis, crust-formation, and hyperpigmentation of skin are common in the chronic stage of scabies, as is the hypertrophy of local lymph nodes. Chronic and severe infestations are complicated with poor appetite and weight loss. The damaged skin is susceptible to secondary bacterial infection. Sarcoptic mange may be fatal if it lasts for a long time. Occasionally scabies may cause severe pruritus with few dermal manifestations. This condition is called scabies incognito and it is usually seen in cases of inadequate treatment, where some scabies mites have been eliminated but the infestation remains.

Sometimes there are severe generalized hyperkeratosis and lichenification of the skin without pruritus. In humans, this condition is called Norwegian scabies. The name is also occasionally used for the similar condition in veterinary medicine. It is common in wild raccoon dogs and foxes, but is has also been described in dogs. In order to become so severe, scabies usually requires a sensitizing factor. In canine cases, sensitizing factors include long-term glucocorticoid treatment, Cushing's syndrome (hyperadrenocorticism), and hypothyroidism.

Diagnosis

Severe itch, lesions in typical sites and a history of contact with potential infestation sources give a reason to suspect scabies. Diagnosis may be confused by the fact that many alternative diagnoses, such as allergic dermatoses of different types and other ectoparasitic infestations, may manifest concurrently.

When suspecting scabies, the inflamed edge of the pinna can be kneaded between the thumb and index finger. Scabies may trigger a reflex, whereby the hind leg of the dog starts to wisp, as if scratching. This so-called pinnal-pedal reflex is typical for dogs suffering from scabies. It is present in 75%–90% of dogs that have scabies and associated lesions in ears.

The diagnosis of scabies can be confirmed by finding *Sarcoptes* mites in a skin scraping sample (Fig. 9.63). The sample should be taken from the skin sites favored by the mite. A thin layer of paraffin or other mineral oil is spread on a scalpel blade. Alternatively, oil can be spread onto the skin before taking the sample. The scrape will contain sebum and keratin, which can be dissolved with 10% potassium or sodium hydroxide. It should be noted that caustic soda kills the mites, and recognizing immobile mites can be difficult in microscopy. A new, red macule is usually an ideal sample site. Damaged skin spots should be avoided. Several samples from sufficient depth should be taken. The yield is moved from the scalpel to the microscopy slide and a drop of paraffin or mineral oil is placed on top. After the sample is covered with a cover slip, it is ready for microscopy. Obtaining a positive scraping is extremely difficult in a case of scabies incognito, whereas lots of mites are found in a case of Norwegian scabies.

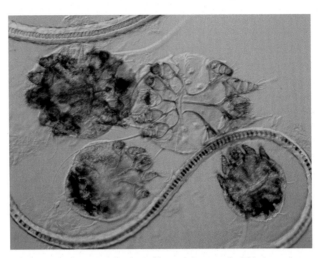

FIG. 9.63 *Sarcoptes* mites in a skin scraping sample. This is an exceptionally large yield. Very often even repeated samplings do not produce a positive finding from an infected dog.

However, typical scabies case is clinically and diagnostically somewhere between these two extremes. Finding a sarcoptic mite confirms the diagnosis, but despite meticulously performed sampling, mites and other confirmatory findings are often not detected in a scraping sample. According to the literature, the chances for success are about 30%–50%. False negatives are common.

Analyzing a skin biopsy seldom brings additional value to diagnostics, since, for instance, eosinophilia, suggestive of parasitic infestation, is found only infrequently in scabies cases (Fig. 9.64). When a dog chews the itchy skin, mites or mite eggs may be swallowed into the alimentary tract.

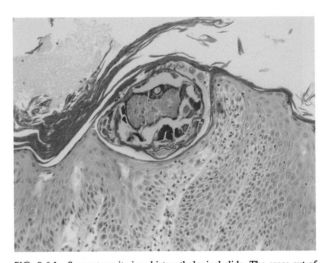

FIG. 9.64 *Sarcoptes* mite in a histopathological slide. The cross cut of the mite is seen under the keratin layer of the skin. Spiky protrusions typical for the species are seen on the dorsal surface of the mite. Parakeratotic hyperkeratosis and epidermal hyperplasia—typical histopathological changes seen in sarcoptic mange—are present in the adjacent epidermis.

This opens up the opportunity to analyze faces with the flotation method for *Sarcoptes* eggs.

Scabies raises the titer of specific antibodies. The infestation can be diagnosed with high confidence from a serum samples with ELISA. The method is considered sensitive and accurate.

In some situations, diagnosis can be based on a therapeutic trial. If such a trial is undertaken, it is important that the dog is treated for a sufficiently long time, as if it had had a confirmed scabies diagnosis. If the pruritus of the dog is found to be nonresponsive to glucocorticoid treatment, this raises the likelihood of scabies diagnosis over allergies.

Canine Scabies Is a Zoonosis

S. scabiei is quick to cause dermatitis in people exposed to mangy dogs. The probability of infestation is up to 50%, according to literature. The risk is so high that, while taking the history of the dog patient, it is wise to ask about possible pruritic skin symptoms in people that have had contact with the dog. Human dermatologists are often baffled by the fact that typical symptoms of *S. scabiei* var. *hominis* infestation, including mite burrows in interdigital skin, wrists, and external genitals, are usually not seen in cases where the canine itch mite is the causative organism. The affected person has often pruritic, erythematous, and papulomatous lesions in skin sites that have been in contact with the dog—most commonly on the arms and abdominal skin (Fig. 9.65). The human lesions are limited and spontaneously cured in 2–6 weeks, as long as canine scabies is treated and the person is not reinfected. An interesting twist to the speculation of "who infected who" is the fact that *S. scabiei* var. *hominis* can infect the dog and cause pruritic dermatitis.

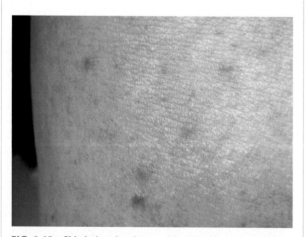

FIG. 9.65 Skin lesions in a human skin caused by canine sarcoptic mange. Typical symptoms of human scabies, such as mite burrows in interdigital skin, wrists and external genitals, are usually not seen in cases, where the canine sarcoptic mite is the causative organism. The affected person has often pruritic, erythematous and papulomatous lesions in skin sites that have been in contact with the dog. (*Photo by Leena Saijonmaa-Koulumies, reproduced with permission.*)

Treatment and Prevention

It is important for the treatment of scabies as well as for treatment trials that all in-contact dogs are handled and that an effective drug is given in correct doses and for a sufficiently long time. An incomplete treatment may lead to scabies incognito. If the treatment trial is carried out without a confirmed diagnosis and the pruritic signs persist, the veterinarian and the owner may erroneously assume that the chance of scabies has been ruled out.

Veterinary medical products registered for the treatment of scabies contain either macrocyclic lactones or isoxazolines. The former include selamectin, moxidectin, and milbemycin oxime. Among the isoxazolines, sarolaner has a registered claim against sarcoptic mange. Based on published studies, other isoxazolines have an efficacy as well.

Drugs of the avermectin group, ivermectin and doramectin, have also been used to treat scabies. They are given either by repeated injections or orally. These substances are not registered for dogs because of the risk of adverse effects especially in dogs of collie breeds. Since adverse effects have also been described in other breeds, the use of avermectins should be avoided. High temperatures are lethal for the Sarcoptic mites and, e.g., exposure to 49°C temperature kills mites within 10 min. The mites may survive in freezing temperature for several days, but 1.5 h in −25°C resulted in 100% mortality. Hence, both high and low temperatures can be used to kill mites in fomites such as contaminated stuffed toys and beddings.

FURTHER READING

Alekseev A, Chunikhin S: The experimental transmission of the tick-borne encephalitis virus by ixodid ticks (the mechanisms, time periods, species and sex differences), *Parazitologia* 24:177–185, 1990.

American Association of Veterinary Parasitologists: *Otodectes cynotis*, 2014. http://www.aavp.org/wiki/arthropods/arachnids/astigmata/otodectes-cynotis/ (Accessed May 2018).

Arlian LG, Morgan MS: A review of Sarcoptes scabiei: past, present and future, *Parasit Vectors* 10:297, 2017.

Atwell R: *Tick paralysis in the Merck veterinary manual*, ed 10, Whitehouse Station, NJ, 2010, Merck & Co., pp 1204–1210.

Atwell R, Campbell F, Evans E: Prospective survey of tick paralysis in dogs, *Aust Vet J* 79:412–418, 2001.

Belova O, Burenkova L, Karganova G: Different tick-borne encephalitis virus (TBEV) prevalences in unfed versus partially engorged ixodid ticks—evidence of virus replication and changes in tick behavior, *Ticks Tick-Borne Dis* 3:240–246, 2012.

Bornstein S: *Sarcoptes scabiei infections of the domestic dog, red fox and pig. Clinical and serodiagnostic studies*, (Doctoral thesis), Uppsala, 1995, Swedish University of Agricultural Sciences.

Bowman A: *Tick paralysis*, 2014. http://www.aavp.org/?s=tick+paralysis (Accessed June 2018).

Bredal W: The prevalence of nasal mite (Pneumonyssoides caninum) infection in Norwegian dogs, *Vet Parasitol* 76:233–237, 1998.

Bredal W, Vollset I: Use of milbemycin oxime in the treatment of dogs with nasal mite (Pneumonyssoides caninum) infection, *J Small Anim Pract* 39:126–130, 1998.

Bredal W, Gjerde B, Kippenes H: Pneumonyssoides caninum, the canine nasal mite, reported for the first time in a fox (Vulpes vulpes), *Vet Parasitol* 73:291–297, 1997.

Burgess I: Sarcoptes scabiei and scabies. In Baker J, Muller R, editors: *Advances in parasitology* (vol. 33), London, 1994, Academic Press, pp 235–292.

Cannon M: *Tick paralysis.* http://www.ava.com.au/sites/default/files/Envenomation_Tick%20Paralysis_MCannon.pdf. (Accessed June 2018).

Chen C: A short-tailed demodectic mite and Demodex canis infestation in a Chihuahua dog, *Vet Dermatol* 6:227–229, 1995.

Chesney C: Short form of Demodex species mite in the dog: occurrence and measurements, *J Small Anim Pract* 40:58–61, 1999.

Dantas-Torres F: The brown dog tick, Rhipicephalus sanguineus (Latreille, 1806) (Acari: Ixodidae): from taxonomy to control, *Vet Parasitol* 152:173–185, 2008.

Dantas-Torres F: Biology and ecology of the brown dog tick, Rhipicephalus sanguineus, *Parasit Vectors* 3:26, 2010.

Deplazes P, Eckert J, Mathis A, von Samson-Himmelstjerna G, Zahner H: *Parasitology in veterinary medicine,* ed 1, Wageningen, 2016, Wageningen Academic Publishers.

des Vignes F, Piesman J, Heffernan R, Schulze T, Stafford IIIK, Fish D: Effect of tick removal on transmission of Borrelia burgdorferi and Ehrlichia phagocytophila by Ixodes scapularis Nymphs, *J Infect Dis* 183:773–778, 2001.

Desch C, Hillier A: Demodex injai: a new species of hair follicle mite (Acari: Demodecidae) from the domestic dog (Canidae), *J Med Entomol* 40:146–149, 2000.

Duclos D, Jeffers J, Schanley K: Prognosis for treatment of adult-onset demodicosis in dogs: 34 cases (1979–1990), *J Am Vet Med Assoc* 204:616–619, 1994.

European Scientific Counsel Companion Animal Parasites (ESCCAP): *Control of ectoparasites in dogs and cats,* Guideline 3, ed 6, March 2018. https://www.esccap.org/uploads/docs/gm7zb43y_0720_ESCCAP_Guideline_GL3_update_v6.pdf. (Accessed May 2018).

Ferrer L, Ravera I, Silbermayr K: Immunology and pathogenesis of canine demodicosis, *Vet Dermatol* 25:427–465, 2014.

Folz S: Canine scabies (Sarcoptes scabiei) infestation, *Comp Cont Pract Vet* 6:176–180, 1984.

Fondati A: Efficacy of daily oral ivermectin in the treatment of 10 cases of generalized demodicosis in adult dogs, *Vet Dermatol* 7:99–104, 1996.

George D, Finn R, Graham K, et al: Should the poultry red mite Dermanyssus gallinae be of wider concern for veterinary and medical science? *Parasit Vectors* 8(178), 2015.

Gray J, Stanek G, Kundi M, Kocianova E: Dimensions of engorging Ixodes ricinus as a measure of feeding duration, *Int J Med Microbiol* 295:567–572, 2005.

Greene C: *Infectious diseases of the dog and cat,* ed 4, St. Louis, 2012, Elsevier-Saunders.

Gunnarsson L: *Nasal mite infection of the dog: prevalence, diagnosis and treatment* (Doctoral thesis), Uppsala, 2000, Swedish University of Agricultural Sciences.

Gunnarsson L, Zakrisson G, Lilliehook I, Christensson D, Rehbinder C, Uggla A: Experimental infection of dogs with the nasal mite Pneumonyssoides caninum, *Vet Parasitol* 77:179–186, 1998.

Gunnarsson L, Zakrisson G, Egenvall A, Christensson D, Uggla A: Prevalence of Pneumonyssoides caninum infection in dogs in Sweden, *J Am Anim Hosp Assoc* 37:331–337, 2001.

Gunnarsson L, Zakrisson G, Christensson D, Uggla A: Efficacy of selamectin in the treatment of nasal mite (Pneumonyssoides caninum) infection in dogs, *J Am Anim Hosp Assoc* 40:400–404, 2004.

Hall-Mendelin S, Craig S, Hall R, et al: Tick paralysis in Australia caused by Ixodes holocyclus Neumann, *Ann Trop Med Parasitol* 105:95–106, 2011.

Herrmann C, Gern L: Search for blood or water is influenced by Borrelia burgdorferi in Ixodes ricinus, *Parasit Vectors* 8:6, 2015.

Hillier A, Desch C: Large-bodied Demodex mite infestation in 4 dogs, *J Am Vet Med Assoc* 220:623–627, 2002.

Hodzic E, Fish D, Maretzki C, De Silva A, Feng S, Barthold S: Acquisition and transmission of the agent of human granulocytic ehrlichiosis by Ixodes scapularis ticks, *J Clin Microbiol* 36:3574–3578, 1998.

Holm B: Efficacy of milbemycin oxime in the treatment of canine generalized demodicosis: a retrospective study of 99 dogs (1995–2000), *Vet Dermatol* 14:189–195, 2003.

Johnstone I: Doramectin as a treatment for canine and feline demodicosis, *Aust Vet Pract* 32:98–103, 2002.

Karbowiak G: The occurrence of the Dermacentor reticulatus tick—its expansion to new areas and possible causes, *Ann Parasit* 60: 37–47, 2014.

Katavolos P, Armstrong P, Dawson J, Telford S III: Duration of tick attachment required for transmission of granulocytic ehrlichiosis, *J Infect Dis* 177:1422–1425, 1998.

Kidd L, Breitswerdt E: Transmission times and prevention of tick-borne diseases in dogs, *Compend Contin Educ Pract Vet* 25:742–750, 2003.

Kraft W, Kraiss-Gothe A, Gothe R: Otodectes cynotis infestation of dogs and cats: biology of the agent, epidemiology, pathogenesis and diagnosis and case description of generalized mange in dogs, *Tierarztl Prax* 16:409–415, 1998.

Krupka I, Straubinger R: Lyme borreliosis in dogs and cats: background, diagnosis, treatment and prevention of infections with Borrelia burgdorferi sensu stricto, *Vet Clin Small Anim* 40:1103–1119, 2010.

Kwochka K, Kunkle G: The efficacy of amitraz for generalized demodicosis in dogs: a study of two concentrations and frequencies of application, *Compend Contin Educ Pract Vet* 7:8–17, 1985.

Le Net J-L, Fain A, George C, Rousselle S, Theau V, Longeart L: Straelensiosis in dogs: a newly described nodular dermatitis induced by Straelensia cynotis, *Vet Rec* 150:205–209, 2002.

Lemarie S, Hosgood G, Foil C: A retrospective study of juvenile- and adult-onset generalized demodicosis in dogs (1986–91), *Vet Dermatol* 7:3–10, 1996.

Lord C: Brown dog tick, Rhipicephalus sanguineus Latreille (Arachnida: Acari: Ixodidae). In *Featured creatures*, Gainesville, FL, July 2014, University of Florida Institute of Food and Agricultural Sciences, Department of Entomology and Nematology. http://www.entnemdept.ufl.edu/creatures/urban/medical/brown_dog_tick.htm. (Accessed May 2018).

Louly C, Soares S, Silveira D, Neto O, Silva A, Borges L: Differences in the susceptibility of two dog breeds of dogs, English cocker spaniel and beagle to Rhipicephalus sanguineus (Acari: Ixodidae), *Inter J Acar* 35:25–32, 2009.

Medleau L, Ristic Z, McElveen D: Daily ivermectin for treatment of generalized demodicosis in dogs, *Vet Dermatol* 7:209–212, 1996.

Miller W, Scott D Wellington J: Clinical efficacy of milbemycin oxime in the treatment of generalized demodicosis in adult dogs, *J Am Vet Med Assoc* 2003:1426–1429, 1993.

Moriello K: Common ectoparasites of the dog; part 2: Sarcoptes scabiei var. canis and Demodex canis, *Canine Pract* 14:25–41, 1987.

Mueller R: Treatment protocols for demodicosis: an evidence-based review, *Vet Dermatol* 15:75–89, 2004.

Pfeffer M, Dobler G: Tick-borne encephalitis virus in dogs—is this an issue? *Parasit Vectors* 4:59, 2011.

Pfister K, Armstrong R: Systemically and cutaneously distributed ectoparasiticides: a review of the efficacy against ticks and fleas on dogs, *Parasit Vectors* 9:436, 2016. https://doi.org/10.1186/s13071-016-1719-7.

Rechav Y, Nuttal P: The effect of male ticks on the feeding performance of immature stages of Rhipicephalus sanguineus and Amblyomma americanum (Acari: Ixodidae), *Exp Appl Acarol* 24:569–578, 2000.

Rikihisa Y: Mechanisms of obligatory intracellular infection with Anaplasma phagocytophilum, *Clin Microbiol Rev* 24:469–489, 2011.

Russel R, Otranto O, Wall R: *The encyclopedia of medical and veterinary entomology,* Wallingford, UK, 2013, CABI.

Saari S, Nikander S: Ruskea koiranpunkki (Rhipicephalus sanguineus), *Suomen Eläinlääkäril* 98:72–77, 1992 (in Finnish).

Saari S, Nikander S: Cheyletiella yasguri—koiranpennun kävelevä hilse, *Suomen eläinlääkäril* 99:613–618, 1993 (in Finnish).

Saari S, Eklöf A, Salminen T, Nikander S: Tunnistatko kapisen koiran—Tarkastelun kohteena syyhypunkki (Sarcoptes scabiei), *Suom Elainlaakaril* 107:432–440, 2001 (in Finnish).

Sainz Á, Roura X, Miró G, et al: Guideline for veterinary practitioners on canine ehrlichiosis and anaplasmosis in Europe, *Parasit Vectors* 8:75, 2015.

Sastre N, Ravera I, Villanueva S, et al: Phylogenetic relationships in three species of canine Demodex mite based on partial sequences of mitochondrial 16S rDNA, *Vet Dermatol* 23:509–514, 2012.

Seixas F, Travassos P, Pinto M, Correia J, Pires M: Dermatitis in a dog induced by Straelensia cynotis: a case report and review of the literature, *Vet Dermatol* 17:81–84, 2006.

Stekolnikov A, Santibáñez P, Palomar A, Oteo J: Neotrombicula inopinata (Acari: Trombiculidae)—a possible causative agent of trombiculiasis in Europe, *Parasit Vectors* 7:90, 2014.

Sweatman G: Biology of Otodectes cynotis, the ear canker mite of carnivores, *Can J Zool* 36:849–862, 1958.

Taylor M, Coop R, Wall R: *Veterinary parasitology,* ed 4, Oxford, 2016, Blackwell Publishing Ltd.

Wagner R, Wendlberger U: Field efficacy of moxidectin in dogs and rabbits naturally infested with Sarcoptes spp., Demodex spp. and Psoroptes spp. mites, *Vet Parasitol* 93:149–158, 2000.

Waisglass S: Demodicosis, *Vet Focus* 25:10–18, 2015.

Willis S, Arrese M, Torrance A, et al: Pneumonyssoides species infestation in two Pekingese dogs in the UK, *J Small Anim Pract* 49:107–109, 2008.

Chapter 10

Crustacea and Pentastomids (Tongueworms)

LINGUATULA SERRATA, Canine Tongueworm

- Worm-like limbless crustaceans found in the nasal cavity and paranasal sinuses of the dog.
- Tongue-shaped, up to 130 mm in length and 20 mm in width, transversely striated.
- The dog is usually infected by eating ruminant offal or slaughter waste.
- Infestation is often subclinical but may manifest and cause nasal discharge, sneezing, pronounced respiratory sounds, and coughing.
- The diagnosis is based on finding typical eggs in fecal or nasal cavity samples.

Identification

The canine tongueworm (*Linguatula serrata*) is classified, despite its name and vermiform looks, as a crustacean. The name tongueworm, as well as the Latin genus *Linguatula*, stem from the flat, tongue-resembling looks of the worm.

Adult parasites reside in the nasal cavity of the dog. The adult female *Linguatula* is 80–130 mm long and about 1 cm wide at the thickest part (Fig. 10.1). The male can grow up to 2 cm length and 3–4 mm in width. The general shape of *Linguatula* is that of a paddle. The front end is wide and flat. The rear end is narrow and cylindrical. The chitin surface is segmented. The mouth and four grabbing hooks can be seen in the anterior end of *Linguatula* (Fig. 10.2).

The eggs exiting from the dog are embryonated and 90 × 70 μm in size (Fig. 10.3). Nymphal stages, infectious for the dog, can be found in the intermediate host (Fig. 10.4). They are under 1 cm long and morphologically resemble adults. They have grabbing hooks, a segmented chitin surface, and a row of barbs can be seen in each segment.

Life Cycle

Adult and preadult *Linguatula* live in the nasal cavity and paranasal sinuses of dogs and other canids. They attach to the mucous membranes with their hooks and use blood and tissue fluids for nutrition. The female can preserve the sperm originated from a single copulation for the rest of its life. The female is an effective egg producer. The eggs end-up voided to the environment either through the alimentary canal of the dog or in sputum or nasal discharge. Many species can act as intermediate hosts of *Linguatula*. The intermediate host is infected when embryonated eggs enter to its intestine. The first-degree early larvae, or nauplius larvae, have limb-like protrusions. The larvae penetrate the gut wall with their stylet-like mouthparts and migrate to different parts of the body, including lymph nodes, liver, and lungs. The larva develops into the nymphal stage, infectious to the dog, which curls into the shape of letter C and encapsulates. The dog is most commonly infected by eating ruminant offal or slaughter waste. The parasitic cyst breaks down in the intestine and the nymphs migrate to the nasopharynx to mature. It takes them about half a year to reach adulthood. An illustrated lifecycle of *Linguatula serrata* is presented in Fig. 10.5.

Distribution

L. serrata has a worldwide distribution but is prevalent especially in the subtropics. It is commonly found in the Middle East, where up to 50% of stray dogs can be infected in some areas.

Importance to Canine Health

Most *Linguatula* infections are subclinical. The linguatulosis may manifest in the upper respiratory organs causing nasopharyngitis and nasal discharge. The discharge may be bloody. The irritation caused by the parasite may lead to sniffling and, due to congested airways, pronounced respiratory sounds.

Canine Parasites and Parasitic Diseases. https://doi.org/10.1016/B978-0-12-814112-0.00010-6

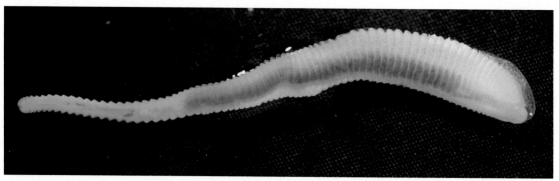

FIG. 10.1 Despite its worm-like appearance, *Linguatula* is classified among crustaceans. A female *Linguatula*, about 80–130 mm long, with distinct transverse striations, is depicted. *(Specimen from Dr. M. Tavassoli, Urmia University, Faculty of Veterinary Medicine, Iran.)*

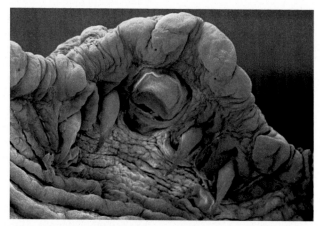

FIG. 10.2 The anterior end of *Linguatula* has a head-like protuberance with a mouth and four grasping hooks. The photo shows *L. arctica*, a close relative of *L. serrata*. *(Reproduced with permission from Nikander S, Saari S: A SEM study of the reindeer sinus worm (L. arctica), Rangifer 26:15–24, 2006.)*

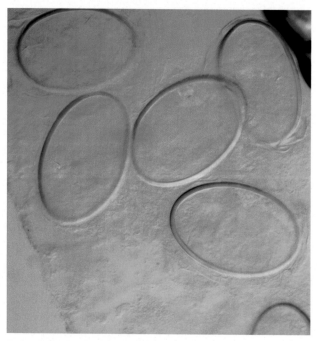

FIG. 10.3 Eggs of *Linguatula* in the uterus. Their size is 90 × 70 μm and they are embryonated when reaching the environment. *(Specimen from Dr. M. Tavassoli, Urmia University, Faculty of Veterinary Medicine, Iran.)*

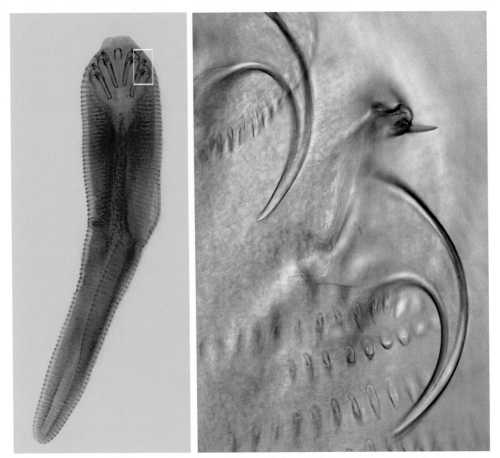

FIG. 10.4 The dog is infected with *Linguatula* by eating organs of an intermediate host, infected with *Linguatula* nymphs. They are under 1 cm long and morphologically bear a close resemblance to adults. They have grabbing hooks, segmented chitin surface, and a row of barbs can be seen in each segment. An enlargement of the area in the rectangle is depicted in the detail photo. *(Specimen from Dr. M. Tavassoli, Urmia University, Faculty of Veterinary Medicine, Iran.)*

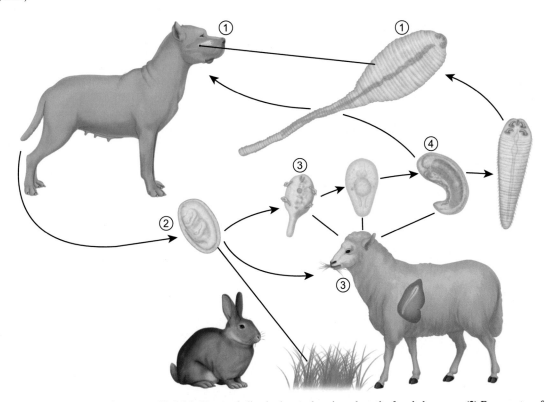

FIG. 10.5 Life cycle of *Linguatula serrata*. (1) Adult *Linguatula* live in the nasal cavity, where the female lays eggs. (2) Eggs are transferred to the environment either through the alimentary canal of the dog or in sputum or nasal discharge. (3) Many animal species may act as intermediate hosts for *Linguatula*. The intermediate host is infected when embryonated eggs come to its intestine. The nauplius larvae, hatching from the eggs, have limb-like protrusions. (4) The larvae penetrate the gut wall and migrate to different parts of the body. The larva develops into the nymphal stage, infectious to the dog, and encapsulates. (5) The dog is most commonly infected by eating ruminant organs. The parasitic cyst breaks down in the intestine and the nymphs migrate to the nasopharynx to mature. This takes about 6 months.

Diagnosis

The diagnosis of linguatulosis is based on finding eggs in fecal or nasal cavity samples. Since eggs are secreted infrequently, false negative findings are common. Adult *Linguatula* can be seen in the endoscopy of upper airways.

Treatment and Prevention

There are no registered medical products for the treatment of *Linguatula* infection, and published information on treatment options is scarce. *Linguatula arctica*, a close relative of *L. serrata* and a parasite of reindeer, is known to be sensitive to macrocyclic lactones. Thus, it is likely that macrocyclic lactones are effective against canine linguatulosis. For prevention, it is important to keep dogs away from slaughter waste originating in potential intermediate hosts.

Morphology of *L. serrata*

Pentastomids are a group of peculiar parasites which, despite their flat and worm-like appearance and lacking jointed appendages, belong to the phylum Arthropoda. Typical arthropod features are, e.g., chitinous cuticle, muscle striation and its attachment to cuticle, sensory sensillae, shape and structure of permatozoa, paired embryonic appendages and developmental ecdysis. Based on reproductive behavior and molecular biological analysis, pentastomids are classified as a group of modified crustaceans.

The adult female *Linguatula* is 80–130 mm long and about 1 cm wide at the thickest part. The male can grow up to 2 cm length and 3–4 mm in width. The general shape of *Linguatula* is that of a paddle. The front end is wide thin and flat. The rear end is narrow and cylindrical. The chitin surface is segmented. The head-like protuberance with a mouth and four heavily sclerotized hooks can be seen in the anterior end of *Linguatula*. The mouth is located anteroventrally between the proximal parts of the inner hooks.

The eggs exiting from the dog are embryonated and 90 × 70 μm in size. Nymphal stages, infectious for the dog, can be found in the intermediate host. They are under 1 cm long and morphologically resemble adults. They have grabbing hooks, a segmented chitin surface, and a row of barbs can be seen in each segment.

L. serrata is a Zoonotic Parasite

L. serrata is a zoonotic parasite. The most common cause of human linguatulosis is when eggs of canine nasal discharge or feces somehow end up in a person's mouth and intestinal canal. The larval stages hatch in the intestine and start to migrate, finding their way to the liver or lymph nodes, for instance, where they form a capsule. The larval stage continues developing in the tissues and grows larger through moltings. Although the larval migration may damage tissues and the growth of larval cysts may cause pressure damage and hypersensitivity reactions in the tissues, this sort of infection is usually subclinical. Humans may also receive the *Linguatula* infection by eating uncooked or poorly prepared tissues of an infected intermediate host, e.g., a sheep or goat. The third-stage larvae released from tissues migrate into the nasopharynx. They cause an acute, self-limiting nasopharyngeal inflammation, which can be accompanied with retching, sneezing, eating difficulties, and facial swelling. It is very rare that adult tongue worms are found in the human nasopharynx.

FURTHER READING

Acha P, Szyfres B: Pentastomosis. In Acha P, Szyfres B, editors: *(toim): Zoonoses and communicable diseases common to man and animals (parasitosis)* (vol. 3, No. 550), Washington, DC, 2003, Scientific and Technical Publication, Pan American Health Organization, pp 345–380.

Behrman K. *Linguatula serrata.* http://animaldiversity.org/accounts/Linguatula_serrata. (Accessed March 2018).

Nikander S, Saari S: A SEM study of the reindeer sinus worm (*Linguatula arctica*), *Rangifer* 26:15–24, 2006.

Rezaei F, Tavassoli M, Mahmoudian A: Prevalence of *Linguatula serrata* infection among dogs (definitive host) and domestic ruminants (intermediate host) in the North West of Iran, *Vet Med* 56:561–567, 2011.

Riley J: The biology of pentastomids. In Baker J, Muller R, editors: *Advances in parasitology* (vol. 25), London, 1986, Academic Press Inc. Ltd/Published by Elsevier Ltd, pp 45–128.

Soulsby EJL: *Helminths arthropods and protozoa of domesticated animals,* ed 7, London, 1982, Bailliere Tindall, pp 497–498.

Tavassoli M, Javadi S, Hadian M: Experimental infection and study of life cycle of *Linguatula serrata* in dogs, *J Facult of Vet Med Univ of Tehran, Iran* 56:1–3, 2001.

Chapter 11

Diagnostics

Many sorts of samples are used to make a parasitological diagnosis. Common samples that are delivered to a parasitological laboratory for identification are entire parasites or feces for microscopical analysis. Samples may also be secretions, as well as tissue, hair, and scraping samples. Blood and serum can be analyzed for diagnosis. Detecting the parasite directly is possible for many blood parasites. Indirect diagnosis can be carried out by analyzing host's antibodies against the parasite. Sampling is often done considering the clinical signs of the animal and, thus determining, which parasite is sought for. This chapter describes the most common methods of parasitological diagnostics.

TAKING AND HANDLING A FECAL SAMPLE

Fecal sample is perhaps the most typical parasitological sample. The optimal fecal sample is sufficiently large and taken directly from a canine rectum by the veterinarian. Ideally, it is analyzed immediately after sampling without storage or delivery. This is rarely accomplished. In practice, the animal owner or handler usually takes and sends the fecal sample.

The sample should be taken from fresh feces. It is preferable that the part taken as a sample has not been in contact with the ground to avoid contaminants. It is important to obtain a large enough quantity of feces, because parasitological methods rarely correspond for example bacteriological techniques in sensitivity, and many different procedures may sometimes be needed to reach a diagnosis. If the suspected parasite produces eggs or cystic forms intermittently into feces, it is feasible to take several samples. Samples of three adjacent days are often requested by the laboratory. If the object of interest can be seen with a naked eye, such as a proglottid of a cestode, it should always be sent along with the fecal sample and preferably packed separately.

The sample should be delivered for analysis without delay. Packing should be done carefully to prevent any leakage and air should be removed from a plastic bag by pressing it out. Ordinary fecal analyses allow for mailing the sample, even if the mail is delivered in room temperature. Since subzero temperatures are unsuitable for parasitological samples, they should not be exposed to outside conditions during mailing in cold winters. It is wise to organize the sampling so that storage time is minimized. Veterinarians and laboratories give advice on suitable sampling and delivery.

STORING A FECAL SAMPLE

If it is necessary to store a fecal sample, the correct temperature is refrigeration in about +4°C. Even if the fecal sample is packed meticulously, it must not be stored with food. When tightly packed, most parasite eggs withstand storage in refrigeration for a week without a notable change in the analysis results.

A frozen sample is unsuitable for parasitological diagnostics. For instance, it does not provide reliable results when analyzed with Baermann technique and also eggcounts will fall due to breakage of some eggs. A fecal sample can be stored for scientific research for a longer time in 70% ethanol or 10% formaldehyde. The solution of sodium acetate, acetic acid, and formaldehyde (SAF) is available commercially and is useful for storing and delivering fecal samples. However, it kills any larvae present in the feces, making thus stored samples unsuitable for analysis with the Baermann technique. It is generally important to consider the possible diagnostic methodology before deciding on the storage conditions.

VISUAL ANALYSIS OF A FECAL SAMPLE

Since canine feces may contain zoonotic pathogens, laboratory staff handling the samples must have adequate protective clothing, use gloves, and wash hands after work. The analysis of a fecal sample always starts with a visual examination for the presence of large parasites or their parts, e.g., cestode proglottids. The appearance of the feces is also noted: does it contain mucus, blood, or foreign objects? Is the feces abnormally soft or colored? Many intestinal parasites may cause diarrhea. This increases the liquid proportion, making the sample more diluted. This may lower the sensitivity of the analysis. After visual observation, a more specific investigation is undertaken, depending on what the focus of the analysis is in light of the dog's history.

Canine Parasites and Parasitic Diseases. https://doi.org/10.1016/B978-0-12-814112-0.00011-8

DIRECT MICROSCOPY OF PARASITE EGGS OR OOCYSTS IN A FECAL SAMPLE

One of the most traditional parasitological methods is the direct microscopy of feces, looking for worm eggs and larvae or protozoal cysts and their more active stages. The prerequisite for finding them is that the parasites are in a reproductive phase, meaning that the prepatent period is over. Because the sensitivity of direct microscopy is poor, methods are used to concentrate the eggs in the sample, for instance, by sedimentation or flotation. The former means that they are made to fall on the bottom of the sample and the latter that they rise to the surface of high-specific-gravity solution. Both methods utilize the difference in specific gravity of the eggs and the surrounding liquid. Despite concentrating the eggs, the methods of the traditional fecal assay are somewhat insensitive and results are dependent on the examiner's skills. In addition, direct conclusions about the parasitic burden cannot be made based on the quantity of eggs, since the number of eggs is not linear with the number of worms. Nevertheless, the quantitative analyses do form a foundation to the assessment of the infection severity. Traditional fecal assays have retained their role along with more modern diagnostic methods, thanks to being easy, inexpensive, and suitable for the analysis of many parasite species.

PASSIVE TEST-TUBE FLOTATION

Only very basic equipment is needed for analyzing worm eggs and oocysts (Fig. 11.1). About a teaspoonful of feces (2–3 g) is thoroughly mixed with slightly over 20 mL (about 1:10) of a flotation solution with a high specific gravity. For example, saturated NaCl, $ZnSO_4$, $MgSO_4$, and sugar, among many others, have been used as flotation solutions. Their specific gravity differs, and it is important to know which kind of solution is being used. The mixture is poured through a filter (e.g., a tea sieve). A test tube is filled with the filtered liquid to the top, full to the brim, so that no foam or air bubbles remain on the surface. A cover slip is placed on top of the tube so that it fully touches the solution and allowed to stay at room temperature for about 10–45 min, depending on the height of the tube and consequently the floating distance. Twenty minutes is a suitable incubation time for a test tube of standard dimensions. If the tube is incubated too long, delaying microscopy, liquid starts to evaporate from the edges of the tube, which causes the flotation salts to crystallize on the glass, and will eventually prevent the microscopic analysis of the sample. After the incubation, the cover slip is lifted from the tube onto the objective slide so that the drop containing parasite eggs at the lower side of the slip is between the two slides. The liquid should spread over the entire area of the cover slip. If needed, more liquid can be pipetted from the very

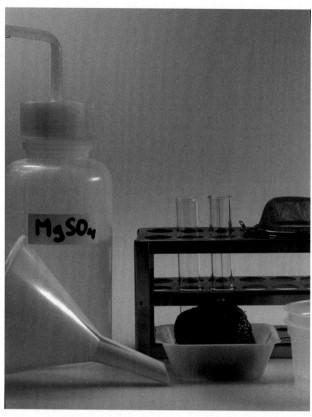

FIG. 11.1 Analyzing a fecal sample with the flotation method requires only basic equipment. In addition to the microscope and the sample, only a disposable vessel, mixing spatula, tea sieve, funnel, test tube, flotation solution, and microscope slides are needed.

top surface of the tube to the border of the slides, from where it will be sucked into the gap between them. The sample is screened with 100-fold (10× objective, if the ocular is 10×) multiplication consistently over the whole cover slip area. This magnification is sufficient for the differentiating of worm eggs as well as coccidia oocysts (Fig. 11.2). If a detail needs closer scrutiny, magnification can be increased for local observation. Results obtained with this method are not quantitative even if the amount of feces and flotation solution are known and the eggs are counted. The performance of the method is illustrated in the information box at the end of the chapter (page 240).

CENTRIFUGATION FLOTATION

Centrifugation flotation is a method more sensitive than passive test tube flotation, but requires more equipment. It is flotation augmented with centrifugation, or sedimentation-flotation. Its first stage is to mix the feces with water (about 1:10), sieve through a tea-sieve or equivalent, and centrifuge the mixture. The supernatant is discarded. The fecal sediment is then mixed well

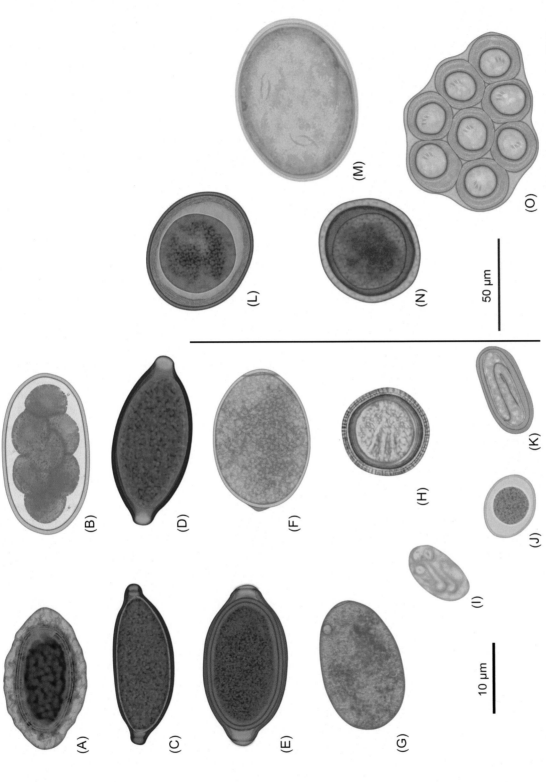

FIG. 11.2 Eggs and protozoal cystic stages of canine parasites. (A) *Dioctophyma renale*; (B) *Ancylostoma* sp., *Uncinaria stenocephala*; (C) *Eucoleus* sp.; (D) *Trichuris vulpis* (E) *Pearsonema plica*; (F) *Diphyllobothrium latum*; (G) *Paragonimus* sp.; (H) *Taenia* spp.; (I) *Giardia*; (J) *Isospora* sp.; (K) *Spirocerca lupi*; (L) *Toxascaris leonina*; (M) *Linguatula serrata*; (N) *Toxocara canis*; (O) *Dipylidium caninum*.

with the flotation solution, and the tube is filled close to the brim with the mixture and centrifuged 3–5 min at $300–500 \times g$. The tube is placed in a holder and filled to the brim with additional flotation solution, and a cover slip is placed on top so that its entire lower surface is in touch with the liquid. After a few minutes of incubation, the cover slip is viewed with microscopy similarly as in the passive tube flotation method. In some centrifuges, the tubes may be whirled with the cover glass already on the tube and viewed without incubation. This requires that the tubes reach a 90 degrees angle during centrifugation (swinging bucket) and that the acceleration can be adjusted gradually. The speed must not be excessive. Some instructions for this method leave out the stage of mixing the sample with water and use the directly flotation solution instead.

SEDIMENTATION

Sedimentation methods are especially suitable for heavy worm eggs, which do not float easily with the methods based on flotation. These include, for instance, eggs of several trematodes. Larvae can also be analyzed with sedimentation. Water is a suitable sedimentation liquid. Feces and water are mixed thoroughly, and the mixture is filtered and allowed to stay in a tube or a larger vial, preferably in a funnel-shaped one. Ten minutes is a sufficient time for incubation in a standard test tube. Sedimentation may be speeded up with centrifugation. The supernatant is carefully removed, not all the way to the bottom, and mixing with water and waiting are repeated a few times in order to remove the remaining feces as thoroughly as possible. Fecal remains interfere with microscopy. After the final incubation, the sediment is viewed using a the microscope with 100-fold magnification for parasites. If the sediment is plentiful, this may require preparing several samples for microscopy. A urinary sample can also be handled with sedimentation without mixing it with water.

STAINING TISSUES AND PARASITES

The sensitivity of detecting certain parasites in feces can be improved by staining methods. A drop of methylene blue (1% solution) after flotation or sedimentation may help visualizing the eggs. *Giardia* and cryptosporidium cysts are easier to see in a sample stained with Lugol's iodine solution than from a sample without a stain. Lugol's iodine stains the nuclear structures and glycogen. The modified Ziehl-Nielsen or auramine phenol stain is used in the diagnostics of cryptosporidium cysts. The former stains acid-resistant cysts red and the later makes the cysts shine yellow in fluorescence microscopy.

Parasites can be sought in a histological tissue section processed in the standard manner. The shortcoming of a histological section is that, even in cases where the parasite is included in the biopsy, it is usually visible only as a thin cut-off, which does not necessarily contain diagnostically relevant structures. A quantitative assessment of the infection would often be useful, while the presence of a single parasite does not necessarily indicate that the signs are caused by the parasitosis. On the other hand, a histopathological examination frequently gives valuable information on the tissue lesions and inflammation associated with the parasite.

When examining tissue sections, hematoxylin and eosin (H&E) stain, the standard staining method of histopathology, is usually adequate for detecting parasites. However, protozoa, such as *Giardia* on the intestinal villi and Leishmania amastigotes inside macrophages, are more clearly seen in Giemsa-stained tissue samples.

Immunohistochemistry and immunofluorescence are immunological methods based on the specific adherence of an antibody to parasitic antigens, visualized by a color reaction. A stain with specific affinity to the parasite facilitates detecting parasites in the biopsy and supports the identification of family or species. Immunohistochemistry is especially useful for visualizing and highlighting protozoa in tissue specimens.

QUANTITATIVE METHODS AND FECAL EGG COUNT REDUCTION TEST (FECRT)

Quantitative flotation methods are useful, when the fecal sample is assessed for the severity of the infection. A known quantity of feces and flotation solution are analyzed in a counting chamber, the parasite eggs or protozoal oocysts are counted, and a conversion factor is used to calculate how many eggs or oocysts are in a gram of feces. This result can be contrasted to the reference values found in literature in order to assess the severity of the parasitic infection. Unfortunately, reference values are rarely available for dogs, because they are typically treated always when a parasite infection is diagnosed, regardless of the number of eggs.

Dogs' fecal samples can be analyzed, for example, with a McMaster chamber, more typically used for handling of equine and ruminant samples (Fig. 11.6). The method has several modifications. When using the chamber, the theoretical minimum detection limit for the used method should be known. Egg numbers that are smaller than the detection limit will not be detected. Laboratories that perform quantitative tests should state the detection limit when providing results.

FLOTAC and Mini-FLOTAC are among the most common of commercially available counting chambers. It provides especially good visibility in microscopy, since only the most superficial layer of the solution in the chamber, containing eggs and oocysts, is taken for viewing. It is necessary to become well acquainted with the method first.

If resistance against an antiparasitic drug is suspected, the FECRT can be used to analyze if the egg count diminishes as expected after deworming. This method is commonly used to investigate the fecal samples of horses and ruminants, but it can also be used for pets' samples, pending the discovery of better methods. The test is recommended to be conducted on groups of animals (e.g., in a kennel). Analysis of an individual animal can at most be considered indicative. A fecal sample, positive for parasite eggs, is taken from a dog immediately before it is treated with the dewormer of interest. The number of eggs per 1 g of feces is determined, e.g., in a McMaster chamber. A new quantitative sample is taken 2 weeks after the treatment. The egg count is expected to drop to zero or close to it. The egg count must diminish at least about 95% (depending on the parasite and the deworming substance) from the count of the medication day. If this is not the case, a resistant parasite colony is suspected to be prevalent in the canine population.

This method of resistance analysis is sensitive to medication errors. The dog under investigation must be weighed so that an accurate dose can be given. The drug must be given so that the dog takes the entire dose. It is preferable that the drug is given by a veterinary healthcare professional, when resistance is investigated. If the egg count is very low before the test, analyzing for resistance is of no value, because the egg counts vary daily and between tests. In these cases, the variation becomes so significant that it may lead to erroneous conclusions about resistance.

DETECTING LARVAE WITH THE BAERMANN METHOD

When the parasite's reproduction strategy is to secrete live larvae, not eggs, to the environment, the Baermann method is suitable for fecal analysis (Fig. 11.3). These parasites include some canine respiratory tract nematodes and the intestinal nematode *Strongyloides stercoralis*. The easy and inexpensive Baermann method is highly recommended diagnostic protocol for the coughing dogs to confirm or rule out the role of lungworms in cases presented with chronic coughing.

Since the Baermann method is based on active larval movement, it is important to consider the welfare of the larvae during transport and storage. The sample must, for instance, not be frozen. The sample must be carefully collected; it must be fresh and not contaminated by earth nematodes. If it is necessary to take the sample from stools on the ground, only the upper part should be taken, not the part that has had contact with the ground.

The sample is placed inside a pouch made of gauze of several layers. A filter paper of tea bags can also be used, if available. A large amount of feces is needed for Baermann, much more than in the flotation methods, for instance.

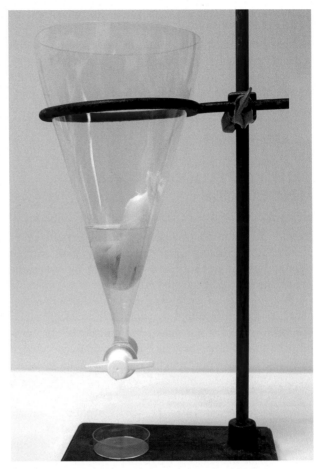

FIG. 11.3 The principle of the Baermann method: the fecal sample is placed into a water-filled funnel in a gauze pouch. Nematode larvae migrate through the gauze into the water and sink to the bottom of the funnel, from where they can be collected for microscopy.

If stools are plentiful, 25 g of feces is a good amount, but the assay sensitivity improves with larger sample. If one has to do with less, the sample should be weighed so that the sensitivity of the test can be assessed afterwards. The gauze pouch is placed in a funnel filled with tap water so that it does not touch the funnel bottom, but is almost entirely covered with water. The sample is incubated the minimum of 2 h or preferably overnight. The microscopic larvae in the feces actively wriggle through the gauze into the water and sink to the bottom, from where they can be collected for microscopy with a pipette. They can also be further concentrated by centrifuging in a small volume or water from the bottom of the funnel. The larvae are easily visible in microscopy, being actively mobile; however, they are not visible to the naked eye. The species can be identified based on the larval dimensions and especially the morphology of the tail. This usually requires help from a parasitologist. Polymerase chain reaction (PCR) methods have also been developed for species identification and antigen-based tests for specific lungworms.

If the species of the larva needs to be determined and the sample is expected to be delivered within a few days, it is best to send the isolated larvae in a small transport tube in water or in physiological saline. For longer storage, 70% ethanol is suitable medium, especially if PCR is used for species identification. If there are few larvae, it is a good idea to send a stool sample at the same time with the larvae to the laboratory so that, if needed, the laboratory can isolate more larvae from the feces.

DETECTING BLOOD PARASITES BY MORPHOLOGY

Circulating parasites can be examined in a full blood sample, after processing accordingly. The microfilariae of nematodes are visible in a blood smear even without staining. Microfilariae are also clearly visible when the sample has been stained with Diff Quick or May-Grünwald Giemsa, for instance, commonly used for a differential leucocyte count and cytological samples and hence, readily available in most of the small animal practices. The visibility of microfilariae may be enhanced and concentrated by lysing the erythrocytes in the sample with, for instance, Knott's solution and centrifugation, after which methylene blue will further augment prominence of microfilaria. The morphological features used for identifying the microfilaria include length, position of nuclei and whether they are sheathed by a sock-like membrane (see information box at the end of this chapter, page 242). Intercellular circulatory protozoa, e.g., *Babesia*, are made visible by staining. So-called small and large *Babesia* can be distinguished morphologically from a stained blood smear. Large *Babesia* fill over one-eighth of the interior of an erythrocyte, while the small ones fill less. *Babesia* should be looked for especially in the edges of a smear. The analysis is specific, but its sensitivity is poor.

DETECTING ANTIBODIES AND ANTIGENS

A parasitic infection can occasionally be diagnosed indirectly by analyzing serum for antibodies, which the host produces in response to the parasite. Antibody production takes place after infection. It takes time for the titer to increase to a detection level, usually at least 2 weeks. Some individual host animals have a poorer ability to generate antibodies than others. Since especially IgG-antibody level stays high for a long time, it is difficult to draw conclusions about whether the infection is acute or whether the antibodies are the result of an old contact with the parasite. It should always be noted that an analysis of antibodies measures the immune response to exposure, not the presence of a parasite. Antibody analysis is an easy, reliable, and inexpensive method for prevalence studies and other population-level analyses. It is a useful method also for

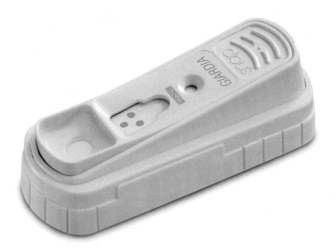

FIG. 11.4 Pet-side rapid tests are nowadays routinely used in veterinary clinics also for parasitological diagnostics. *(Reproduced with permission from IDEXX Laboratories.)*

supporting individual diagnosis, especially in uncommon parasitic diseases, but the limitations of the method must be kept in mind. The most common method for analyzing antibodies in clinical samples is enzyme-linked immunosorbent assay (ELISA), in which the serum antibodies are detected by joining them with the parasite antigen and visualizing the union with a measurable enzymatic color reaction. Parasitic antigens can be analyzed with ELISA as well. The reaction employs a ready-made antibody against the parasite, to which the parasite's antigen attaches. Many in-clinic rapid tests are also based on these antigen-antibody binding methodologies (Fig. 11.4).

The choice of sample for antigen analysis depends on where the parasite lives in the body. A blood sample is suitable for parasites with a life cycle in blood. Fecal sampling is widely used and convenient in parasitology, and it is possible to develop fecal antigen tests for diagnosing intestinal parasites. An example is the common animal-side fecal antigen test for *Giardia*. The antigen test is a direct method detecting parasite structures, not the immune response of the host. Since also parts of dead parasites are antigenic, the method does not give information on the viability of parasites. This should be borne in mind, if antigen analysis is used for investigating the efficacy of treatment, for example. The result may be positive, although the detected antigen consists merely of dead parasites or their remnants. It is also important to remember that parasites and their close relatives may cross-react in an antibody as well as an antigen test.

DETECTION OF PARASITIC DNA

Parasitic DNA in the sample is a direct sign of the presence a parasite. Sampling is directed according to the parasite's life cycle: fecal sample suits for intestinal parasites, blood for circulating parasites, and so on. The DNA in the sample is first released from inside the cell. In several cycles of alternating temperatures, the DNA strands are separated from each other (denaturation), then purpose-designed primers are attached to the open strands (annealing), and finally with the aid of enzyme the DNA sequence sought for is copied between the primers to the extent that it can be detected by specific techniques (elongation). Generally, PCR reveals nothing about the viability of the parasite. When it works, it is very sensitive, but reaction-inhibiting substances of some sample materials, such as feces, may interfere with the assay, and this has to be controlled. Some parasitic stages that survive environmental conditions well, e.g., cysts and eggs, may have a very robust outer shell. To access their DNA, extra procedures may be needed. The sample volume needed for PCR is very small. This is not only a benefit: does a negative result obtained from a small sample mean that there is no parasite in the host, or should a bigger sample be analyzed? This problem can be controlled in some cases by concentrating the potential proportion of the parasite before the PCR analysis. The extremely high sensitivity of the method may also be problematic for the interpreter of the results: what is the clinical relevance of a positive finding?

Molecular applications are also used for identifying the species of parasites, not only showing their presence (Fig. 11.5). It is possible that the parasite has already been found and classified to a certain group, but morphological analysis cannot distinguish the exact species. In this case, molecular biological methods are needed. Recognizing the species of morphologically identical parasites may be useful, for instance, when considering whether the parasite can infect other host animals, including humans, or when there are differences in the pathogenesis of similar parasites. Sometimes species-specific diagnosis is helpful for investigating the infection source or the distribution of certain species. Molecular methods can also be used for identifying parasitic characteristics on occasion, such as resistance against treatments.

Differential Diagnosis of Coccidian Oocysts

Dogs unfortunately often eat stools of other animals. Few parasites of herbivorous animals are infectious to dogs, but canine coprophagia has the potential to cause problems for parasitic diagnostics. Parasite eggs and oocysts found in herbivore feces are transferred through the canine intestine and are visible as parasitic findings, when the feces is analyzed in a laboratory. The researcher must be able to decide whether the finding is due to a canine infection or an accidental finding of parasites of another species passing by. Hare droppings often contain coccidian oocysts of the *Eimeria* genus, while coccidians of the dog are of *Isospora* (Cystoisopora) genus. Once they have sporulated, the oocysts are morphologically distinct. There are four sporocysts inside a sporulated *Eimeria* oocyst, parasitizing lagomorphs and ruminants, for example. Inside each are two sporozoites and some *Eimeria* oocysts also have a plug (micropyle). In contrast, the oocysts of *Isospora* genus have two sporocysts, with four sporozoites inside each. There is no micropyle. Sporulation can be triggered in a laboratory by leaving the sample for a few days in room temperature. Contact with air starts the sporulation, but at the same time, the sample should not be allowed dry. Sporulation can be augmented with 2% potassium dichromate solution.

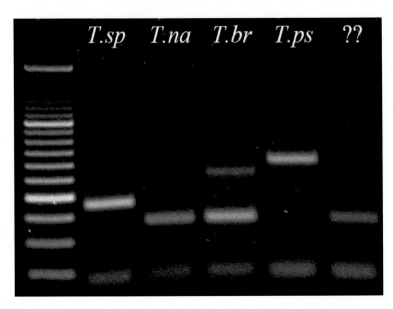

FIG. 11.5 Polymerase chain reaction (PCR) facilitates species identification when morphological differences are subtle. Genetic differences can be visualized, for instance, by distinguishing the amplified specific DNA strands by their size on agarose gel. The agarose gel in the photo has been used to study trichinellosis. The sample under study is at the right lane and the molecular weight marker in the *left*. The amplified DNA strands of four *Trichinella* species (*T. spiralis, T. nativa, T. britovi*, and *T. pseudospiralis*) are at the center lanes. The sample was identified as *T. nativa*.

Simple Flotation Method for Detecting Worm Eggs

1. Place one teaspoonful of feces into a disposable cup.

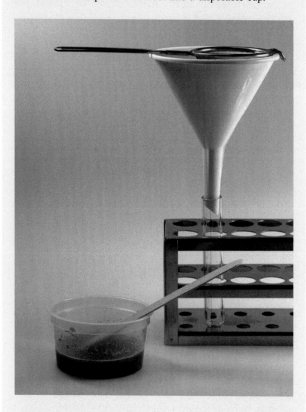

2. Add flotation solution with a high specific gravity, e.g., saturated MgSO solution about 10:1.

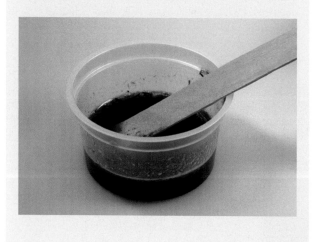

Simple Flotation Method for Detecting Worm Eggs—cont'd

3. Mix carefully. Pour the suspension with a funnel through a tea sieve or double gauze into a test tube.

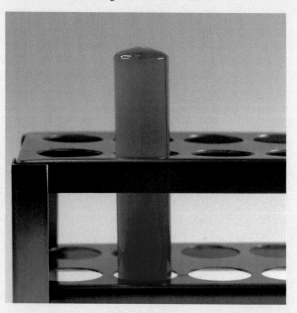

4. Add flotation solution to the tube so that it is filled to the brim and the liquid surface is convex. Avoid air bubbles.

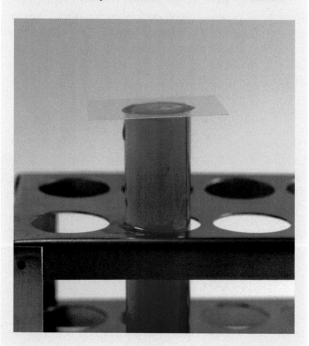

Simple Flotation Method for Detecting Worm Eggs—cont'd

5. Cover immediately with a cover slip.

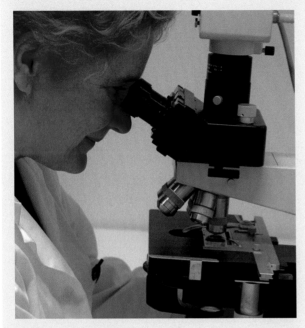

6. After about 20–45 min, move the cover slip carefully on a microscope slide. The sample is ready for viewing with a microscopy with 100× magnification.

Sedimentation-Flotation Method for Detecting Worm Eggs

1. Place one teaspoonful of feces into a disposable cup.
2. Add water about 10:1 while continually mixing to make a slurry.
3. Pour the suspension through a tea sieve or double gauze into another vessel and then to a test tube or directly to the tube, leaving large particles in the filter.
4. Centrifuge the tube for about 3 min at about 300 × g.
5. After centrifuging, the supernatant, containing fecal pigments and particles, is sucked off. Discard this.
6. Fill the tube with flotation solution and mix the sediment on the bottom, containing worm eggs, into the solution thoroughly.
7. Centrifuge the tube again for about 5 min.
8. Take a sample carefully with a glass rod, metal loop, or pipette from the liquid surface. Place this onto a microscope slide, cover it with a cover slip, and view in a microscope with 100× magnification.

Instead of taking the sample from the surface, the tube can be filled to the brim with flotation solution and cover the tube with a cover slip. After some minutes of incubation, lift the cover slip onto a microscope slide and analyze it.

A Modified McMaster Method for Quantitation of Parasite Eggs

1. Place 4 g of feces into a vessel, e.g., a disposable cup.
2. Add 26 mL of flotation liquid, e.g., saturated $MgSO_4$ solution so that the combined volume of the solution and the feces is 30 mL.
3. Mix thoroughly.
4. Filter the sample though a double gauze layer or a tea sieve into another vessel.
5. Mix the filtered sample meticulously and pipette the mixture before the flotation starts into both McMaster chamber (Fig. 11.6) so that the chambers fill totally. If bubbles are seen in the chamber, empty it and refill.
6. The sample is ready for microscopy in a few minutes. Since vaporization of the liquid and crystallization of the salt start to interfere with microscopy, the samples should be analyzed soon after pipetting.
7. The microscope should be focused on the upper level of the liquid in the chamber, where the eggs are concentrated thanks to flotation. Small air bubbles tend to appear at the same level.
8. Observe the sample with 100× magnification (if the oculars magnify 10×, turn on the 10× objective to acquire 100×). Count all worm eggs and protozoan oocysts within the grid and combine the numbers from both squares. The number of eggs/oocysts in 1 g of feces = 25 times the counted number.

(The space under each counting square is 0.15 mL. Counting the worm eggs in the area of both squares produces a number indicating the number of eggs in 0.30 mL of the liquid under observation. This volume is 1/100 of the total volume of the sample. Thus, multiplying the obtained number 100-fold gives the total number of worm eggs in the whole sample. Since the sample originally contained 4 g feces, this number must still be divided by four.)

Several modifications are in use; this is one of them.

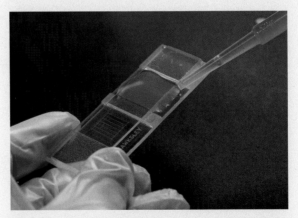

FIG. 11.6   The use of McMaster chamber is based on the flotation, with the added benefit of being able to quantify the parasites in the sample. Worm eggs can be identified morphologically and the number of egg per gram of feces can be assessed.

Baermann Method for the Diagnosis of Lungworms and *S. stercoralis* Larvae

1. Place 25 g feces into a gauze pouch and fasten the pouch into the rim of a glass or metal funnel. (A rubber tube with a clamp may be attached to the bottom of the funnel.)
2. Fill the funnel with water so that the pouch, containing feces, is submerged. Incubate the sample at room temperature overnight or at least 2 h. During incubation, the microscopic larvae emerge from the fecal mass, pass through the gauze into the water, and sink to the bottom of the funnel (Fig. 11.3).
3. Next day collect a sample from the bottom of the funnel. This may be concentrated by pipetting 10–15 mL of the solution from the funnel bottom to a test tube. Centrifuge the tube or allow it to stand for about 30 min.
4. Most of the supernatant is sucked off. Pipette the sediment from the bottom of the test tube as a sample.
5. A stereomicroscope is preferred for viewing the sample, because it allows screening larger volumes. A regular light microscope can also be used, but the potential larval portion of the sample has to be sedimented well to diminish the sample volume. The larvae can be seen in an unstained sample thanks to their active movement, but Lugol or Gram-staining dyes may help in visualization.

Knott's Solution for Analysis of Microfilaria

1. Add 10 mL of 2% formaldehyde into 1 mL of EDTA-blood and mix. The solution lyses the erythrocytes and the sample can be sent to a parasitological laboratory for further analysis. If you want the mixture to be normotonic after the hemolysis, add 2 mL of 5.4% NaCl saline.
2. Centrifuge for 5 min at 300–400 × g.
3. Discard the supernatant. The pellet that remains in the tube can be stained with an equal volume of 1:1000 methylene blue solution before microscopy or making an air-dried smear on a microscopy slide, which is then stained with May-Grünwald Giemsa.
4. View the sample in microscopy at 100 × magnification.

	Dirofilaria immitis	*Dirofilaria repens*	*Acanthoceilonema reconditum*
Length	About 300 μm	About 370 μm	About 270 μm
Thickness	About 6 μm	About 9 μm	About 4.5 μm
Head	Slightly cone shaped; head has a large "empty" zone without nuclei	Round; head has an "empty" zone, smaller than that of *D. immitis* microfilaria, with one eye-like pair of nuclei	Blunt; a hook-like structure pressed close to the head
Tail	Straight	Straight	Often hooked
Motility	Wriggles in one place	Wriggles in one place	Advances wriggling
Staining with acidic phosphatase	Two distinct stained locations (at the level of secretion and anal orifices)	One distinct stained location (at the level of the anal orifice)	One distinct stained location at the level of secretion orifice. Diffuse staining of whole microfilaria caudally from mid-point.

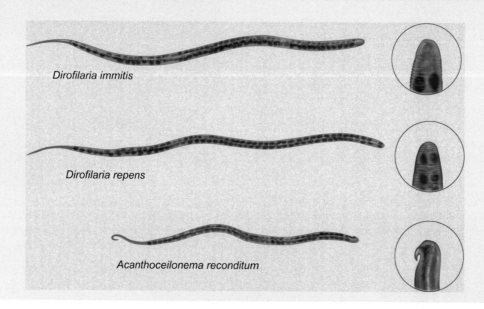

Dirofilaria immitis

Dirofilaria repens

Acanthoceilonema reconditum

Pseudoparasites

When analyzing fecal samples microscopically, it is important to learn to recognize the most common helminth eggs, because almost all samples contain other structures that can be confused for eggs (Fig. 11.7). The most common so-called pseudo-parasites are air bubbles, pollen particles, fungal spores, plant fibers, and other detritus originating in vegetation. A sample taken from the ground is more likely to contain all sorts of contaminants than one taken from the rectum. Distinguishing pseudo-parasites from true eggs or oocysts is facilitated when the microscope ocular lens is equipped with a calibrated scale.

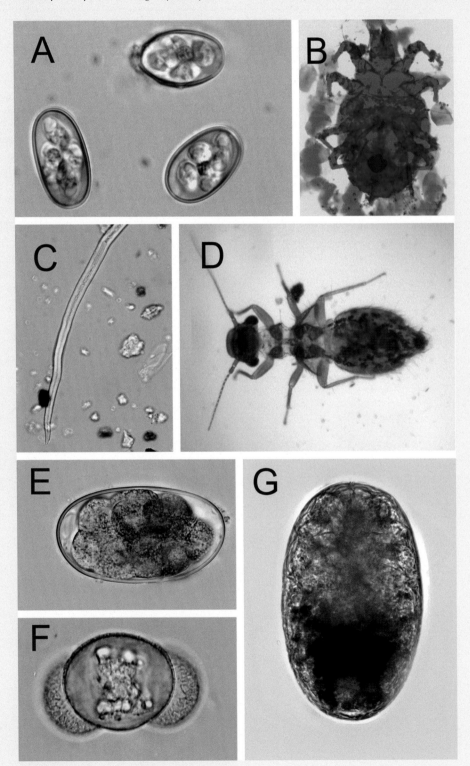

FIG. 11.7 See legend on next page

Continued

Pseudoparasites—cont'd

FIG. 11.7 Pseudoparasites commonly encountered in diagnostic parasitology: (A) coccidian oocysts (*Eimeria* sp.) of an herbivore. When found in a dog's sample, no intervention is needed. They can be distinguished from canine coccidians on the basis of four sporocysts, found inside a sporulated oocyst. In canine coccidian oocysts (*Isospora* spp.), there are two sporocysts after sporulation. The origin of *Eimeria* oocysts found in canine intestine are usually the droppings of a hare or sheep, eaten by dogs; (B) stained urine sediment and a storage mite. The sample has been contaminated at sampling; (C) plant fiber resembling a nematode; (D) a booklouse (*Liposcelis* sp.). Booklice are found in small numbers in households. They use organic material for nutrition and are infrequently found in dogs' fur. Booklice have no relevance as ectoparasites. A sudden increase in booklouse numbers may suggest a moisture problem in the house; (E) worm egg of an herbivore, belonging to the Strongylida suborder. It is difficult to distinguish it morphologically from canine hookworm eggs. Herbivorous animal's helminth eggs end up in canine from the dog's habit of eating stools of especially lagomorphs, ruminants, or equines; (F) pollen particle of a pine. This is a common pseudo-parasite finding in fecal analysis; and (G) an egg of a nonparasite mite, found in a fecal sample. The preforms of legs are faintly visible through the eggshell.

When an object suspected to be a parasite is found, its dimensions can be compared to those in the literature. For instance, an inexperienced parasitological researcher may interpret the sample's round air bubbles as roundworm eggs. In contrast to the morphology of roundworm eggs, the bubbles have a smooth surface and their size varies a lot. The fiber structures of plant stems, leaves, and roots may resemble nematode larvae.

Plant structures are usually transparent and their contents lack the typical structures of nematodes. The rough rule is that a particle suspected to be a parasite, although plentiful in the sample, is probably not a parasite, unless its structure and dimensions match with those in the literature. Finding a totally new parasite in dogs is highly unlikely.

In summer, flies quite quickly lay eggs on canine stools, and it is common that fly larvae, hatching from the eggs, may be misinterpreted as parasites.

Many dogs practice coprophagy. The stools they eat may contain intestinal parasites, their larvae, eggs, or oocysts, typical for the host species. These parasites are rarely harmful to the dog's health, but they pass through the dog's intestine and can be seen in feces when analyzed. They should be identified as pseudo-parasites.

Common pseudo-parasites seen in parasitology laboratories are arthropods found in dog's fur, suspected to be canine ectoparasites. For example, booklice (Psocoptera), resembling sucking and chewing lice, and plant and storage mites, resembling parasitic mites, can be found in dogs' fur.

Lactophenol Solution for Clarifying Ectoparasite Samples

Mix 20 mL glycerin, 10 mL lactic acid, 10 mL melted phenol crystals, and 10 mL water. Preserve in room temperature protected from light. The sample under examination is covered with a drop of lactophenol and a cover slip is placed upon it.

Clarification usually takes about 1 day. Lactophenol should be handled wearing gloves. The vapors should not be inhaled. Any splashes should be immediately be washed from the skin with copious water. Phenol is mutagenic (Fig. 11.8).

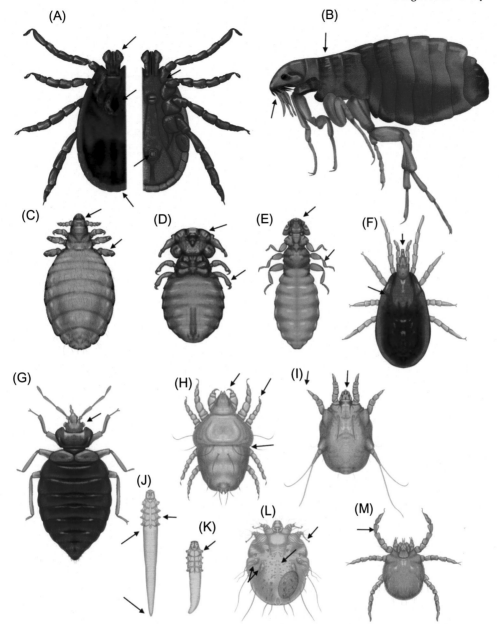

FIG. 11.8 The most common ectoparasites of dogs with some key morphological features highlighted. Please note that the ectoparasites illustrated here are not drawn to scale and hence, the sizes are not comparable. (A) Typical ixodid tick. Eight legs: Identification is based on the shape of head, shape of proximal part of the first pair of the legs, ornamentation, location of anus, and festoons. (B) Flea (*Ctenocephalides felis*): Flea has six legs and is laterally flattened and possesses strong and well-developed third pair of legs. Identification to the species level is based on comb-like chitin spikes, stenidiae. The genal comb is at the low edge of the head, and the pronotal comb at the neck. The number of stenidiae or the lack of them can be used for species identification. (C) *Linognathus setosus* (sucking louse): Note the dorso-ventrally flattened body, six legs and a head that is narrower and thorax, a well-developed claw and the thumb-like protrusion of each leg form an effective gripping structure. (D) *Trichodectes canis* (chewing or biting louse): Dorso-ventrally flattened body with six legs; the head is shaped like a rounded trapezoid and is wider than the length and its middle body. The head is shaped like a rounded trapezoid. The well-developed mouthparts specialized for chewing and grasping hairs are located in the ventral side of the head. Each leg has one claw, and each claw is matched by two stick-like structures. (E) *Heterodoxus spiniger* (Tropical chewing louse): Dorso-ventrally flattened body with six legs. The antennae protected in holes at the sides of the head, leaving only the tip visible. Two claw-like structures in the tip of each leg. (F) Dermanyssidae and Macronyssidae mites: There are a lot of mites resembling these mites. Many of them are nonhost specific ectoparasites of birds and rodents. Similar mites are seen among nonparasitic mites as well. The identification is based on the shape of cuticular plates and the morphology of piercing mouthparts. (G) *Cimex lectularius* (bed bug) dorso-ventrally flattened reddish brown insect: It has long antennae, consisting of four segments. Raspberry-like compound eyes are clearly seen on both sides of the body. The front of the middle part of the body appears sunken in the middle, so that the louse's head is partly surrounded by the thorax. (H) *Cheyletiella yasguri*: Eight-legged mite with the slight narrowing (wasp waist) of the mid-body. Well-developed jaw extremities, with prominent and curved palpal claws at the end. Branched, comb-like structures in the end of its legs. (I) *Otodectes cynotis* (Ear mite) Four leg pairs, which extend beyond the profile of the abdomen, except the atrophied fourth leg pair of the female. The anus is located at the rear. Sucker-type structures (pulvillae), shaped like a wine glass, at the tip of all legs. (J) *Demodex injai*: Elongated, cigar-shaped body the ring-like segmentation of opisthosoma (the caudal part of the body) and very short legs with clawnail-like hooks at the tips. An exceptionally long opisthosoma. (K) *Demodex canis*: Elongated, cigar-shaped body the ring-like segmentation of opisthosoma (the caudal part of the body) and very short legs with clawnail-like hooks at the tips. (L) *Sarcoptes scabiei* (Scabies mite): The mite is oval and has four pairs of legs. The third and fourth pairs are located so ventrally that they do not extend beyond the mite's silhouette. The two first pairs have a sucker in the end of a long and straight shaft. Triangular chitin spikes on the dorsal surface. Anus is terminally located. (M) *Neotrombicula* sp.: Only six-legged larval stages of these mites are parasites; orange or reddish in color.

FURTHER READING

Deplazes P, Eckert J, Mathis A, von Samson-Himmelstjerna G, Zahner H: *Parasitology in veterinary medicine,* ed 1, Wageningen, 2016, Wageningen Academic Publishers.

European Scientific Counsel Companion Animal Parasites (ESCCAP): Control of ectoparasites in dogs and cats. https://www.esccap.org/uploads/docs/gm7zb43y_0720_ESCCAP_Guideline_GL3_update_v6.pdf. (Accessed May 2018).

Schrey C, Trautvetter E: Canine and feline heartworm disease—diagnosis and therapy, *Waltham Focus* 8(2):23–30, 1998.

Taylor M, Coop R, Wall R: *Veterinary parasitology,* ed 4, Oxford, 2016, Blackwell Publishing.

Zajac A, Conboy G: *Veterinary clinical parasitology,* ed 8, Chichester, 2012, Wiley-Blackwell.

Chapter 12

Therapy and Control

There are multitudes of antiparasitic products available for dogs. The optimal one should be chosen for each situation for each individual dog. It is essential to ensure that the active substance of the drug is in fact effective against the parasite in question. The suitability of the product has to be considered, because, for instance, the dog's breed, age, reproductive state, or suckling may limit the use of some products. In addition, the choice should be optimized as for the administration route and the duration of effect. Before administration, the dog must be weighed to determine the correct dose. The dog must get the full dose, and underdosing must be avoided. Parasite control is not just medical treatment. For example, collecting and discarding dog stools from urban environment should be the duty of every dog owner, in order to diminish the infection pressure of internal parasites. In some parasite infections, the treatment must also be accompanied with other procedures in the dog's environment, such as cleaning.

The same deworming and prevention procedures are not suitable for every individual dog. There are certain general risk factors that elevate the probability of helminth infections in dogs and should be taken into account when deciding the worm control program or the frequency of fecal sampling. Often control of parasites is intended to take care of not only canine health, but also human welfare, if the parasite in question is zoonotic (Fig. 12.1). The resistance of parasites against antiparasitic drugs should also be considered. The limitations of parasitic diagnostics have to be recognized so that we know when treatment is necessary, even in the absence of specific diagnosis.

In this chapter, we present the most common antiparasitic medications intended for canine use. Some of them are not registered for dogs, some are prescription free, and some require a veterinary prescription; these vary between countries. Always check the accurate national legislation and local guidelines for the treatments. The substances are listed according to their primary indication, but many may have other indications too.

ANTIPROTOZOAL AGENTS

There are various kinds of medicines used in protozoan treatment, some of which are more familiar from other than parasitic indications, such as antibiotics.

Toltrazuril

Toltrazuril has been used historically as a coccidiostat against coccidia infections of production animals. It is known to be efficacious against canine *Isospora* infections as well. Since toltrazuril, unlike sulfonamides, acts well against both merogony and gametogony phase coccidia, it has the benefit of interrupting or greatly reducing oocyst secretion.

Sulfonamides and Trimetoprim

Sulfonamides and trimetoprim are primarily used as antibiotics, but they are effective against some protozoal species as well. The effect is based on the interference with cellular folic acid synthesis.

Only organisms that produce folic acid are sensitive to the action of sulfonamides and trimethoprim. This is the reason why mammalian cells are impervious to these substances. When treating for coccidiosis with sulfonamides and trimethoprim, oocyst production can be reduced, but usually not stopped.

Nitroimidazoles (Metronidazole)

Of canine protozoal infections, giardiasis and amoebiosis can be treated with substances of the nitroimidazole group. The efficacy of metronidazole has been limited at best, and resistance has also now been reported.

Clindamycin

The antibiotic clindamycin is commonly used for the treatment bacterial infections, but it can be used in Toxoplasma infections too.

Antimony Compounds (*N*-Methylglucamine Antimoniate)

Meglumine antimoniate is used in *Leishmania* treatment and it interferes with the energy metabolism of the protozoan.

Canine Parasites and Parasitic Diseases. https://doi.org/10.1016/B978-0-12-814112-0.00012-X

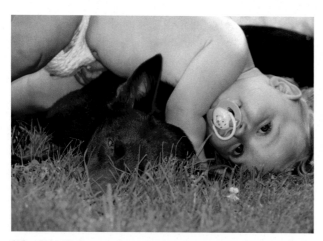

FIG. 12.1 Canine parasite control often also aims at minimizing human health risks. Dogs live in close contact to humans and may carry zoonotic parasite species.

Benzimidazoles (Fenbendazole)

Fenbendazole (50 mg/kg once per day for 5 days) is in many countries the primary treatment of *Giardia* infections in dogs.

Imidocarb

This antiprotozoal agent is used in *Babesia* treatment as injections administered 2 weeks apart.

Pyrazolopyrimidines (Allopurinol)

Allopurinol is a leishmanial drug that is often combined with meglumine antimoniate or miltefosine. It interferes with the nucleic acid and protein synthesis of *Leishmania*.

Alkylphophocolines (Miltefosine)

Miltefosine is used in *Leishmania* treatment, usually combined with allopurinol. It causes DNA fragmentation, which damages *Leishmania* organisms.

ANTHELMINTICS

The deworming of dogs is usually performed with some of the substances of this group. The dose is usually given orally.

Benzimidazoles (Fenbendazole, Flubendazole, Febantel, Oxfendazole, and Albendazole)

Fenbendazole is a widely used antiparasitic drug of dogs. Febantel is a drug that is metabolized to fenbendazole. Fenbendazole is effective against nematodes, including the migrating stages of canine roundworm, as well as some cestodes. If a bitch is given fenbendazole on day 40 of the pregnancy and the treatment is continued daily until the puppies are 14 days old, puppies have 89% less roundworms than puppies of untreated bitches. This regimen, however, is not for routine use in all pregnant bitches. Fenbendazole is often the primary treatment of *Giardia* infections in dogs. Benzimidazoles interfere with the organization of microtubules inside the parasite cell and inhibit the elimination of cellular waste and absorption of nutrients. Parasite cells become emaciated quite rapidly and the parasite dies. Benzimidazoles are well tolerated and even multiple label doses rarely cause adverse effects. Albendazole has been reported to cause bone marrow suppression in dogs, and it should be used with caution. Resistance has developed against the drugs of the benzimidazole group among equine, ovine and caprine nematodes, but resistance has not been widely reported in worms parasitizing dogs yet.

Tetrahydropyrimidines (Pyrantel, Oxantel)

Pyrantel and its derivative oxantel belong to the tetrahydropyrimidine group. Pyrantel is used as tartrate, citrate, or pamoate (also known as embonate) salts. Tetrahydropyrimidines mimic the action of acetyl choline and cause interference in the action of nerve-muscle junction. The worm undergoes a spastic paralysis. The paralyzed parasite is evacuated from the animal along the gut contents. The drugs have a wide effect against adult nematodes and their L4 stages. The absorption from the intestine is negligible, which makes the effect local and directed to the intestinal forms of the parasites. Oxantel is designed especially for its efficacy against whipworms (*Trichuris*), to which pyrantel has less effect. Anthelmintic resistance against pyrantel has been reported among *Ancylostoma caninum* and *Toxocara canis*.

Praziquantel, Epsiprantel

Praziquantel and epsiprantel are specifically used for the control of cestodes and trematodes of dogs. They are rapidly absorbed through the surface of the worm (tegument) and interfere with the calcium permeability of the cell wall. The cell wall gets depolarized, the muscles contract and the tegument simultaneously breaks down. The worm dies and is removed in feces.

Emodepsid

Emodepsid is a cyclic octadepsipeptid used to control nematodes. Emodepsid acts presynaptically by stimulating secretin receptors, causing the worm to be paralyzed and to die. To gain efficacy against tapeworms, in some veterinary products emodepsid is combined with praziquantel.

Isothiocyanates (Nitroscanate)

Nitroscanate have effect on both nematodes and cestodes. The mode of action is not well known, but it is assumed to be related to the uncoupling of oxidative phosphorylation in mitochondria and through that interfering ATP synthesis and causing problems to the worm movement and other functions.

ENDECTOCIDES

Sometimes there is a demand of simultaneous control of both endo- and ectoparasites. The form of the medication may be oral, injection, or transcutaneous spot-on substance.

Macrocyclic Lactones and Their Derivatives (Selamectin, Ivermectin, Milbemycin Oxime, Moxidectin, Eprinomectin, and Doramectin)

Macrocyclic lactones are used for the control of internal as well as external parasites. They are effective in small doses against a large group of nematodes, including their migrating stages, and act against many arthropods. There is wide variation in the efficacy against fleas, and generally the group's efficacy against ticks is insufficient. Macrocyclic lactones are lipophilic, and are stored in body fat, from where they are gradually released. This is the reason for the relatively long duration of action, and they can be used to prevent new parasite infections. The administration route varies depending on the active substance. It can be oral, subcutaneous, or transcutaneous.

Macrocyclic lactones act by interfering with the transfer of nerve impulses in the glutamate-dependent chloride ion channels, causing the parasite to become paralyzed and die. Because cestodes lack this system of nerve impulse transfer, the drugs of this group are inefficient against them. The vertebrate blood-brain barrier prevents entry from large molecules into the central nervous system, making them quite impervious to macrocyclic lactones: the drug is toxic to the parasite, not the host. However, ivermectin causes severe adverse reactions to certain dogs. Collie breeds and their relatives are especially sensitive. They have a deletion mutation affecting the coding of p-glycoprotein (MDR1-gene) that acts as a transport protein at the blood-brain barrier. Due to the gene error, certain substances accumulate in the brain causing problems. Ivermectin, at low doses, has been registered in some countries for the prevention of heartworm disease. Its use in dogs should be limited to this indication because of the adverse reaction risk and because there are better tolerated alternatives available.

The most common macrocyclic lactones in canine use are selamectin, moxidectin, and milbemycin oxime. They can be used in all dog breeds, but in many countries, their use requires a veterinary prescription. Diminished efficacy of macrocyclic lactones has been found in the prevention of heartworms.

ECTOCIDES

In regions with heavy seasonal or constant flea-exposure, routine ectoparasite treatment is common in dogs. Ticks are another reason for a long-term ectocide use. Protection of dogs from blood-sucking vector insects may be necessary in countries that are endemic for heartworm and *Leishmania*. Ectoparasite treatment can be given orally, by injection, or transcutaneously as a spot-on or a collar.

Pyrethroids (Deltamethrin, Flumethrin, and Permethrin)

Pyrethroids act on the sodium channels of the nerve cell walls, slowing down nerve repolarization. This is fatal for the parasite. Drugs of this group of substances have been used for a long time as pesticides as well as in the control of flying insects. Apart from the action of killing arthropods, the pyrethroids have some repellent efficacy. The products are used externally either as a spot-on or a medicinal collar, which releases small amounts of active substance to the skin for a long time. The drugs of this group are mostly used in tick prevention and to prevent the sand flies that act as vectors for *Leishmania*. Most pyrethroids are toxic to cats. This should be remembered if the treated dog has close contact with a cat.

Phenylpyrazoles (Fipronil, Pyriprol)

Phenylpyrazoles have an insecticidal as well as arachnicidal effects. The substances attach to the chloride channels regulated by the gamma-aminobutyric acid (GABA) and stop the chloride ions from passing through cell membranes. The central nervous system of the parasite fires up uncontrollably and the parasite dies as a result. Fipronil has been long the world's most used ectoparasite treatment in dogs and it is also used as an agricultural pesticide. The drugs of the phenylpyrazole group are primarily used in flea and tick control. Fipronil-resistant strains have been reported among fleas.

Imidacloprid

Imidacloprid is an insecticidal chlorinated nicotin derivative. It binds into nicotinic acetylcholine receptors and blocks cholinergic transmission. As a result, the insect is paralyzed and dies. Imidacloprid's binding to mammalian receptors is minute and the blood-brain barrier stops access of the substance to the mammalian central nervous system. Imidacloprid is a widely used insecticide. In veterinary medicine, it is usually combined with another substance to boost toxicity against the early stages of the flea's life cycle.

Garlic Is Not an Antiparasitic Agent Suitable for Dogs

Alternative medicine, which operates beyond natural sciences, has also been introduced to canine parasite control. Examples include different herbal treatments, homeopathy, and resonance therapy. The efficacy and safety of these modalities are either not scientifically proven or have been found lacking. In the best case, the treatments do not harm the dog. The worst-case scenario is that the diagnosis is erroneous, the dog is left without effective treatment, and the treatment is harmful for the dog. For instance, large doses of antiparasitic drugs, sometimes given by nonveterinarians, constitute inadequate care. By law in many countries, only a qualified veterinarian can make a diagnosis and decide about treatment and other care of an animal.

In alternative treatment modalities that rely on herbal treatments and in the associated internet discussion, garlic often features as an antiparasitic drug. Garlic may have pharmacological actions and some beneficial uses in human medicine, but there is no evidence of its efficacy in the control of canine parasites. In addition, it is known that a dose of 5 g/kg causes the lysis of red blood cells and anemia. Garlic is not in any way suitable for parasite control in dogs, not even as a feed supplement. In human studies, garlic has not been shown to be efficacious, for instance, as a tick prevention, even in very large doses.

Some plants are claimed to purge mucus from the intestinal surface and parasites with it. If feed supplements will increase mucus production in the gut, some parasites may be flushed out mechanically, but even at its best, this sort of treatment only has the potential to slightly reduce the parasite population.

Many plant-based substances have, however, effects against parasites. For instance, pyrethrum, extracted from chrysanthemums, is still used as an insecticide. Countless plants have been analyzed in search of beneficial substances for parasitological use. It is likely that useful substances will be found and scientifically tested in the future for the benefit of domestic animals.

S-Methoprene

Methoprene is an insect growth regulator. It blocks the immature stages of the parasite (eggs, larvae, and pupae) from maturing. In veterinary medicine, *S*-methoprene is almost always combined with a substance that is effective against adult fleas. Thanks to its mode of action, methoprene has almost no effect on mammals.

Amitraz

Amitraz causes the nervous system of an ectoparasite to become overactive. This is lethal for the parasite. Amitraz has been used for the control of mites (especially *Demodex*), ticks, and biting and chewing lice. It has a repellent action. Nowadays amitraz has been widely replaced with other easier to use substances.

Lufenuron

Lufenuron is given orally or by injection. It binds to fat tissue and is gradually released from it. It affects the chitin synthesis of insects and interrupts their life cycle. Adult individuals survive, because their chitin structure is complete, but they are unable to produce viable eggs. Lufenuron is most often used in combination with a drug that is effective against adult fleas.

Isoxazolines (Afoxolaner, Fluralaner, Lotilaner, and Sarolaner)

Isoxazolines are insecticidal and arachnicidal substances that can be given orally, or topically as spot-ons, and act systemically in the blood circulation. The requirement for a killing action is that the arthropod is exposed to the drug, when it sucks blood. Isoxazolines have a very long-lasting duration of activity: up to 12 weeks. They are commonly used for the control of ticks and fleas, but they are active against many other parasites, including the ear mite, *Sarcoptes*, and *Demodex*. Isoxazolines selectively affect the arthropods' chloride ion channels and nervous impulses mediated by GABA, causing the death of the parasite.

VACCINES

The most convenient way to protect a dog from parasitoses would be vaccination. For metazoan parasites (helminths and arthropods) a vaccine is difficult to design, because of their complexity. For the protozoans *Babesia* and *Leishmania*, there are commercial vaccines available. The vaccination interferes with the serological diagnosis of these diseases.

WORM CONTROL FOR DOGS

The most important causes for routine deworming of dogs are nematodes (mainly *T. canis* and especially in warm regions *A. caninum*) and cestodes. The distribution of parasite species varies between countries, and therefore it is not possible to give recommendations that suit every geographical location. In addition, the local authorities might require specific instructions to be followed. Sometimes the motivation to deworming the dog might be human health rather than canine, this applies to the zoonotic parasites particularly. There are certain general risk factors that elevate the probability of helminth infections in dogs and should be taken into account when deciding the worm

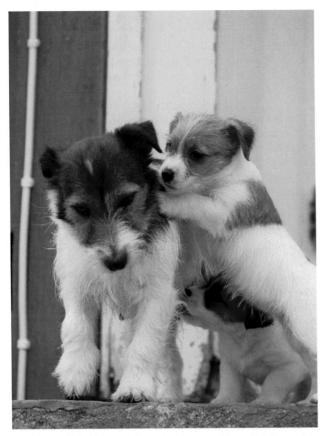

FIG. 12.2   Puppies are at specific parasite risk due to their incomplete immunity and the direct infection route from the dam to puppy. *(Reproduced with permission from Aino Pikkusaari.)*

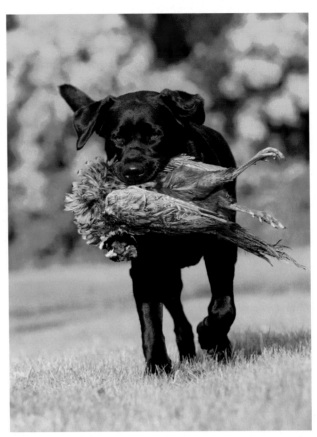

FIG. 12.3   Hunting is considered one of the parasite risks for dogs. The hunting dog has access to carcasses of the cestode intermediate hosts and may also be exposed to other parasites even without the owner noticing it. *(Reproduced with permission from Aino Pikkusaari.)*

control program or the frequency of fecal sampling (Figs. 12.2 and 12.3).

According to European guidelines for canine worm control (https://www.esccap.org/), dogs living in families with young children or dogs allowed to roam free unsupervised are recommended to be dewormed often. This regimen is designed mainly to reduce *Toxocara* and also *Echinococcus* infection risk for humans. Research results have indicated that in order to diminish roundworm prevalence in a certain population, more than four annual deworming doses are needed. The age, living conditions, use, and background of the dog should be considered. In addition to the background information, fecal testing is the key for deciding the required frequency of treatment and which parasites need to be controlled.

Dogs should be treated with the correct drug dose, which requires weighing of the animal. For oral treatment, it is essential that the dog actually ingests the full dose. If there is a reason to suspect lack of efficacy, the case should be analyzed by experts. Isolated cases of canine helminth's resistance against drugs have been reported in Australia, Brazil, and the United States, but resistance is still rare. The investigation of the suspected cases often reveals that a reinfection has happened or there has been poor treatment

compliance in the form of underdosing. Resistance risk should, nevertheless, be kept in mind when deciding the deworming regimen. Frequently repeated treatments select for resistance among the worm population and may erode the efficacy of antiparasitic drugs.

Deworming a Dog: General Guidelines

(Check the legislation and local recommendations in your country first.)

Puppy

A drug effective against nematodes is given when the puppy is 2, 4, 6, 8, and 10 weeks old. The dam is also treated simultaneously until the weaning. If there is a need to monitor treatment efficacy, fecal samples can be analyzed at vaccination times, when the puppy is 3 and 4 months old. The result is taken into account in treatment decisions. If the owner is reluctant to have testing done, treatment is continued every month up to the age of 6 months, and thereafter according to the individual risk profile.

Adult dog with no specific risk

Routine dewormings for nematodes and cestodes (or fecal examination) 1–2 times per year are recommended in Europe

---

Continued

Deworming a Dog: General Guidelines—cont'd

(https://www.esccap.org/) for adult dogs without any specific parasite risks. If the dog meets other dogs from outside the own household, treatment four times per year is recommended; if the dog is allowed to roam free, as many as 12 treatments may be necessary.

Routine treatments may be replaced with fecal parasite monitoring, whenever possible. Then treatments, if any, are based on the test results: is deworming necessary? Which parasites need controlling? Treatments or tests are conducted more frequently if risks for parasites are high. If consecutive negative results are obtained, longer intervals between testing can be considered. Monitoring, however, is done at least once a year, even if the risk is proved low and every time there is a suspicion of a parasite infection. In the absence of test results, the drug and the treatment frequency are decided with regard to the risk profile. The need for tests and treatments can increase because of traveling, systemic diseases causing immunodeficiency, immunosuppressive medication, or stress.

Kennel dog

The breeder and the veterinarian cooperate to create a parasite control plan for a kennel. This requires that the parasites prevalent in the kennel and the dogs' risk profile are determined. Roundworms and protozoan *Giardia* are often a challenge in the kennel environment. Ectoparasites should also be noted in the plan.

Traveling dog

The medication of a traveling dog is planned taking into account the parasite burden in the destination. The owner should study these matters well in advance so that, for instance, heartworm prevention can be commenced early enough. Countries where the cestode *Echinococcus multilocularis* is not endemic may require that the dog is treated with a suitable anticestode drug before importation. The treatment must be documented according to the authorities' guidelines. The ectoparasite epidemiology varies from country to country and should be considered as well.

Hunting dog

Cestodes must be controlled with effective treatment every month during the hunting season or otherwise when the dog has free access to eat the intermediate hosts or their offal. Because many of the nematodes may also infect dogs via infected meat, nematodes should be dispelled simultaneously.

Parasite Control Program for Kennels

Large kennels should cooperate with a veterinarian to tailor a parasite control program, which considers not only antiparasitic treatments but also other factors related to parasite infection pressure. This enhances the health of the dogs, and may also save money, when problems are prevented and routine medications diminished.

The history of the kennel may include information regarding past parasite problems, which may need attention.

Parasite Control Program for Kennels—cont'd

If dogs have been exposed to exceptional parasite risks, for instance when traveling, in dog shows, hunting, or being fed with raw food, these should be taken into account in the control program.

Planning a control program is started by examining the individual fecal samples of all dogs. This gives a good idea about the situation regarding intestinal parasites. If positive samples are found, these individuals are treated and, if considered appropriate, also the in-contact dogs. Two weeks after treatment, new samples are obtained from the treated dogs to ensure the efficacy of the medication. The egg count should be zero. Thereafter the situation is monitored in intervals defined by the veterinarian. If the sample of all dogs is negative, the interval of sampling can be increased. Small puppies tend to be the most sensitive and show signs of parasitosis already during the prepatent period. This is why they are dewormed against roundworms in biweekly intervals. In case of diarrhea of a puppy, fecal sampling should be done and protozoans (especially *Isospora*, *Cryptosporidium* and *Giardia*) should be tested too.

The kennel premises and the traffic of the dogs should be analyzed in terms of of parasite risk. The working processes of staff and cleaning routines should be observed. If there is a suspicion of contamination in outside pens, soil samples can be analyzed. The soil of a badly contaminated pen can in some circumstances be changed to reduce infection pressure. The soil material effects on the durability of the environmental forms of parasites—moisture is beneficial to them.

Any outbreaks of parasite infection should be handled immediately and vigorously. Long-term treatment and, depending on the parasite, various environmental procedures are often necessary.

Temperature and Moisture Influence on the Survival and Development of Parasites

Erroneously in countries with a cold winter and snow, dog owners might think that the cold temperature kills all the parasites from the ground. If the snow cover is thick, the temperature does not fall much below zero in the ground layer. Dropping and rising temperatures with freeze-thaw cycles however damage the egg or oocyst shells and are fatal to them. Moisture is essential to the parasites in general and the conditions of moisture and temperature together are involved in the development of parasites in the environment. *T. canis* eggs are known to develop fully at 10°C, but the development is slower than at 20°C. *Toxocara* eggs that were kept at 1°C and −2°C for 6 weeks stayed unembryonated, but when they were transferred to temperatures of 15–30°C, they were able to develop to the larval stage. This means that after winter, when the temperature rises again, the over-wintered eggs are able to turn infective. In the absence of critical environmental conditions, *Toxocara* eggs may stay viable for 5 years. Tapeworm *E.*

Temperature and Moisture Influence on the Survival and Development of Parasites—cont'd

multilocularis eggs are well adapted to low temperatures: in a study they survived at 4°C for 478 days and at −18°C 240 days, so winter is no problem for them either. For the protozoan cysts or oocysts, the winter is more deadly. *Giardia* and *Cryptosporidium* were not able to survive Norwegian winter in a study conditions. *Cryptosporidium* oocysts were shown to be more tolerant, however.

The freeze-tolerance of parasites is also of interest when potentially infected meat is used as food. For dogs raw-food diet (BARF) aims to offer as natural food as possible. The commercial raw dogfood is often sold frozen, which diminishes the parasite risks. However, there are certain parasites that can tolerate low temperatures in meat well. The most extreme example is *Trichinella nativa*, which has been reported to survive in frozen (−18°C) fox muscle for 4 years. The animal species has an effect on the survival. In sheep muscle, larvae of *Trichinella spiralis* and *Trichinella pseudospiralis*, species that are not known for their freeze-resistance, survived freezing at −18°C for 4 weeks. However, in pig musculature *T. spiralis* is eliminated from the food chain in certain situations by freezing (e.g., 20 days at −15°C).

The age of the metacestode larvae also influences in *Taeniae*'s survival in the frozen meat, but as an example, 100% of *Taenia saginata* metacestodes were killed at −20° C in 120h.

There are several studies of the freeze-tolerance of Toxoplasma tissue cysts. To be safe, at least 3 days at −20°C, so that all the tissue is in that temperature, should be sufficient.

Of fish-borne parasites, *Diphyllobothrium latum* is killed when the fish is thoroughly frozen at −10°C. There are varying results of different Trematode metacercariae, but as a rule of thumb, more than 1 week's thorough freezing at −20°C kills many species of them.

The upper temperature limit for survival of the different stages of parasites vary, but if food-safety is considered, thorough cooking to a temperature of 67°C is sufficient, if every part of the food reaches this temperature.

Memo for Traveling With Dogs

- Study the requirements for dog importation and the parasite risks in the destination.
- Check the current legislation of you own country for returning with a dog.
- Discuss the parasite risks and the treatments with your veterinarian well ahead of the trip.
- Give the possible preventive medication meticulously and check the dog daily for external parasites.
- If the dog gets sick after travel, be sure to tell your veterinarian about the traveling history.

Parasite Risks for a Dog Traveling in Europe

E. multilocularis

This zoonotic cestode is common in Europe, especially in wild canids, except in Nordic countries. Countries where it is not endemic may require the dog to be treated with praziquantel or epsiprantel before importation. The treatment must be recorded according to the authorities' instructions.

Dirofilaria immitis

Southern and parts of central Europe are endemic for heartworm. Killing adult heartworms is difficult and dangerous, and prevention is therefore encouraged. Dirofilariasis is prevented by a treatment that continues for the whole duration of the stay in the endemic areas. The treatment eliminates the L3 and L4 stage larvae that are injected into the dog when the mosquito sucks blood. Most common drugs used belong to the macrocyclic lactone group, e.g., milbemycin oxime, moxidectin, or selamectin. The same drugs are probably effective against the less harmful *Dirofilaria repens*.

Babesia

Babesia infections and the ticks that act as vectors for canine *Babesia* are common in southern and central Europe. Prevention is achieved by protecting the dog against the ticks. It is also important to remove any attached ticks immediately.

Leishmania infantum

Dog owners traveling in southern European areas endemic for *Leishmania* should protect their dogs against sandfly stings with insecticides and keep the dogs inside at dusk, when the flies are most active. Products containing permethrin and deltamethrin have an indication for sandfly protection. Leishmaniosis is especially common in Mediterranean countries. Elsewhere dogs can receive a nonvectorborne autochthonous infection without ever visiting the areas of true *Leishmania* prevalence.

FURTHER READING

American Association of Veterinary Parasitologists, AAVP: http://www.aavp.org. (Accessed February 2018).

Azam D, Ukpai O, Said A, Abd-Allah G, Morgan E: Temperature and the development and survival of infective *Toxocara canis* larvae, *Parasitol Res* 110:649–656, 2012.

Borges J, Skov J, Bahlool Q, et al: Viability of cryptocotyle lingua metacercariae from atlantic cod (*Gadus morhua*) after exposure to freezing and heating in the temperature range from −80°C to 100°C, *Food Control* 50:371–377, 2015.

Bowman D: Heartworms, macrocyclic lactones, and the specter of resistance to prevention in the United States, *Parasit Vectors* 5:138, 2012.

Deplazes P, Eckert J, Mathis A, Samson-Himmelstjerna G, Zahner H: *Parasitology in veterinary medicine*, Wageningen, 2016, Wageningen Academic Publisher.

Djurković-Djaković O, Milenkovic V: Effect of refrigeration and freezing on survival of *Toxoplasma gondii* tissue cysts, *Acta Vet* 50:375–380, 2000.

Epe C: Intestinal nematodes: biology and control, *Vet Clin North Am Small Anim Pract* 39:1091–1107, 2009.

European Scientific Counsel Companion Animal Parasites: ESCCAP guidelines: http://www.esccap.org. (Accessed February 2018).

Fan P: Viability of metacercariae of *Clonorchis sinensis* in frozen or salted freshwater fish, *Int J Parasitol* 28:603–605, 1998.

Hilwig R, Cramer J, Forsyth K: Freezing times and temperature required to kill cysticerci of *Taenia saginata* in beef, *Vet Parasitol* 4:215–219, 1978.

Jesus A, Holsback L, Selingardi M, Cardoso M, Cabral L, Santos T: Efficacy of pyrantel pamoate and ivermectin for the treatment of canine nematodes, *Semina Cienc Agrar* 36:3731–3740, 2015.

Kapel C, Pozio E, Sacchi L, Prestrud P: Freeze tolerance, morphology, and RAPD-PCR identification of *Trichinella nativa* in naturally infected arctic foxes, *J Parasitol* 85:144–147, 1999.

Keegan J, Holland C: A comparison of *Toxocara canis* embryonation under controlled conditions in soil and hair, *J Helminthol* 87:78–84, 2013.

Kopp S, Kotze A, McCarthy J, Coleman G: High-level pyrantel resistance in the hookworm *Ancylostoma caninum*, *Vet Parasitol* 143:299–304, 2007.

Nijsse R, Mughini-Gras L, Wagenaar J, Ploeger H: Recurrent patent infections with *Toxocara canis* in household dogs older than six months: a prospective study, *Parasit Vectors* 9:531, 2016.

Robertson L, Gjerde B: Effects of the Norwegian winter environment on *Giardia* cysts and *Cryptosporidium* oocysts, *Microb Ecol* 47:359–365, 2004.

Traversa D: Pet roundworms and hookworms: a continuing need for global warming, *Parasit Vectors* 5:91, 2012.

Theodoropoulos G, Kapel C, Webster P, Saravanos L, Zaki J, Koutsotolis K: Infectivity, predilection sites, and freeze tolerance of *Trichinella* spp. in experimentally infected sheep, *Parasitol Res* 86:401–405, 2000.

Veit P, Bilger B, Schad V, Schäfer J, Frank W, Lucius R: Influence of environmental factors on the infectivity of *Echinococcus multilocularis* eggs, *Parasitology* 110:79–86, 1995.

Wikgren B-J, Nikander P: Cause of death of plerocercoids of *Diphyllobothrium latum* at low temperatures. *Memo Soc Fauna Flora Fenn* 40: 1963–1964.

Wolstenholme A, Evans C, Jimenez P, Moorhead A: The emergence of macrocyclic lactone resistance in the canine heartworm, *Dirofilaria immitis*, *Parasitology* 142:1249–1259, 2015.

Chapter 13

Immunology

Immunology is greatly involved in the clinical appearance of parasite infections. The same infection level can cause markedly different outcome in different dogs due to their individual immunological response. Immunology is constantly under research to help us better understand the host-parasite relationship and to design diagnostics, cure or prevention to parasite infections. Here the basics of immunological reactions typical to parasite invasions are introduced.

IMMUNOLOGICAL VIEW ON PARASITOLOGY

The definition of parasitism includes a presumption that the parasite lives at the expense of the host and causing harm to it. Historically, natural selection has favored parasites, which stimulate the host's immune defense as little as possible. The success of the parasite in the dog, as well as what clinical signs of parasitism are expressed, depend greatly on the mechanisms that the host uses to cope with the infection. They also depend on the solutions the parasite has for avoiding the host's defense. Most canine parasites are able to maintain their physiological and reproductive functions regardless of the dog's effective immune defense. Many parasites, especially worms, can survive long times in the host by inhibiting or evading the dog's immunity. Despite the apparent inactivity of the host organism, the presence of the parasite always triggers some sort of active immunological process in the host.

Parasites and the immune defense against them have significance beyond parasitic diseases. Parasites modulate the immune defense in a way that influences the autoimmune diseases, idiopathic inflammatory disease and hypersensitivity reactions, for instance. These conditions have lately increased in humans as well as dogs in western countries, when, at the same time, the parasite infections have decreased. In order to understand these rapid changes, we need to learn more about parasitic immunology.

PARASITES EVADE CANINE IMMUNE DEFENSE

Many parasite species have a complex life cycle that can involve also intermediate hosts with their own immune systems. Once the parasite gets to the definitive host, it has to still survive the migration phase in the host, mature and reproduce. All these stages happen while defying the host's immune defense. Parasites have developed various evasion mechanisms to avoid detection. For example, worms can disguise themselves under a shield built of the molecules of the host. They may also change their surface molecules in molting or secrete chemical substance and enzymes, which interfere with the host's immune defense.

CANINE IMMUNE SYSTEM

Dog defends itself against outside insults with two major mechanisms: the general defense mechanisms and the immune defense. The general defense mechanisms make it difficult for the parasites to invade the system and to stay there. Many of these features are physical and chemical. For instance, intestinal parasites must cope with the challenges of low pH at beginning of the alimentary tract, digestive enzymes, intestinal flow, gut peristalsis, mucous secretion, and the regeneration of the epithelium.

The host immunity reacts to the presence of parasites with two major ways. Even without prior contact to the parasite, it defends itself with innate immunity. On the other hand, the adaptive immunity develops after the host has had contact to a certain parasite species long enough to activate this system. Both innate and adaptive immunity can be divided into two branches: humoral and cell-mediated immunity.

The major player of the humoral immunity is the complement system. Complement contains a group of circulatory and surface bound proteins that have a duty of both recognize pathogenic organisms and protect host structures against complement activation. The proteins of complement participate in a chain reaction, where the first activated protein triggers the activation of the next one, which further activates the next appropriate protein in the chain. The chain reaction accumulates as it proceeds. The complement cascade can be triggered by, for instance, microbial carbon hydrates, a surface material that has been recognized as foreign or antibodies attached to the microbial surface. The final product of the chain reaction is the Membrane Attack Complex (MAC), which forms transmembrane channels leading to the destruction of the pathogenic organism.

Canine Parasites and Parasitic Diseases. https://doi.org/10.1016/B978-0-12-814112-0.00013-1

Complement-mediated cell membrane destruction has minor importance in parasitic infections, because most parasites are too large and robust to be sufficiently damaged by the activated complement. Complement activation also leads to the release of inflammation mediators, which attract phagocytes to the site. Phagocytes are responsible for the cell-mediated branch of the immunity. They are capable of ingesting pathogens that invade the organism. There are two main types of phagocytes: monocytes and granulocytes. Both are white blood cells, or leucocytes, and they have the ability to migrate through blood veins to infected tissue when needed. The transfer to tissues takes place at the infection site, attracted by substances secreted by leucocytes. This sort of inflammation mediators include the break-down products of complement, C3a and C5a, prostaglandins and leukotrienes, lipid mediators produced by phagocytes and mast cells. Granulocytes are further separated into basophilic, neutrophilic, and eosinophilic granulocytes. The connective tissue is especially rich with mast cells, which contain many granules for heparin, histamine, and protease storage. Mast cells can release the contents of the granules into the tissue fluid or blood. The main responsibility for defense against parasite infections belongs to eosinophilic granulocytes, mast cells and basophilic granulocytes. They produce enzymes that are toxic for parasites, and nitrogen and oxygen radicals that damage the parasite's membrane structures.

Most canine parasites are too large and thick skinned to be targets for the phagocytic cells of the organism. Granulocytes, as well as monocytes, which mature to macrophages while migrating into tissue, recognize the pathogen by its surface structures or the antigenic molecules it secretes. For example, the structure of bacterial cell membrane differs significantly from the cell membrane of the canine cells, enabling the cells to distinguish the invaders from the own structures and target only foreign cells for destruction. The phagocyte first recognizes the pathogen with the aid of the receptor proteins on its surface. It can recognize foreign structures for instanced with the toll-like receptor (TLR) and complement receptors, once the target is first marked (or opsonized) with complement factors produced during complement activation. As the result of the identification, the pathogen to be phagocytosed lands in the pit formed on the surface of the phagocyte. Gradually the phagocyte wraps itself around the pathogen completely and surrounds it with its membranes. Surrounded by the phagocyte's membranes, the pathogen forms a phagosome. The pathogen is destroyed by an injection of pH-lowering hydrogen ions inside the phagosome. Enzymes are simultaneously secreted to breakdown the invader's structures.

The cell-mediated immunity described above has a special role in protozoal infections, but the nature has also created defense mechanisms for protozoa. Leishmaniosis is a classic example. When the sand fly has transferred *Leishmania* promastigotes into the canine skin while sucking blood, the protozoa are quickly ingested by phagocytes. Normally the cells effectively kill the intruder they have eaten. However, *Leishmania* has adapted to live as an intracellular parasite. It multiplies in the phagosomes of the macrophage, until the macrophage is torn open and the protozoa are released into the surroundings of the cell. Soon they are eaten by yet other phagocytes. *Leishmania* has several mechanisms to make the macrophage, one of the most important weapons of immune defense, its reproduction plant. Substances secreted by *Leishmania* slow down the phagosome growth, resulting in the inhibition of nitrogen oxide production and the weakening of the macrophage's reactions to several inflammation mediators. In addition, the macrophage's skill of introducing an identified foreign antigen, a crucial feature of immune defense, is significantly impaired. There is substantial variation in what happens in the battle between the *Leishmania* and the macrophage in individual dogs. In an ideal situation for the dog, the macrophage recognizes the protozoan it has ingested, receives support from type 1 helper lymphocytes (Th1), and the protozoan is killed in the phagosome. This is known as Th1-responce. In a successful immune response, the macrophage transports the killed protozoan to a lymph node and together with dendritic cells activate naive, antigen-specific Th-cells which then offer appropriate signals for antigen-specific B lymphocytes to be activated. This triggers the humoral part of adaptive immunity, protecting the organism from future infections, in the form of IgG antibody production. However, *Leishmania* prevails in some dogs. It effectively multiplies in the phagosomes while interfering with the macrophage's skill of introducing antigens to immune defense. *Leishmania* infect more and more macrophages, which transfer the infection from the skin to lymph nodes, spleen and elsewhere in the organism. Typical to this situation is that the lymphocyte response is of type Th2, and the macrophage cannot get sufficient assistance from helper T lymphocytes to enforce the defense.

IMMUNE RESPONSE CAUSED BY PARASITES

Although parasites' morphology and life cycles vary widely between species, the host response against them—especially in worm and ectoparasite infections—is generally quite similar. The dominant type of immune reactions is the Th2 response by T helper cells, often combined with copious production of certain interleukins (IL-4, IL-5, IL-9, IL-10, and IL-13) together with a strong response of immunoglobulin E (IgE), mast cells and eosinophilic granulocytes. This immune reaction explains many pathological changes and pathogenicity of most parasites. The same immune reactions naturally also defend the host animal, for instance by preventing—or at least fighting—reinfection. IgE is produced as a result of the host's humoral immune response, usually against the secretory antigens generated by the parasite. IgE is capable of binding into several parasites. Eosinophilic granulocytes, mast cells, macrophages, and platelets have, in contrast, Fcε receptors (FcεR) for IgE on their surface. IgE antibodies recognize the parasite and bind to it. Eosinophils, macrophages and platelets, attracted to the site, cover the parasite by grasping into the IgE molecules with their receptors. The oxidizing agents, nitrogen oxide and enzymes, released from the granules of eosinophilic granulocytes, damage and destroy the parasite. As a sign of the potency of eosinophils, the adjacent tissues of the host itself do not escape without damage. Mast cells have an important role in this process. The antigens secreted by the parasite and the associated IgE response cause the disruption of the mast cell granules, releasing different vasoactive molecules, such as histamine, leukotrienes, and prostaglandins. They cause cramps in smooth muscles and increase vascular permeability, leading into edema. Chemokines attract eosinophilic granulocytes to the site. The reaction may develop into a cascade of events, leading, for instance, into the elimination of an entire parasite population from the intestine.

ROLE OF THE HOST AND DIFFERENT IMMUNE RESPONSES IN PARASITIC INFECTION

The ability of parasites to cause sickness and pathological lesions in the host animal varies widely. For instance, the dog's age, gender, hormone balance, and genetic features may involve factors, which have a decisive effect on whether the infection is possible at all. Parasites are traditionally considered a problem of young animals, but the ability to control parasite infection varies greatly among adult animals as well. It is known especially from equine and ruminant studies that when a large number of fecal samples are examined and the animals come from similar circumstances, some individuals have many worm eggs in the feces, although they appear to be perfectly healthy. In the same population, many individuals have hardly any worm eggs in the stools, despite constant exposure. In addition, the population may include individuals, who clearly have the appearance of a heavily worm-affected animal, despite a small number of eggs. They can get a severe worm infection with a number of parasites, which would not cause signs in other animals of the group. Furthermore, some animals may carry large numbers of worms, which do not seem to cause any harm to the host. It is clear that the absolute number of parasites in itself is not the decisive factor in the severity of the disease. The host resistance against the parasite invasion is more important, that is, the ability of the host to restrain the number of parasites.

The host's tolerance to the infection is the ability of the host to cope with parasites without severe clinical signs.

The background of the individual variation in parasitic immunity is poorly known in the dog. Studies conducted in humans and mice can cautiously be adapted to dogs as well. It is known that Th1 and Th2 lymphocytic responses regulate each other. Th2 response that supports the activity of eosinophils has an essential role in the immune defense against parasites. Regulator T-cell (T$_{reg}$) response, which is responsible for controlling the mutual relationships of Th1 and Th2 responses and the strength of the response, is closely related to the lymphocyte response. Dominant immune response profiles have been identified in parasite infections affecting humans and mice. Individuals with balanced Th1/Th2 response with T$_{reg}$ in harmony are capable of vigorously resisting parasitic infections. Individuals with a modified Th2 response profile, in contrast, have an effective Th2 and T$_{reg}$ response, but a decreased Th1 response. A modified Th2 response profile is favorable for many worms, and individuals with this profile often carry reproductive adult worms. The third recognized profile type is the uncontrolled Th1 response. An overexpressed Th1 response and a weak T$_{reg}$ response are typical for this reaction type. In a worm infection, this reaction type is manifested as severe inflammatory reactions. Individual variation in parasitic immunity is illustrated in Fig. 13.1.

Intestinal parasites and host animals have had millions of years to develop their coexistence. Up to recent times, the presence of intestinal parasites in animals has been self-evident. It seems that the elimination of parasites from the organ's ecosystem may, in some individuals, upset the balance of Th1 and Th2 responses. As a result, the immune defense may become active when it is not wanted.

During the last decades, the prevalence of different autoimmune diseases and idiopathic inflammatory diseases has increased in industrialized countries. These include chronic inflammatory bowel disease (IBD), especially Crohn's disease, ulcerative colitis, and indeterminate colitis. IgE-mediated hypersensitivity reactions have increased as well. A similar tendency is seen in canine populations. The change has been too rapid to be genetic only. A number of scientific articles have charted regions where worm infections are common in humans. When the maps depicting the prevalence of IBD have superimposed upon the worm burden maps, the affected regions are practically mirror images of each other, i.e., those countries with high numbers of worm infections in humans have low prevalence of IBD, and vice versa.

Many mouse studies have shown that worm infections either prevent or slow down the development of many other inflammatory diseases. A severe worm infection and an associated Th2 response, for example, can weaken the immune response of a vaccination, because the overexpressed Th2 response weakens the Th1 response. Similarly,

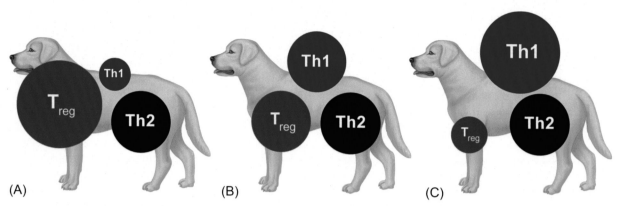

FIG. 13.1 Immune responses associated with parasitic infections. *(Modified from Maizels R, Yazdanbakhsh M: Immune regulation by helminth parasites: cellular and molecular mechanisms, Nat Rev Immunol 3:733–744, 2003. A. Modified Th2 response B. Balanced Th1/Th2 response C. Uncontrolled Th1 response.)*

it has been observed that a parasite infection in mice delays the tissue transplant rejection reaction and greatly dampens the defense reaction against Helicobacter. These observations have led researchers to consider if it is possible to prevent, treat, or even cure inflammatory diseases with a controlled worm infection or by artificially activating immune reactions caused by them. Results from animal experiments have suggested that endoparasites may prevent, for instance, MS disease and autoimmune rheumatic disorders. Human studies have indicated that worms may have therapeutic benefits in, for instance, IBD, Crohn's disease, ulcerative colitis and MS disease.

Many aspects of parasites' pathogenicity and the immune response caused by parasites remain unknown. For example, the pathogenesis of canine demodicosis is still mostly enigmatic, despite the prevalence of the disease. It appears that the veterinary profession as well as dog owners will have to alter their attitude towards many parasites, and to replace the traditional attitude of "good versus evil" with a more favorable position towards parasites.

FURTHER READING

Fitzsimmons C, Falcone F, Dunne D: Helminth allergens, parasite-specific IgE, and its protective role in human immunity, *Front Immunol* 5:1–12, 2014.

Hedman K, Heikkinen T, Huovinen P, Järvinen A, Meri S, Vaara M, editors: *Infektiosairaudet—Mikrobiologia, immunologia ja infektiosairaudet*, vol. 3, Duodecim, 2013, Helsinki (in Finnish).

Loke P, Lim Y: Helminths and the microbiota: parts of the hygiene hypothesis, *Parasite Immunol* 37:314–323, 2015.

MacDonald A, Ilma Araujo M, Pearce E: Minireview: immunology of parasite helminth infections, *Infect Immun* 70:427–433, 2002.

Maizels R, Yazdanbakhsh M: Immune regulation by helminth parasites: cellular and molecular mechanisms, *Nat Rev Immunol* 3:733–744, 2003.

Maizels R, McSorley H, Smyth D: Helminths in the hygiene hypothesis: sooner or later? *Clin Exp Immunol* 177:38–46, 2014.

McKay D: The therapeutic helminth, *Trends Parasitol* 25:109–114, 2009.

Osada Y, Kanazawa T: Parasitic helminthes: new weapons against immunological disorders, *J Biomed Biotechnol* 2010:743758, 2010.

Sorci G, Cornet S, Faivre B: Immune evasion, immunopathology and the regulation of the immune system, *Pathogens* 2:71–91, 2013.

Glossary

Acarisidic Lethal to ticks and mites

Acetabulum The ventral sucker of a trematode

Alae Wing-like cuticular structures

Amastigote The flagella-free stage of certain protozoa

Anterior In the front

Anthelmintic Worm medicine, dewormer

Baermann method Laboratory method for finding fecal nematode larvae, based on sedimentation

Basis capituli The base of tick's head

Blastomere Cell produced by cleavage (cell division) of the zygote after fertilization

Bothrium, plur. bothria Longitudinal grooves on the scolex of cestodes

Caudal Towards the tail

Ciliate Group of protozoans with hair-like organelles, cilia

Coccidiosis Diarrheal disease caused by coccidia protozoans (commonly Isospora or Eimeria)

Coenurus A matacestode stage of taeniidae, with one or more scolexes in a fluid-filled cyst

Coprophagy Eating feces

Copulatory bursa Widening of the tail of a male nematode, aids in copulation. Nematodes are classified on the basis of the presence or non-presence of bursa

Coracidium Ciliated first-stage aquatic embryo of pseudophyllidae cestodes with aquatic cycles

Ctenidia A comblike structure consisting of cuticular spines which occurs in rows on the head of flea

Cuticula, Cuticle Layered outer surface of nematodes

Cysticercoid A metacestode stage of taeniidae, small enough to fit inside an arthropod intermediate host

Cysticercus A metacestode stage of taeniidae with one protoscolex inside a cyst

Definitive host Host animal, in which the parasite's sexual reproduction takes place

Dorsal Back side of the body, opposed to ventral

Endemic Present in a region or population

Endectocide Antiparasitic pharmaceutical product used to control nematodes and arthropods

Feco-oral infection Fecal pathogen is passed on by eating

Festoon A feature of hard tick species, when the rear edge of the tick appears with pie-crust pattern

Flagellate A protozoan with one or more whip-like appendages, flagellae

Flotation Method of concentrating worm eggs on the surface of a liquid with high specific gravity

Gametogonia Sexual reproduction of coccidians

Genal ctenidium Row of chitin spikes in the lower edge of flea's head

Gubernaculum Structure guiding spiculas in a male nematode

Hemimetabolism Incomplete metamorphosis

Holometabolism Complete metamorphosis

Hydatid cyst Metacestode stage of taeniidae, a fluctuating cyst containing many protoscoleces

Hypobiosis Adaptation of life cycle, a dormant phase, in which the life cycle stops for an unfavorable season

Insecticide A compound lethal to insects

Intermediate host Host animal necessary for some parasites' life cycle, the site of asexual reproduction

Larva migrans Migrating larva of a nematode

Lateral Towards the side

Life cycle Series of changes a parasite undergoes, including host animals

McMaster chamber A device for counting eggs and oocysts from feces for making a quantitative diagnosis

Merogony Asexual reproduction of coccidian protozoans

Metacestode stage Larval stage found in intermediate hosts of taeniidae cestodes, infectious for the definite host

Microfilaria Early larval stage in the life cycle of certain parasitic nematodes

Micropyle Pore in the coccidian oocyst covered with a plug

Miracidium Free-living motile larva of trematode, covered with cilia, released into aqueous environment

Myiasis Infection with a fly larva

Nymph Early stage of acari life cycle, resembles an adult, still infertile

Oncosphere Six-hooked larval stage inside a tapeworm egg

Oocyst Offspring of a coccidia protozoan as a result of sexual reproduction

Operculum Lid covering a pore of certain parasite eggs

Paratenic host Accidental host, not needed for the parasite's life cycle to progress

Patent period Period when the parasite lives and reproduces in the host and can be detected

Phagocytosis Process by which a cell engulfs a solid

Platyhelminthes Flatworms

Prepatent period Interval between infection onset and the moment when the parasitic reproduction starts and it can be detected in the host

Proboscis Elongated appendage of the head, tubular mouthparts used for feeding and sucking

Promastigote Flagellar stage of some protozoa

Pronotal ctenidia Row of chitin spikes in flea's neck

Protist Kingdom of eukaryotic organism that is not an animal, plant or fungus

Protoscolex Juvenile scolex of a cestode inside a metacestode cyst

Pseudoparasite Finding resembling a parasite or a stray parasite in a wrong host

Pulvillus Cushionlike pad at the tip of the foot on insects and mites

Qualitative Referring to quality or characteristics, not the number

Quantitative Referring to measurable amount

Reservoir Group of organisms or environment acting as a source of infections

Scolex Head of cestode

Scutum Dorsal shield of a tick

Sedimentation Method of concentrating worm eggs on the bottom of a sample

Sensilium Dorsally located, a saddle-shaped sensory organ on the flea

Spermatheca Sperm storage in a female flea

Spicula Sexual organ of a male nematode

Spiracle Air vent

Sporocyst Cyst containing sporozoites inside an oocyst that has become infectious through sporulation

Sporozoite Infectious coccidian forms inside a sporulated oocyst

Sporulation Change of oocyst to infectious and containing sprorocysts

Stigmata Air vent of arachnida

Strobilocercus Taeniidae metacestode form resembling a worm

Strobila Segmented trunk of a cestode

Tegument Spongy surface of flatworms

Transplacental infection Pathogen is passed through the placenta to the fetus

Trichography Diagnostic technique based on the microscopy of plugged hairs

Vector Arthropod carrier of infection

Ventral Towards the abdominal side of the body, opposed to dorsal

Zoonosis Disease capable of passing between humans and animals

Index

Note: Page numbers followed by *f* indicate figures, and *t* indicate tables.